D0086424

ANESTHESIA
UNPLUGGED

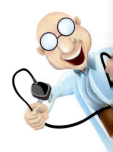

NOTICE

Medicine is an ever-changing science. As new research and clinical experience broaden our knowledge, changes in treatment and drug therapy are required. The authors and the publisher of this work have checked with sources believed to be reliable in their efforts to provide information that is complete and generally in accord with the standards accepted at the time of publication. However, in view of the possibility of human error or changes in medical science, neither the editors nor the publisher nor any other party who has been involved in the preparation or publication of this work warrants that the information contained herein is in every respect accurate or complete, and they disclaim all responsibility for any errors or omissions or for the results obtained from use of the information contained in this work. Readers are encouraged to confirm the information contained herein with other sources. For example and in particular, readers are advised to check the product information sheet included in the package of each drug they plan to administer to be certain that the information contained in this work is accurate and that changes have not been made in the recommended dose or in the contraindications for administration. This recommendation is of particular importance in connection with new or infrequently used drugs.

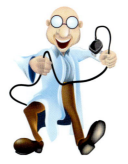

ANESTHESIA UNPLUGGED

A Step-by-Step Guide to Techniques and Procedures

Christopher Gallagher, MD

Associate Professor, Department of Anesthesiology,
State University of New York at Stony Brook, Stony Brook, New York

Ricardo Martinez-Ruiz, MD

Assistant Professor, University of Miami, Jackson Memorial Hospital,
Department of Anesthesiology, Miami, Florida

David Lubarsky, MD, MBA

Professor and Chair, University of Miami, Jackson Memorial Hospital,
Department of Anesthesiology, Miami, Florida

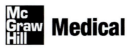

New York   Chicago   San Francisco   Lisbon   London   Madrid
Mexico City   Milan   New Delhi   San Juan   Seoul   Singapore   Sydney   Toronto

The McGraw·Hill Companies

Anesthesia Unplugged
A Step-by-Step Guide to Techniques and Procedures

Copyright © 2007 by The McGraw-Hill Companies, Inc. All rights reserved. Printed in China. Except as permitted under the United States Copyright Act of 1976, no part of this publication may be reproduced or distributed in any form or by any means, or stored in a data base or retrieval system, without the prior written permission of the publisher.

1 2 3 4 5 6 7 8 9 0   CTP/CTP   0 9 8 7 6

ISBN 13: 978-0-07-145816-0
ISBN 10: 0-07-145816-6

This book was set in Janson by Techbooks.
The editors were Joseph Rusko and Heather Cooper.
The production supervisor was Sherri Souffrance.
The text designer was Alan Barnett.
Project management was provided by Techbooks.
China Translation and Printing was printer and binder.

This book is printed on acid-free paper.

Library of Congress Cataloging-in-Publication Data

Anesthesia unplugged/[edited by] Christopher Gallagher, Ricardo Martinez-Ruiz,
David Lubarsky.
    p. ; cm.
  Includes index.
  ISBN 0-07-145816-6 (alk. paper)
    1. Anesthesia.   I. Gallagher, Christopher J.   II. Martinez-Ruiz, Ricardo.   III.
Lubarsky,
  David A.
    [DNLM: 1. Anesthesia. WO 200 A579556 2006]
  RD81.A542 2006
  617.96–dc22

                                                              2006048230

To our patients.
Get well soon!

My sincere thanks to the entire University of Miami—Jackson Memorial Hospital Anesthesiology Department. They did the procedures, wrote the chapters, got the pictures, and, most importantly, took good care of our patients.

A special thanks to Richard Elf and Bruce Weisenberger, senior medical students who served as my "enforcers," bugging the chapter authors to "turn the darn thing in." Granted, slashing tires and breaking thumbs is a bit excessive, but one does what one must.

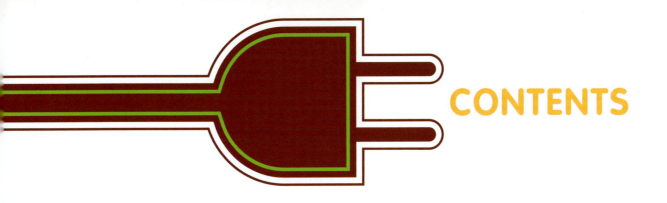

CONTENTS

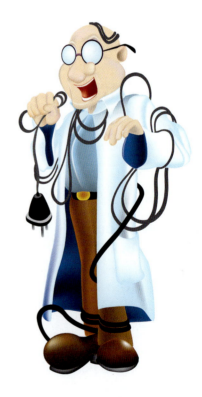

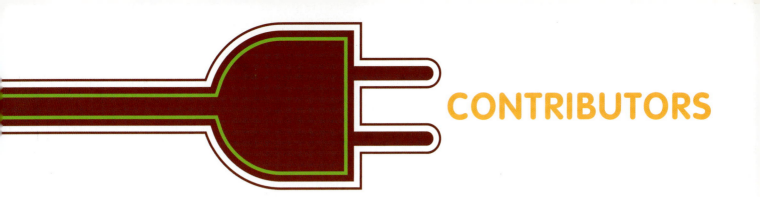

CONTRIBUTORS

Karim Abouelenin
Assistant Professor, University of Miami, Jackson Memorial Hospital, Department of Anesthesiology, Miami, Florida
The Anesthesiologist's Party Piece: The IJ
The Surgeon's Bailiwick: The Subclavian

Emilio Alarcon, MD
Assistant Professor, University of Miami, Jackson Memorial Hospital, Department of Anesthesiology, Miami, Florida
A Sympathetic Ear and a Sympathetic Block

Neil Anand, MD
Fellow, University of Miami, Jackson Memorial Hospital, Department of Anesthesiology, Miami, Florida
Living Better with Electricity: Pacing

Mike Barron, MD
Associate Professor, University of Miami, Jackson Memorial Hospital, Department of Anesthesiology, Miami, Florida
EEEEK! Do We Dare? The Brachial A-line

Ady Bermudez, MD
Resident, University of Miami, Jackson Memorial Hospital, Department of Anesthesiology, Miami, Florida
Armed and Dangerous: The Arm Block

Dan Castillo, MD
Asst Professor, University of Miami, Jackson Memorial Hospital, Department of Anesthesiology, Miami, Florida
Living Better with Electricity: Pacing

Gilbert Chidiac, MD
Assistant Professor, University of Miami, Jackson Memorial Hospital, Department of Anesthesiology, Miami, Florida
Positioning is Everything

Lebron Cooper, MD
Assistant Professor, University of Miami, Jackson Memorial Hospital, Department of Anesthesiology, Miami, Florida
"The Lung's Not Down, You Idiot!" Lung Isolation

Chadi Dahabra, MD
Resident, University of Miami, Jackson Memorial Hospital, Department of Anesthesiology, Miami, Florida
The Rodney Dangerfield of Lines: The IV

Christian Diez, MD
Resident, University of Miami, Jackson Memorial Hospital, Department of Anesthesiology, Miami, Florida
The Vanilla Ice Cream of Intubation: Laryngoscopy

Brantley Dollar, MD
Resident, University of Miami, Jackson Memorial Hospital, Department of Anesthesiology, Miami, Florida
The Anesthesiologist's Party Piece: The IJ

Marco Foramiglio, MD
Resident, University of Miami, Jackson Memorial Hospital, Department of Anesthesiology, Miami, Florida
Positioning is Everything

Christopher Gallagher, MD
Associate Professor, Department of Anesthesiology, State University of New York at Stony Brook, Stony Brook, New York
The Rodney Dangerfield of Lines: The IV
The Mask of Zorro: Mask Ventilation
The Crown Jewel of Intubations: Awake Fiberoptic
Roomsmanship
Simulators

Ramiro Gumucio, MD
Resident, University of Miami, Jackson Memorial Hospital, Department of Anesthesiology, Miami, Florida
Oh, the Little Darlin's: Kiddie Caudal

Fernando Gavia, MD
Resident, University of Miami, Jackson Memorial Hospital, Department of Anesthesiology, Miami, Florida
The Mask of Zorro: Mask Ventilation

Steven Gayer, MD
Associate Professor, University of Miami, Jackson Memorial Hospital, Department of Anesthesiology, Miami, Florida
Ophthalmic Anesthesia: More Than Meets the Eye

Rebecca Gilbert
Resident, University of Miami, Jackson Memorial Hospital, Department of Anesthesiology, Miami, Florida
Wiretapping: The Retrograde Wire Intubation

Jay Grossman, MD
Assistant Professor, University of Miami, Jackson Memorial Hospital, Department of Anesthesiology, Miami, Florida
Echo, Echo, Echo: Transesophageal Echocardiography

Amy Gruen, DO
Resident, University of Miami, Jackson Memorial Hospital, Department of Anesthesiology, Miami, Florida
Mending Fences: The Blood Patch

James Halliday, MB, BCh, FCARS (I)
Professor, University of Miami, Jackson Memorial Hospital, Department of Anesthesiology, Miami, Florida
Oh, the Little Darlin's: Kiddie Caudal

Ricardo Irizarry, MD
Resident, University of Miami, Jackson Memorial Hospital, Department of Anesthesiology, Miami, Florida
Transportation Made Somewhat Less Deadly

Michael Jarrell, MD
Resident, University of Miami, Jackson Memorial Hospital, Department of Anesthesiology, Miami, Florida
Roomsmanship

Sarah Kafi, MD
Resident, University of Miami, Jackson Memorial Hospital, Department of Anesthesiology, Miami, Florida
Lego-Land: Lower Extremity Nerve Blocks

Jas Katariya, MD
Assistant Professor, University of Miami, Jackson Memorial Hospital, Department of Anesthesiology, Miami, Florida
Getting a Case Going at a Greater-than-Glacial Pace

Jonathan Katz, MD, DMD
Resident, University of Miami, Jackson Memorial Hospital, Department of Anesthesiology, Miami, Florida
Echo, Echo, Echo: Transesophageal Echocardiography

Stephanie Katz, DO
Resident, University of Miami, Jackson Memorial Hospital, Department of Anesthesiology, Miami, Florida
Oh Damn, CSF! The Epidural

Samir Kulkarni, MD
Staff Anesthesiologist, University of Miami, Jackson Memorial Hospital, Department of Anesthesiology, Miami, Florida
Getting a Case Going at a Greater-than-Glacial Pace

Allison Lee, MD
Assistant Professor, University of Miami, Jackson Memorial Hospital, Department of Anesthesiology, Miami, Florida
Mix and Match: The Combined Spinal-Epidural
Mending Fences: The Blood Patch

Jong Y. Lee, MD
Assistant Professor, University of Miami, Jackson Memorial Hospital, Department of Anesthesiology, Miami, Florida
Wiretapping: The Retrograde Wire Intubation

Michael Lewis, MD
Associate Professor, University of Miami, Jackson Memorial Hospital, Department of Anesthesiology, Miami, Florida
The Zirconium Jewel of Sort-of-Intubation: The LMA

David Lindley, DO
Resident, University of Miami, Jackson Memorial Hospital, Department of Anesthesiology, Miami, Florida
A Sympathetic Ear and a Sympathetic Block

Ana Lipska, MD
Resident, University of Miami, Jackson Memorial Hospital, Department of Anesthesiology, Miami, Florida
The Beat to Beat Faucet: The Radial A-line

Roger Marks, MD
Assistant Professor, University of Miami, Jackson Memorial Hospital, Department of Anesthesiology, Miami, Florida
The Beat to Beat Faucet: The Radial A-line

Ricardo Martinez-Ruiz, MD
Assistant Professor, University of Miami, Jackson Memorial Hospital, Department of Anesthesiology, Miami, Florida
Root Beer Float? No, Floating a Swan

Christina Matadial, MD
Assistant Professor, University of Miami, Jackson Memorial Hospital, Department of Anesthesiology, Miami, Florida
Oh Good, CSF! The Spinal
Oh Damn, CSF! The Epidural

Carlos Mijares, MD
Assistant Professor, University of Miami, Jackson Memorial Hospital, Department of Anesthesiology, Miami, Florida
Nasogastric Tube's Away!

Andres Missair, MD
Resident, University of Miami, Jackson Memorial Hospital, Department of Anesthesiology, Miami, Florida
Mix and Match: The Combined Spinal-Epidural

Nicholas Nedeff, MD
Resident, University of Miami, Jackson Memorial Hospital, Department of Anesthesiology, Miami, Florida
"The Lung's Not Down, You Idiot!" Lung Isolation

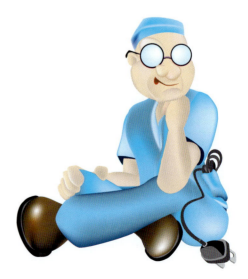

Craig Nelson, MD
Staff Anesthesiologist, University of Miami, Jackson Memorial Hospital, Department of Anesthesiology, Miami, Florida
The Bastard Step-Child: The Femoral
An Ever-Present Friend in Time of Need: The Femoral

Fani Nhuch, MD
Resident, University of Miami, Jackson Memorial Hospital, Department of Anesthesiology, Miami, Florida
Fix Bayonets: The Surgical Alternative

James S. Oleksa, MD
Resident, University of Miami, Jackson Memorial Hospital, Department of Anesthesiology, Miami, Florida
Root Beer Float? No, Floating a Swan

Howard Palte, MD
Assistant Professor, University of Miami, Jackson Memorial Hospital, Department of Anesthesiology, Miami, Florida
Armed and Dangerous: The Arm Block
Lego-Land: Lower Extremity Nerve Blocks

Christina Rankin, MD
Resident, University of Miami, Jackson Memorial Hospital, Department of Anesthesiology, Miami, Florida
Simulators

Kiley Reynolds, DO
Resident, University of Miami, Jackson Memorial Hospital, Department of Anesthesiology, Miami, Florida
An Ever-Present Friend in Time of Need: The Femoral

Bryan Robbins, MD
Fellow, University of Miami, Jackson Memorial Hospital, Department of Anesthesiology, Miami, Florida
The Vanilla Ice Cream of Intubation: Laryngoscopy

Goeffrey Sanders, MD
Resident, University of Miami, Jackson Memorial Hospital, Department of Anesthesiology, Miami, Florida
EEEEK! Do We Dare? The Brachial A-line

Jeffery Schubert, DO
Resident, University of Miami, Jackson Memorial Hospital, Department of Anesthesiology, Miami, Florida
Oh Good, CSF! The Spinal

John Sciarra, MD
Assistant Professor, University of Miami, Jackson Memorial Hospital, Department of Anesthesiology, Miami, Florida
Don't Buck Up the End of the Case: The Smooth Wake Up

Richard Silverman, MD
Assistant Professor, University of Miami, Jackson Memorial Hospital, Department of Anesthesiology, Miami, Florida
Fix Bayonets: The Surgical Alternative

David Sinclair, MD
Assistant Professor, University of Miami, Jackson Memorial Hospital, Department of Anesthesiology, Miami, Florida
Transportation Made Somewhat Less Deadly

Codruta Soneru, MD
Resident, University of Miami, Jackson Memorial Hospital, Department of Anesthesiology, Miami, Florida
Don't Buck Up the End of the Case: The Smooth Wake Up

Shantanu Srinivasan, MD
Resident, University of Miami, Jackson Memorial Hospital, Department of Anesthesiology, Miami, Florida
Nasogastric Tube's Away

Jennifer Vaughn, MD
Resident, University of Miami, Jackson Memorial Hospital, Department of Anesthesiology, Miami, Florida
The Bastard Step-Child: The Femoral

Benjamin Yu, MD
Resident, University of Miami, Jackson Memorial Hospital, Department of Anesthesiology, Miami, Florida
The Surgeon's Bailiwick: The Subclavian

Ahmed Zaky, MD
Resident, University of Miami, Jackson Memorial Hospital, Department of Anesthesiology, Miami, Florida
The Crown Jewel of Intubations: Awake Fiberoptic

PREFACE

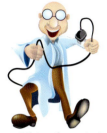

We tinker in anesthesia. Whether it's a Swan-Ganz catheter or an ankle block, we tinker with needles and tubes and catheters. Anesthesia people are procedure people, pure and simple.

This, then, is instruction in said tinkering. We'll show you the main anesthesia procedures—lines, blocks, and intubations.

How have we laid out this book? We start with venous access, starting with a peripheral venous line, then going round the body for other avenues—internal and external jugular, subclavian, and femoral. A Swan-Ganz catheter floats through a vein, so this, too, is included in the vein section.

Next we look at arterial lines, radial, brachial, and femoral.

The airway—a real party piece among anesthesiologists—next comes under the glare of our spotlight. We start with mask ventilation, then proceed to the LMA, direct laryngoscopy, awake fiberoptic intubation, retrograde wire intubation, and finally the surgical airway.

Anesthesiologists have endured insults for years, and one of those insults is actually true. We are back-stabbers! Spinals, epidurals, combined spinal-epidurals, blood patches, and kiddie caudals all fall into the next section, puckishly named, Et tu, Brute? A Stab in the Back.

If there's one thing that separates the good from the great anesthesiologists (at least in the surgeons' eyes), it's being efficient in the OR. The next section, Efficiency-ville, looks at that very topic. You'll read about Getting a Case Going, The Smooth Wake-Up, and Roomsmanship. Not your usual anesthetic procedures, but important arrows in the anesthesiologist's quiver. This section will also look at other "overlooked" aspects of doing a case, placing an NG tube, positioning, and transport. Who hasn't heard of a transport horror story?

Regional anesthesia, depending on what you want to block, could occupy an entire textbook by itself. Look around, such textbooks may be staring at you from your shelf right now. We took on the main regional blocks that a regular anesthesiologist should know how to do—upper and lower extremity blocks, eye blocks, and sympathetic blocks.

Captain Kidd may have buried treasure somewhere on a deserted island, and we can't direct you to that chest of doubloons and pieces of eight, but we can direct you to our own treasure chest. Chest procedures, that is. Lung isolation (always a challenge, no matter how long you've been "doing lungs"), pacing, and transesophageal echocardiography are what you'll find in our treasure chest.

The final section looks at medical simulation—the latest, greatest twist on medical education. A slick way to hammer home learning points, with no damage to any patient! Granted, residents and medical students may stumble out of the simulator with a bruised ego, but egos recover.

Who should read this book?

- Medical students with an interest in anesthesiology.
- Anesthesiology residents.
- Student CRNAs.
- Other specialties with an interest in these procedures (Internal Medicine residents need to put in lines, Emergency Medicine Residents have to take on airways and place lines, too).
- Any Intensive Care Unit personnel, because most OR procedures are also ICU procedures.

Keep in mind, this is a "how-to" procedure book, but don't view this book as a way of making procedures "routine." No procedure is routine, for no patient is routine. They each have a story to tell.

Turn the page and see if these stories speak to you.

PART 1

INTRAVENOUS WORLD

CHAPTER 1

The Rodney Dangerfield of Lines: The IV

Christopher Gallagher and Chadi Dahabra

I don't get no respect.

Rodney Dangerfield

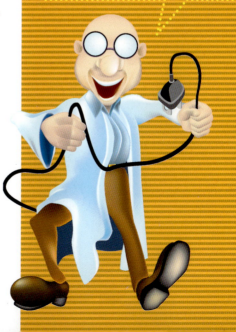

INTRODUCTION

No IV, no anesthetic.
No anesthetic, no job for you.
You need to get in IVs if you are in anesthesia. Both to deliver drugs and to deliver fluids, you need good IVs.

Inadequate venous access or an infiltrated IV can set you up for disaster.
Pediatric cases are often started by mask induction without an IV, but the IV is placed post-induction.

INDICATIONS

Need to deliver fluids or drugs

CONTRAINDICATIONS

- None

EQUIPMENT

- IV catheter (have extras in case you miss)
- Alcohol wipe
- Tourniquet
- Small syringe with local anesthetic (1% lidocaine plain)
- Small needle on the local anesthetic syringe
- IV bag and tubing to connect to catheter
- Steri-Drape and tape to secure IV

BEWARE THE FLOOR IV

- Up on the floor, the IV is used for antibiotics and for maintenance IV infusion.
- Up on the floor, the IV is usually not as much the lifeline like it is during anesthesia.
- Patients come from the floor with infiltrated IVs, kinked IVs, and poorly secured IVs.
- Mistrust all floor IVs.
- Put in your own IV if you are ever in doubt.

PHILOSOPHY OF IVS

- You will *never* regret having one IV too many.
- You will *always* regret having one IV too few.

- A 16 gauge runs as well as a 14 gauge (most resistance occurs in the long-tubing line).
- A 16 gauge is as easy to put in as an 18 gauge.
- Better to be happy with a 16 gauge that got in, than to be angry with a 14 gauge that did not.
- You're anticipating monstrositous blood loss, do yourself a big favor and just put in a central line.
- A central line that is long and skinny is *not* a *volume* line. So, if you put in a 7-Fr triple lumen with three 18-g ports, that is *not* a volume line. A volume line is **big** and allows a **lot** of blood to get pushed through it. So, a 9-Fr introducer is a *volume* line. Big, big, big.
- Hidden IVs do terrible things, like infiltrate during anesthetic induction.
- Whenever possible, keep IVs in sight.
- Watch IVs like a hawk during transfer, for IVs love to get pulled out.
- Never lose an IV for lack of tape.

IV HISTORY AND PHYSICAL

- Do a quick IV history.
- Chemotherapy patient? IV drug addict? Morbidly obese? History of difficult stick? If yes, then give yourself plenty of time to get the IV and have backup plans, such as a central line.
- Do a quick IV physical.
- Arms smooth as marble, swollen from obesity or anasarca? Again, consider options such as a central line if peripheral just looks impossible.
- One central line stick is less painful than 25 peripheral sticks.

An IV is Not Trivial Pursuit

Do not kid yourself. An IV is not a trivial part of the case, and it's not a given. Horror stories abound.

Halfway through an induction, the patient is half-induced, half-paralyzed, and then you see the IV has blown. Now what do you do? You can forge ahead and try to intubate, but the patient will have enough oomph left to fight you. Do you quick like a bunny run around the side and start another IV? Ask the surgeon to help? The circulator?

A long neuro case with the patient's arms tucked as they lay in the prone position. The patient has lost a lot of blood and you put blood into pressure bags to infuse more quickly. End of case, you move the patient supine and see, to your dismay, that the IV blew *sometime* during the case and now the forearm is completely swollen. Eventually, the patient develops compartment syndrome and requires a fasciotomy.

All this, from an IV!

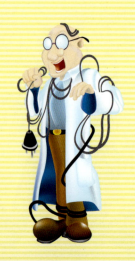

TECHNIQUE

- Place tourniquet—a real one, not a glove. That makes you look amateurish. (Save the gloves for yourself before touching any patient.)
- Place the tourniquet so you will later be able to release it with one hand, that is, don't tie the tourniquet into a knot.
- Hang arm down to have gravity help fill up the vein.
- Have patient pump his fist.
- Look for a vein that has an inverted Y.
- Aim for the crotch of the Y.
- Place a little local anesthetic where you plan on sticking, especially when you are using a cannula size greater than or equal to 16 g
- For right-handers: With your left hand, pull the skin taut as a drum skin.
- Stick the catheter through the skin and into the vein.
- Make sure when you see the flash of blood in the hub of the needle that you advance another millimeter or two to get the catheter into the vein, not just the tip of the needle.
- Without letting go of the skin, use your right hand (the same hand you used to stick the vein) to advance the catheter all the way into the vein.
- Don't pull the needle out yet.
- With your right hand, reach up and undo the tourniquet.
- With your left hand, reach up and compress the vein just above where you placed the catheter, which will prevent blood from running out of the catheter when you take the needle out. Neatness counts!
- With your right hand, pull out the needle, throw it into a nearby sharps container.
- For a left-hander, of course, use the opposite hands to those mentioned above.
- Don't leave a bloody sharp sitting around. Sooner or later, someone will get stuck, and that someone might be you.
- Hook up the IV tubing and secure it to the catheter.
- Place a Steri-Drape, and tape it to secure the IV.
- Open the IV and make sure it runs.
- If the site gets puffy, the IV is infiltrated. Stop the IV, pull the catheter out, and start again.

- An infiltrated IV hurts as well, so you can ask the patient with edematous puffy sites about pain.
- If the site does not get puffy and everything works well, remember to slow down the IV.

HEY WAIT! WHAT ABOUT KIDDIE IVS?

Good news: We can induce general anesthesia with inhaled agents prior to IV cannulation. We have an immobile patient with dilated veins.

Bad news: Not all children are suitable for inhalation induction. Rapid sequence induction is needed, very small infants, hypovolemia, and malignant hyperthermia susceptibility? All these need an IV preinduction, and it can be tough.

IV access can be very difficult in some infants: Multiple previous attempts by other staff, and the bonnie infant with lots of puppy fat.

Indications

- Need to deliver drugs, fluids, or parental nutrition.

Contraindications

- None

Equipment

- EMLA cream when planning awake IV access. (EMLA is a eutectic mixture of local anesthetic that needs at least 30 minutes of contact with skin to be effective; consider it in adults as well).
- Alcohol wipe.
- Tourniquet.
- Local anesthetic: 1% lidocaine if plan is to place awake IV and there is insufficient time for the EMLA to work (30 min minimum).
- IV bag, 100 mL buretrol, tubing.
- Steri-Drape to secure IV.
- 24-g catheter for infants, newborns, full-term, and premature.
- 22-g catheter for others.
- The saphenous vein may be a suitable peripheral site in infants for this gauge catheter.

Warnings: Children arriving at the OR with the IV in place. These need to be carefully checked because there is a very good chance that they have extravasated. Beware the volumetric infusion pump that cheerfully pumps fluid into the infant's subcutaneous tissues.

Peripherally inserted central catheters (PICCs) are *not* intended for fluid bolus or blood administration, as they are too long and narrow gauge.

Technique

- Place tourniquet (again, a real one, not a glove—that makes you look amateurish).
- Place the tourniquet so you will later be able to release it with one hand, that is, don't tie the tourniquet into a knot.
- Hang arm down to have gravity help fill up the vein.
- Look for a vein that has an inverted *Y*.
- Aim for the crotch of the *Y*.
- (For right-handers) With your left hand, pull the skin taut.
- Stick the catheter through the skin and into the vein.
- Make sure when you see the flash of blood in the hub of the needle that you advance another millimeter or two to get the catheter into the vein, not just the tip of the needle.
- Without letting go of the skin, use your right hand (the same hand you used to stick the vein) to advance the catheter all the way into the vein.
- Don't pull the needle out yet.
- With your right hand, reach up and undo the tourniquet.
- With your left hand, reach up and compress the vein just above where you placed the catheter, which will prevent blood from running out of the catheter when you take the needle out. Neatness counts!
- With your right hand, pull out the needle, throw it into a nearby sharps container.
- For a left-hander, of course, use the opposite hands to those mentioned above.
- Don't leave a bloody sharp sitting around. Sooner or later, someone will get stuck, and that someone might be you.
- Hook up the IV tubing and secure it to the catheter.
- Place a Steri-Drape, and tape it to secure the IV.
- Open the IV and make sure it runs.
- If the site gets puffy, the IV is infiltrated. Stop the IV, pull the catheter out, and start again.
- If the site does not get puffy and everything works well, remember to slow down the IV.

Some pediatric pointers

- Overzealous preoperative fluid restriction may result in the *dried prune* syndrome rendering the search for a vein even more difficult. A tourniquet that is too tight will compound this problem, restricting arterial flow **into the limb**.
- A little 50/50 $N2O/O_2$ mixture goes a long way in the older child who may be unhappy about the idea of needles.

Can't see any veins?

Try some of these sites for hidden veins. These can help in adults as well.

- The saphenous: This lies immediately anterior to the medial malleolus.
- It is big and great for those chubby little 6-month olds.
- Between the 4th and 5th metacarpal bone: Look at your own hand there is always a vein there.
- The anatomical snuffbox: Beware, however, as the radial artery may be here.
- The palmar surface of the wrist can be very productive in infants.
- In big cases with multiple lines don't forget to label them, it is not good to get your peripheral, central, and PIC lines mixed up.
- Don't forget to look in the upper arm. There are often veins here that others have not found.
- Transillumination with cold, bright devices to show up the vessels are also available. Blood vessels do not let the light pass through and they appear as dark lines.
- You despair, as you cannot find any venous access. Fear not. A tibial intraosseous needle is an option under such desperate circumstances. They are available in 14, 16, and 18 gauges in the Dieckman variety.
- Use of US (ultrasound) guided technique leads to higher success and less sticks in difficult IV access patients.
- Try also dilating the veins using 2% NTG ointment.

Common problems

- Stopping when you get a flash of blood in the hub—you might only have the tip of the needle in the vein. The catheter itself is a few teeny millimeters up the road and you have to slip that into the vein too.
- Letting go of the skin once you get the blood flash—the skin retracts, and the underlying vein also pops back. Then your catheter tip is no longer in the vein.

One-Handed: The Way to Go

To make the vein hold still and not roll, you pull the skin tight with your non-dominant hand. That way, you pop through skin tight as a drum skin rather than rolling up skin that crinkles like a Shar-Pei.

Now here's the really cool thing:

If you get the flash of blood and then release the skin with the nondominant hand, *the skin springs back … and the damned vein springs back too.* This catheter, which had been in the vein, has now backed out of the vein.

Damnation and hellfire!

Now the trick is that if you keep holding the skin with your nondominant hand, and slide the catheter up with the same hand that placed the IV, the skin doesn't spring back and the vein doesn't spring back either.

You've got it!

Let's go over that again:

Say you're right-handed.

You hold the patient's hand and pull the skin tight with your left hand.

You pop the catheter into the vein with your right hand.

Now, *slide the catheter up without releasing your left hand.*

This takes a little bit of practice. Try it with a catheter a few times. Stick the catheter in some 4 by 4s, and work that little movement with your left hand.

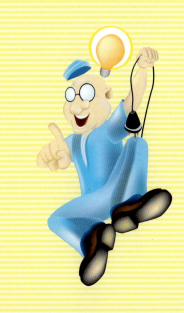

Wherefore Art thou, Vein?

So where do you want to put this wonderful IV, now that you know the trick ?

Hand?

Antecub?

Wrist?

Inside of the wrist?

Forearm?

Foot?

The back of the hand is, pardon the pun, handy. Look for a Y and go for the confluence. That makes for a good insertion. If you stick a vein that looks like an *l* , you can go through the other side: a *Y* is a more favorable geography. When you place the IV in the hand, think of where the end of the catheter goes. If the end of the catheter is where the wrist bends, you can get a positional IV.

Antecub is big, but after the operation, it makes life semi-miserable for patients. They have to keep their arms straight. Now, if you are doing an outpatient case and you're going to pull the IV at the end of the day, then so what? Make your life easy and snap up that antecub. Keep in mind, though, that at the end of the case, when patients are arousing from slumber, they may bend their arms up and cut off the IV, right when you might need it. Picture this: You extubate, the patient goes into laryngospasm, is thrashing, bends his arm up, and now you can't give SUX to break the laryngospasm because the IV can't flow. Isn't that a dainty dish to set before the king?

Wrist? The intern vein is nice because it's unlikely to kink off.

Inside of the wrist? We use that a lot in kiddies, and tend not to think of that for adults, but it is often the only vein you can see in the obese patient. That can really save your tail. You can at least get a little IV in there and get some sedative in the patient. Then everybody breathes easier. Beware that this is a pain-sensitive site.

- Not blocking off the vein when you pull the needle out—blood spills all over your lap and everyone in the room laughs at you.
- Leaving the sharp needle around—bad, bad, bad, bad, bad!
- Failing to secure the IV—and immobilizing the limb with a board. When tots wake up, they are very capable of removing improperly secured IVs.
- Letting the IV run too rapidly—you're so happy you got the IV in that you open up the IV and forget about it while you do other things. Then a minute later you look up, the bag's empty, and the patient is swollen up like the Michelin tire man. Even if it is in the vein, 100 mL of fluid from the buretrol, given rapidly to a 2-kg baby is a very bad idea.

Favorite sites

- Very often we cannot actually see or palpate a vein in the child. This is the case in the chubby 6-month old or the post-premature child whose veins have been used and abused in their protracted stay in newborn ICU.

Try the aforementioned sites as well.

That's it for the younger set!

COMMON GLITCHES

- Going for veins that look like an *l* rather than a *Y*—the *l* vein is harder to hold down and will more likely roll away from you.
- Always be sure to not damage nerves, arteries, or other structures.
- Use sterile technique because any IV can be the source of serious infection.

EXTERNAL JUGULAR

Indication

- Need to deliver fluid or drugs.
- Patient's peripheral IV access is difficult or insufficient.

Contraindications

- Infection at access site.
- Suspected or confirmed fracture of cervical spine.
- Coagulopathy (relative contraindication, as this is the very patient you can't get central access on).

Equipment

- Same as for other peripheral IV access; in addition, you might need a 3-cc syringe.
- Don't bring your tourniquet here. Placing a tourniquet around the neck generates patient complaints.

Technique

- Place the patient in slight Trendelenburg position, which reduces the incidence of venous air embolism, and makes EJ vein more engorged with blood.
- Turn the patient's head away from site of insertion.
- Prep the area with alcohol, iodine or, better, chlorhexidine.
- Viewed by some as modified central line, you are advised to use sterile technique including sterile gloves and gown as well as face mask and cap.

  Infiltrate site of insertion with local anesthetic.
- With one hand, pull the skin taut as a drum skin, try darting movements because, especially here, the vein tries to escape away from the needle.
- Stick the catheter through the skin and into the vein.
- If you don't see the flash of blood in the hub, try connecting the catheter to a 3-cc syringe and gently aspirate. Here, sometimes even if you are in the vein, you might not have spontaneous backflow.
- Also because the vein is superficial, consider bending the IV catheter to avoid going unintentionally too deep.
- When you see a flash of blood in the hub of the needle or in the syringe, continue same steps for regular peripheral IV.

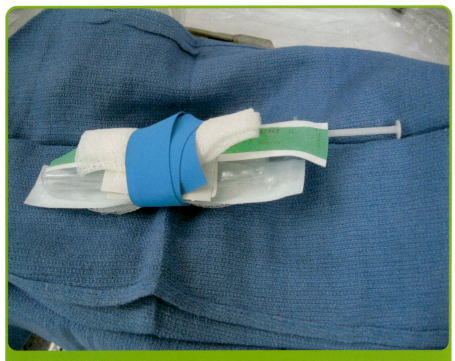

Figure 1. Do yourself a favor and put together a little IV kit so you'll have everything you need right there.

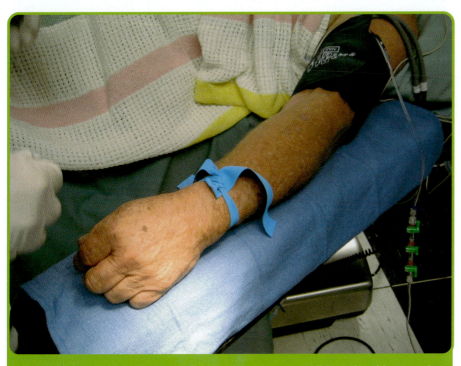

Figure 2. Put the tourniquet on, making sure that you will later be able to undo it with one hand

Forearm? Some big ones can appear there, but you don't see many Ys. It's mostly Is, so you can get frustrated there.

Foot? Placing an IV in the lower extremity in an adult has been likened to bragging about having an ugly spouse.

Just not done.

Bottom line, if you're having tons of trouble peripherally, go central.

Securing that Puppy

Never lose a line for lack of tape. Nor for that matter, never lose an IV for lack of common sense.

Make sure the IV line is well secured (well, just how obvious is that). Let's look at that in more detail:

• Your best first piece of tape is just above the hub of the connection, on the IV tubing. If you are putting an IV in an intoxicated or thrashing patient, you won't have the luxury of wrapping the IV up like The Mummy, so put this piece of tape on first.

• Put something clear on the actual connection site. If you cover up the site with something opaque, then you won't pick up a misconnection.

• When securing the line, get rid of all loose loops of IV tubing. A big loop will catch on blankets and will pull out. Loops are bad.

Bad loops.

Make them go away.

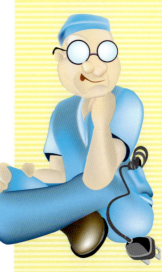

Housekeeping

Now that you have the IV, arrange it so that it works well for you. When you tape it down, tape on the tubing *not* on the connections. Tape the tubing so that there's plenty of play and the IV won't pull out.

Have a stopcock for injecting and have that stopcock easy to get at. Don't have the IV tubing hanging down in never-never land where it can get squished. If you have miles of tubing, loop it up and secure it with "tabbed" pieces of tape. (Tabs make it easy to undo at the end of the case.)

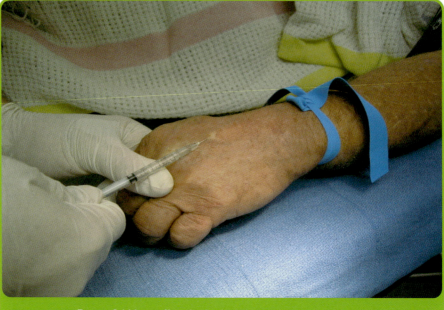

Figure 3. Wipe off with alcohol then put in a little local.

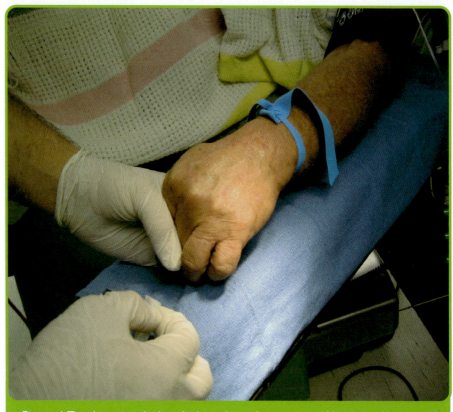

Figure 4. Tap the vein a little, which might make it pop up. Alternatively, you can use warm towels, have the patients pump up their arms, or even wipe a little nitroglycerin on their skin to make the vein dilate.

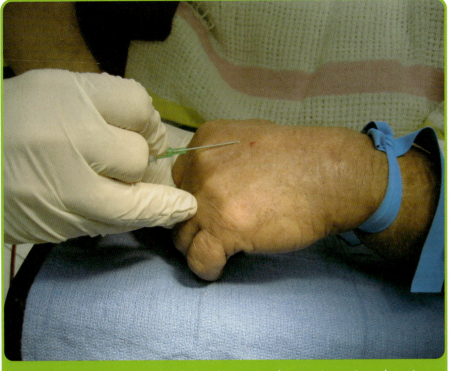

Figure 5. Work on a one-handed technique, so that you insert into the vein and advance with the same hand, that way you don't let the skin spring back, making you lose the vein.

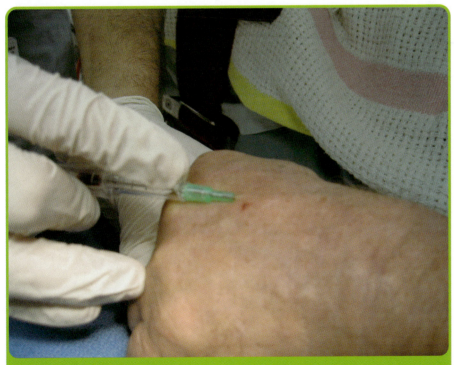

Figure 6. You'll know you're in the vein when you feel a little and you get a flash of blood. Careful! The tip of the needle may be in but you haven't yet advanced the catheter into the vein. Keep the skin taut!

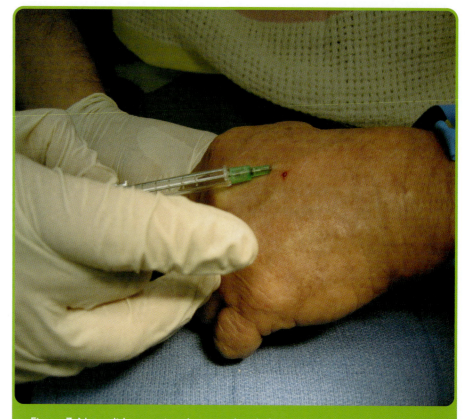

Figure 7. Now, slide up using the same hand, that way you won't lose the vein.

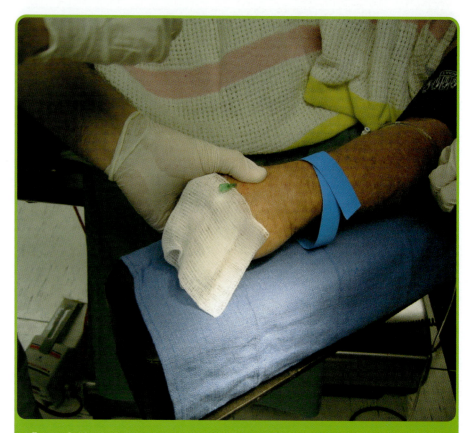

Figure 8. Undo the tourniquet and hold the vein above the catheter, otherwise you will lose blood, and, even worse, you'll lose style points. Image is everything!

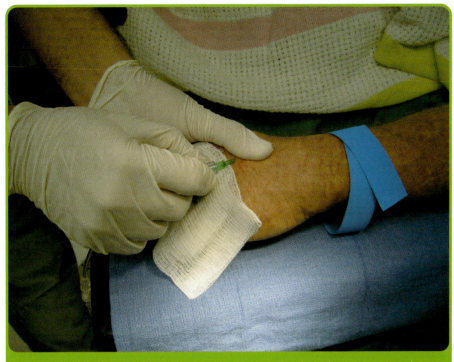

Figure 9. Hook up the IV and make sure it runs. If it doesn't run, you may be in the subq tissue (*damnation*) or you may have forgotten to undo the tourniquet (*oops*) or the blood pressure cuff may be up (*oops again*).

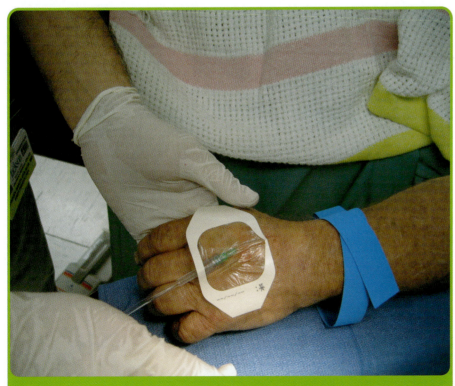

Figure 10. Secure the IV now, making sure you can see everything. Disconnects occur in hidden places, so don't let that happen to you. When you tape the IV in, make sure there are no kinks in the tubing, and also make sure there are no big, open loops that can get hooked. This will result in a yanked-out IV and you will be most unhappy.

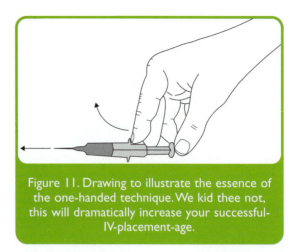

Figure 11. Drawing to illustrate the essence of the one-handed technique. We kid thee not, this will dramatically increase your successful-IV-placement-age.

SUGGESTED READING

Ay caramba! All these references for the lowly IV? Yes, indeedy, do right. There is no such thing as a lowly IV when you can't get one.

Hoffmann KK, Weber DJ, Samsa GP, Rutala WA. Transparent polyurethane film as an intravenous catheter dressing: a meta-analysis of the infection risks. *JAMA* 1992;267:2072–2076.
Plunk a little gauze on that central line before you put on the transparent dressing.

Kagel EM, Rayan GM. Intravenous catheter complications in the hand and forearm. *J Trauma* 2004;56(1):123–127.
This article shows you the many complications of IV access, some of which are thrombophlebitis, hematomas, skin necrosis, cellulitis.

Lenhardt R, Seybold T, Kimberger O, Stoiser B, Sessler DI. Local warming and insertion of peripheral venous cannulas: single blinded prospective randomised controlled trial and single blinded randomised crossover trial. *BMJ* 2002; 24:325(7361):409–410.
They went pretty high tech on this warming business, using a carbon-fiber heating mitt (!) versus the warming blankets that most of us would use. Well, heating works. It is all about vasodilating the veins by different means: NTG, warming, pooling, whatever it takes.

Maki DG, Botticelli JT, LeRoy ML, Thielke TS. Prospective study of replacing administration sets for intravenous therapy at 48- vs 72-hour intervals: 72 hours is safe and cost-effective. *JAMA* 1987;258:1777–1781.

Maki DG, Ringer M. Risk factors for infusion-related phlebitis with small peripheral venous catheters. A randomized, controlled trial. *Ann Intern Med* 1991;114:845–854.
Face it, this chapter is mostly about getting the damned IV in, but we'd be remiss if we spit on the catheters first and stirred up a lot of infections. So it's worth reading this to review the factors that go into IV phlebitis and infections.

Naimer SA, Temira F. Evaluation of techniques for intravenous catheter and tubing fixation. *Mil Med* 2004;169(1):79–81.
Wrap that arm in polyethylene and you'd be able to use that IV to rappel off a cliff and it wouldn't pull out. Most of us won't go nuts and wrap an entire arm in polyethylene to keep an IV in, but this is something to consider in, for example, a military or mass casualty situation where you just can't afford to lose the line, and the patient may require some rough handling during evacuation.

Roberge RJ, Kelly M, Evans TC, Hobbs E, Sayre M, Cottington E. Facilitated intravenous access through local application of nitroglycerin ointment. *Ann Emerg Med* 1987;16(5):546–549.
Oh, the logic of it! This is a why-didn't-I-think-of-that paper. Put a little 2% nitro on the back of the hand, presto-changeo, veins stick up and it's easier to nail the vein. Any side effects from the nitroglycerin absorption? No.

Rogers TL, Ostrow CL. The use of EMLA cream to decrease venipuncture pain in children. *J Pediatr Nurs* 2004;19(1):33–39.

EMLA cream seems like the greatest thing since sliced bread when it comes to putting IVs in kids. And science looked at this statement and confirmed it. You will note this comes from the nursing literature, an oft-forgotten source of useful information for all anesthesia people.

Rohm KD, Schollhorn TA, Gwosdek MJ, Piper SN, Maleck WH, Boldt J. Do we necessarily need local anaesthetics for venous cannulation? A comparison of different cannula sizes. *Eur J Anaesthesiol* 2004;21(3):214–216.

You don't really need to inject local for inserting 18-g or smaller cannulas. Needle stick and local sting hurts as much in this case.

Stein JC, Cole W, Kramer N, Quinn J. Ultrasound-guided peripheral intravenous cannulation in emergency department patients with difficult IV access. *Acad Emerg Med* 2004;11(5):581–582.

Damned useful technique. Once they had trouble putting in an IV, they called in the cavalry (in the form of an ultrasound guide) and lo and behold, they got it. I sure would prefer that to getting stuck over and over and over again, wouldn't you?

Weinstein SM. *Plumer's Principles and Practice of Intravenous Therapy*, 6th ed. Philadelphia: Lippincott; 1997, p 84-109.

Man, a whole book on IVs. Well, the whole thing isn't about placing IVs, these 25 pages look at the placement, the rest of it is about what goes through the IVs.

The Anesthesiologist's Party Piece: The IJ

Karim Abouelenin and Brantley Dollar

INTRODUCTION

When anesthesiologists need central lines, they usually follow the cue of Dracula et al. and go for the jugular, specifically, the internal jugular. The internal jugular is familiar turf to us. On the right side, it's a straight shot into the heart, so most righteously adapted to passage of a Swan-Ganz catheter, should that need arise.

The internal jugular is an ever-present friend in time of need.

THE ESSENCE OF THE INTERNAL JUGULAR APPROACH

- Cannulation of the internal jugular vein (central venous access) is a procedure performed to provide safe vascular access. This facilitates administration of rapid fluid boluses, transfusion of large volumes of blood products, and administration of cardiosupportive and anesthetic drip medications.

- Central venous access is required for cardiac monitoring: It provides central venous pressure measurements (CVP), pulmonary artery catheterization, and helps to provide transvenous cardiac pacing. It's also used as a rescue monitor for aspiration of air emboli (multiorifice) during craniotomy surgery.

- The internal jugular vein is one of the most common sites used for central venous access, especially by anesthesiologists. It has several advantages such as easy visibility, adequacy of bleeding control, and is a reliable technique with high success rate. On the other side, some of the known disadvantages are its close anatomic site to the carotid artery, and high risk of catheter-associated infection (especially in the ICU).

- Understanding the anatomic landmarks of the neck is a critical step in jugular vein cannulation. Different techniques for cannulation have been described such as the anterior, medial, and posterior approaches and, most recently, is the use of ultrasound-guided technique that has the advantage of superior patient safety compared to other approaches.

- Jugular venous cannulation is usually performed intraoperatively before or after anesthesia induction, although most anesthesiologists prefer placement of the central venous catheter after anesthesia induction in order to avoid patient discomfort, and respiratory depression from excessive use of sedative drugs. On the other hand, some anesthesiologists place the catheter before anesthesia induction, which can be done with adequate sedation and close patient monitoring.

- In the ICU, the multiple indications of central venous access among critically ill patients make it one of the most common procedures being done. The procedure is usually performed with adequate sedation and local anesthesia placement.

INDICATIONS

- Rapid infusion of fluids: Major surgery
  Major trauma
- Drug administration: Vasoactive drip medication
  Hyperalimentation
  Chemotherapy
- Prolonged antibiotic therapy
- Central venous pressure monitoring
- Pulmonary artery catheterization
- Transvenous cardiac pacing
- Temporary hemodialysis
- Aspiration of air emboli

RELATIVE CONTRAINDICATIONS

- Previous carotid surgery
- Documented carotid disease
- Superior vena cava obstruction
- Severe trauma of the neck
- Coagulopathic patients

How come vampires always get the jugular? They never seem to miss. You never see them digging around or "going to the other side," or "going subclavian."

Lament of an anesthesiologist who has missed the jugular. More than once.

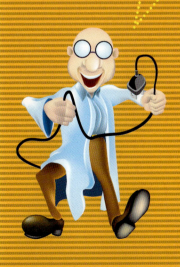

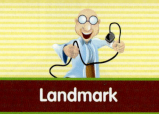

Landmark

There's one landmark here. Forget the triangles and all that crap, there's one landmark that really and truly matters. That landmark is the carotid. Feel the carotid and go just a little bitty bit lateral. That's where the internal jugular is and that, my friends, is that.

Don't believe me? Here's what you do:

The next time the ENT is doing a radical neck dissection, go into the room and look at the neck when they've pulled the skin back. Look right at the IJ and the carotid. There they are, right smack dab side by side. Couldn't be closer. Just like those huge rocks at Macchu Picchu, you couldn't fit a knife blade between them. No kidding. Looking over these vessels during a radical neck dissection is the world's greatest review of the anatomy. Anatomy books are dandy, sure, and by now there must be all sorts of virtual-dissection computer whizbang gizmos, but seeing the vessels in a real live human being hammers home the point.

The vessels are side by side. Feel the pulse in one to know where that is, then go a touch lateral. Bazingo.

ANATOMY OF THE INTERNAL JUGULAR VEIN

- The vein originates at the jugular foramen and runs down in the neck to terminate behind the sternoclavicular joint (medial side of the clavicle), where it joins the subclavian vein.

- It lies alongside the carotid artery and the vagus nerve within the carotid sheath. The vein is initially posterior to, then lateral and then anterolateral to the carotid artery during its descent in the neck. The vein lies most superficially in the upper part of the neck.

- At the level of the thyroid cartilage, the vein lies deep to the sternomastoid muscle. As it passes toward the thorax, it emerges from behind the muscle and comes to lie at the apex of the triangle between the sternal and clavicular insertions of the muscle.

- On both ends of the internal jugular vein there is a bulb, superior and inferior. The inferior jugular bulb contains a bicuspid valve that permits the flow of blood toward the heart.

- On the left side of the neck, the internal jugular vein lies anterior to the thoracic duct. For this reason, the right side is usually preferred to avoid the risk of thoracic duct injury; in addition, the right side offers more direct access to the superior vena cava.

- If you go in on the right, you have a straight shot all the way, but on the left, the vessel takes a right turn once you enter the thorax, so a vigorous push with a dilator could tear through the vessel at this right turn and cause a hemothorax.

IMPORTANT TIPS

- Before starting the procedure always be familiar with central venous catheter types, gauges, length and number of lumens. They vary depending on the purpose of their use: CVP monitoring, drip medications, or large fluid boluses in trauma patients.

- Multilumen catheters are preferred because they allow multiple functions but, at the same time, they carry high risk of infection and increased incidence of vascular perforation. A new popular catheter used for multiple purposes is the large introducer sheath; a short double-lumen catheter that can be inserted through the introducer valve, or even a pulmonary artery catheter that can be inserted via the valve.

- Always review your patient's medical condition, coagulation profile, and select the best safe site according to the indication of catheter placement (catheterization of the right jugular vein is beneficial for cardiac pacing and aspiration of air).

- Always be familiar with the contents of the kit (needles, dilator, central venous catheter, guidewire, local anesthetic), and keep sharps in a safe place away from your moving hands (needle stick injuries are serious).

BEWARE THE CENTRAL LINE FROM A MEDICAL INTENSIVE CARE UNIT

- Just as floor IVs are suspect, suspect central lines from medical units.

- Medical central lines are rarely placed with the same attention to detail that we pay to placing central lines.

- We hover around our central lines and use them for resuscitation, medical people place the line and write orders from afar.

- If a medical line comes down, make sure you can aspirate all the ports, look for kinks, stitches that are out (or were never placed).

- If a medical central line comes down with a pump attached, disconnect and make sure the line is not in an artery (no joke, this is the voice of experience talking).

- If a medical central line comes down and the patient is having ectopy, check the CXR and make sure the wire is still not inside (you think we're kidding? We're not).

- Find out how long ago the line was placed.

- If moss is growing out of the line, consider that the line may have been in long enough.

PROCEDURE AND APPROACH

- Patient should be adequately sedated, receiving oxygen via a mask. ECG, blood pressure monitors, and pulse oximeter are all placed before starting the procedure.

- Many approaches have been applied for internal jugular vein cannulation. Among the most used is the anterior approach that is described in this chapter. This approach is at a higher neck level compared to others with less risk of pneumothorax.

- Positioning the neck is very important for proper anatomic landmark identification and for providing a fast successful procedure. Careful history and exam is also very important, especially among patients with carotid artery disease because concurrent vertebral artery atherosclerosis is common, which can cause inadequate cerebral circulation with excessive neck extension.

- Patient is placed in the supine position, with slight turning of the head to the opposite side (20 degrees) to provide adequate exposure of the procedure site. The neck is slightly extended with a small roll placed under the shoulders. It is important to avoid flexion or excessive neck extension that can alter the anatomic landmark and collapse the vein.

- Before draping, anatomic landmark of the neck (sternocleidomastoid, sternal notch, and the mastoid process) should be felt, because attempts to palpate these landmarks will be difficult with the sterile drape coverage.

- Strict aseptic technique is required, following the CDC guidelines to reduce the risk of infection and catheter colonization:

  - Hand wash before the procedure with aseptic solution.

  - Sterile gloves and mask with shield should be worn when placing the central line in the operating room and in the ICU.

  - Cleanse the skin of the neck covering the area from the earlobe down to the clavicle and the sternal notch with antiseptic solution. Cleansing should be in circles, starting at the point of the stick and circling farther and farther away.

  - Apply a sterile drape over the neck; in the ICU, for long-term catheters, place a larger drape to cover the body.

- Apply the Trendelenburg position once drapes are placed by the help of an assistant. This will prevent the vein from collapsing unless the patient has high central venous pressure, and can't tolerate the Trendelenburg position.

- Carotid pulsations are palpated with the index and middle fingers of the left hand. If pulsations are not felt at all it is safer to use the ultrasound-guided technique.

- The skin and the subcutaneous tissue is infiltrated lateral to the carotid pulse at the level of the thyroid cartilage using a 25- or 26-g needle and 1% lidocaine. Local infiltration is needed only if line placement is done before anesthesia induction or in the ICU.

- A gentle palpation of the carotid pulses using the left fingers is applied. Then proceeding with the 22-g (mounted on a 3-mL syringe) needle at an angle 30 degrees to the skin at the same infiltration site, the needle is inserted at the medial border of the sternocleidomastoid between the two heads of the muscle toward the ipsilateral nipple.

- With gentle negative pressure applied to the needle and within 2-4 cm from the skin, the jugular vein should be encountered by observing venous blood (dark) entry into the vein.

- Although the use of a needle finder adds an extra step, it provides a safe technique by avoiding hematoma formation in a situation of carotid puncture.

- If the vein is not located with the finder needle, withdraw the needle and flush it. Reassess the anatomic landmark and patient position. Then apply the needle again directed slightly lateral to the carotid artery in an orderly fashion until the vein is located.

- After the internal jugular vein is located, the needle finder is kept in place, and a larger 18-g short bevel needle mounted on 5-mL syringe is applied just adjacent to the needle finder with gentle aspiration in the same needle finder track. The vein is located by observing dark venous blood entering with easy aspiration. Then remove the needle finder (22 g).

- With firm fixation of the hub of the 18-g needle by the left index finger and the thumb, the syringe is detached. Very important: Watch venous blood flow slowly and not pulsatile (arterial flow).

- A safe, confirmative technique for venous puncture is the use of a 2-inch, 18-g venous catheter mounted over the 18-g needle. This provides transducing the venous catheter end and observing a CVP tracing on the monitor. Or attaching short venous extension tubing and observing the blood flow pressure, which will distinguish venous from arterial flow. That is, hook up tubing to make sure the blood flow from the "stack vessel" is truly venous and not arterial.

- Seldinger guidewire is passed through the 18-g needle into the vein with the aid of the J-shaped tip, using the right hand while still holding the hub with the

How About That Little Echo Thingie?

Great idea. No less august a group than the Anesthesia Patient Safety Foundation recommends we use the device.

Old time anesthesiologists will snort and say, "I don't need it." And they are right.

Most of the time.

Like most specialty devices, you don't need it, until you **do**. I suggest you use the Site-Rite or similar neck-imaging devices, a few times before you *have to*. (Just as you don't do fiberoptics only when you have to if you hope to keep any proficiency).

But the world's best central line placer, when facing the obese, multiply-stuck, diabetic, short-necked person with no peripheral access, will perhaps embrace the echo locator device.

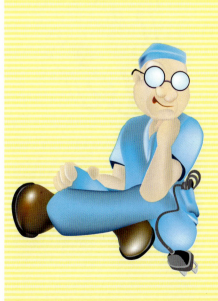

The Wire-Brushing Your Forearm Trick?

Drape and gown up. A recommendation by the Anesthesia Patient Safety Foundation. Anyone who has done anesthesia for a while will admit that, perhaps once or twice, the central line wire has, in the course of wobbling around, brushed against their ungowned forearm.

That is what you call a "Close Encounter of the Nonsterile Kind." So, gown up.

Here's a little real-world tip for when you glove up: When you open the gloves, to keep the sterile paper from folding up and making you look like a dope, just fold the bottom part of the paper underneath. That keeps the paper flat, and you can pull your gloves out easily.

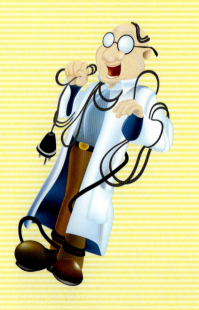

left hand to no more than 18-cm distance, and continuously watching the ECG monitor for arrhythmias. The wire should pass easily through the vein without forcing it.

- If arrhythmias are encountered on the monitor, *immediately* stop passing the wire, and pull it back until arrhythmias disappear.

- *Always* pay attention to the wire and *never* let go of it through the entire procedure.

- The puncture site is then enlarged with a scalpel to facilitate placement of the central venous catheter over the guidewire. Then a firm dilator is placed over the guidewire to dilate the skin and subcutaneous tissue still more, and to provide smooth central venous catheter placement.

- When using large introduce sheath catheters, the dilator and the sheath form one unit. Never bend the free end of the guidewire when placing the sheath and the dilator together.

- Once the dilator is removed, the central venous catheter is placed over the guidewire. Always pay attention to the wire and never let it free from your hand; accomplish this by pulling the wire carefully at the patient's skin until sufficient length of the wire comes out through the catheter port while inserting the catheter at adequate depth. Then hold the free end of the wire with your right hand and withdraw it completely.

- Adequate depth of the central venous catheter is important to ensure placement of the catheter tip at the superior vena cava above the junction with the right atrium.

Right internal jugular vein is about 16 cm to the atrio-caval junction.

Left internal jugular vein is about 19 cm to the atrio-caval junction.

- Aspiration of blood from each catheter port is important to remove air, check venous blood flow, and assure patent ports before the catheter is sutured in place and sterile dressing is applied.

- Confirm the central venous catheter position by ordering a portable chest X-ray. This can be done in the operating room, recovery area, or in the ICU.

The catheter should lie in the SVC, at the level of T 4–T 5 below the clavicle.

FLOURISH AND EXCUSES

- If you zip the line right in with no problems, then say, just loud enough for

everyone in the room to hear, "It usually doesn't take me this long."

- If you can't get it, and you flounder helplessly, then mutter something under your breath about "aberrant anatomy."

COMMON GLITCHES

- Take the time to set up a good working environment, otherwise you end up twisting yourself in knots trying to grab stuff.

- As you press the neck to feel the carotid, you do compress the IJ, making it harder to hit. Once you feel the carotid, ease up on your finger pressure.

- If you miss, and you start getting panicky, you tend to stick all over the place. Be methodical. Go in, pull straight back, change direction a little, go in there. That way you fan all the possible planes and are more likely to hit.

- Don't be in a rush. Take the time to make sure you're not in the carotid.

- Don't get married to one place. If you just cannot get it, go somewhere else.

- If something doesn't seem right, (the wire comes out crooked, one port doesn't flush), then trust your instincts—something probably *isn't* right. Redo the line. You hate to be halfway into a case and find out, damn it, that the line **is** in wrong.

ULTRASOUND-GUIDED CENTRAL VENOUS CANNULATION

Ultrasound-guided approaches to the internal jugular vein resulted in fewer needle passes, reduces the incidence of arterial punctures, and is a more successful technique compared to other approaches. In the near future, the ultrasound technique will become a standard of care for jugular venous cannulation. The medical malpractice crystal ball sees this question in future courtrooms: "Why, doctor, did you *not* use the ultrasound on this patient? Well, speak up! Some of the jurors are hard of hearing."

The jugular vein is identified by

- easy compression with the Doppler probe.

- lack of pulsation.

- enlargement with Valsalva maneuver.

New evidence by ultrasound has shown us

- veins are compressed by the cannulating needle.

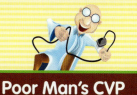

- vein puncture is observed equally with needle withdrawal and advancement.
- in a few patients the internal jugular vein lies over the carotid artery.

COMPLICATIONS OF JUGULAR VEIN CANNULATION

- Carotid artery puncture
- Incidence: 2%-8%.
- High risk of hematoma formation in coagulopathic patients.
- Carotid stick can lead to airway compromise.
- Carotid stick can also lead to pseudoaneurysm or cerebrovascular insufficiency.
- Carotid artery cannulated with a large port catheter?
- AARGH! The ultimate intravascular boo-boo.
- Leave the catheter and consider your options as you bite your lip and wish you'd gone into dermatology.
- If the patient is at low risk of complications, remove the catheter and apply firm pressure for 15 minutes with close neurological, hemodynamic, and airway monitoring.
- If the patient is at high risk of complications, consider intubating the patient before removing the catheter (preventing airway compromise).

- Some authors prefer exploratory operation, as pressure might be ineffective.
- If the cannula is removed, apply firm pressure (remember firm pressure on the carotid artery can precipitate a cerebral event). Consult a vascular surgeon as soon as possible to determine if surgical exploration is needed.
- Vertebral artery puncture
- Pneumothorax
  - High incidence with low approach in the neck.
- Venous air embolism.
  - Occurs with subatmospheric pressure in the venous system when it opens to atmosphere. Paradoxical air embolism is common among patients with patent foramen ovale.
- Nerve injury.
  - Vagus, phrenic, accessory, hypoglossal nerves, and the stellate ganglion.
- Guidewire-inducing arrhythmias.
- Chylothorax from thoracic duct injury, left-side approach.
- Tracheal perforation and endotracheal cuff perforation.
- Venous thrombosis and impaired venous drainage.
- Infection, catheter colonization, and line sepsis
  - Occur as late complications.

Poor Man's CVP

Once you have the wire in, you need to make sure the wire is in the right place. Take just a little extra time to assure that. Here's the way to do it:

If you have a catheter in, hook up a little tubing to it and hold the tubing up. You should see the blood column rise a little bit, consistent with a CVP number. If the blood pulses up, is bright red, has a PaO_2 of 350, and transduces at 120/80, then you may want to reassess whether you are in the venous bed.

If you used the needle as a guide, then take one minute out of your busy day, slide the 18-g catheter down the wire (if you're in the carotid, you've already made an 18-g hole with the needle, so by placing the 18-g catheter, you're not making anything worse), then pull out the wire and do the poor man's CVP maneuver with a short piece of tubing.

Why?

When you place the wire through the needle, you don't have the luxury to look closely at the signal from the hub of the needle. You are so intent on keeping the needle still, that you just take a quick look then ram the wire in before you lose your place.

That can lead to an unrecognized carotid stick.

By taking the extra time to slide the 18-g catheter in, you have a little more luxury time to really look over where you are. That catheter isn't going to jump out of the vessel, so you have time to do the poor man's CVP (or, for that matter, send a blood gas or hook up a real transducer if you want to). The minute it takes you to do that is much less than the time it takes to repair a carotid.

Do You Need to Intubate First?

Clinical aside here:

If you are placing a central line in patients, and you can't get them anywhere near flat, ask yourself this question, "Should I be intubating patients when they are so short of breath?" You might be better off securing the airway first, making sure the patient is stable, and oxygenation is assured before you place that line. It's easy to get focused on *the line* and forget *the patient*.

If they need ventilatory support, well, give them ventilatory support. You are not a CVP technician, you are a physician, evaluating the whole picture.

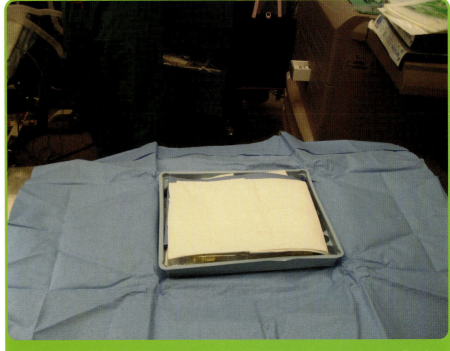

Figure 1. Give yourself plenty of room and lay out the kit nice and neat. Don't jam yourself into a corner or you'll contaminate something.

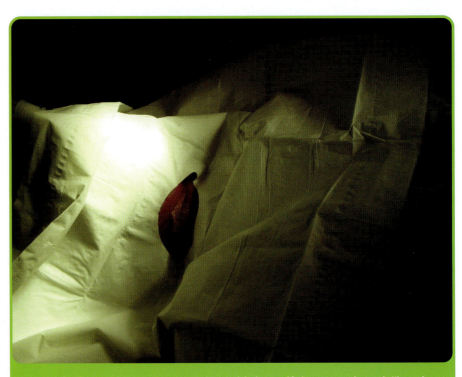

Figure 2. Prep, drape and get some good lighting. If the patient's neck "bunches up", then have someone reach down, pull down on the chest, and stretch things out. "Create a neck" where there was no neck.

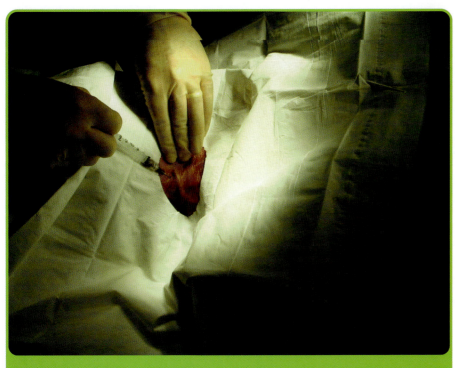

Figure 3. After you put in some local, then go in with a finder. Better to hit "big red" with a little finder needle than hit it with an 18 g catheter. (Note, some people argue against use of a finder needle.)

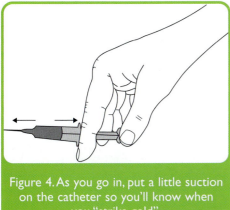

Figure 4. As you go in, put a little suction on the catheter so you'll know when you "strike gold".

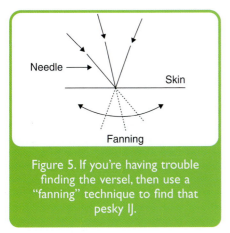

Figure 5. If you're having trouble finding the versel, then use a "fanning" technique to find that pesky IJ.

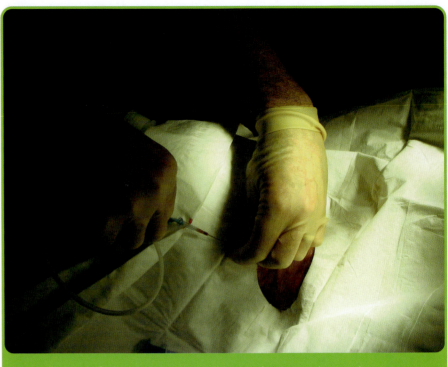

Figure 6. Once you get the needle or catheter in, advance the wire, watching for arrhythmias.

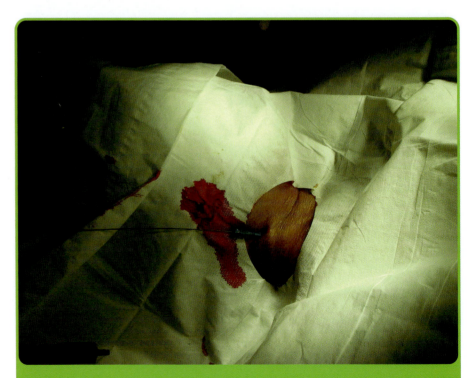

Figure 7. But wait! Once that wire is in, don't make the mistake of saying, "Aha! I KNOW I'm in the right place." Instead, say to yourself, "The wire is now *somewhere*, and I have to prove it's in the right place before I put the big hogger in there." So put the catheter back down the wire (this whole thing takes about 45 seconds), then withdraw the wire, hook up some tubing, and do the "Poor man's CVP."

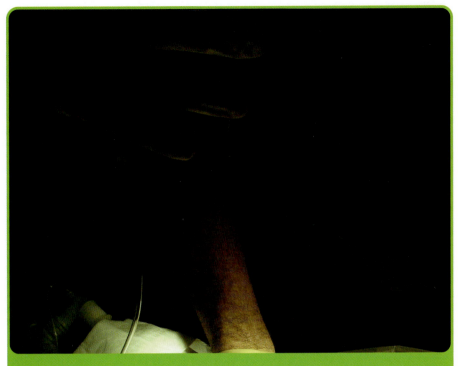

Figure 8. Look at the tubing, the blood is going up just a little ways, giving you a CVP of, say 6 cm. Certainly this is not pulsatile, bright blood. So you've determined where you are and now you can proceed to the big monster.

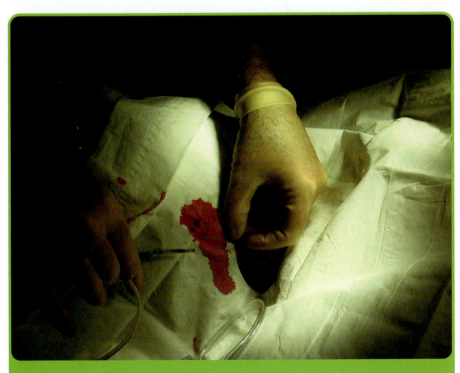

Figure 9. So now put the wire back in.

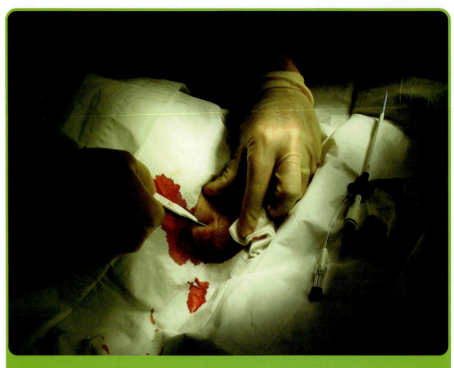

Figure 10. Now it's time for the knife stick. Lay that blade flat on the wire, making sure the sharp part of the blade is facing away from the carotid.

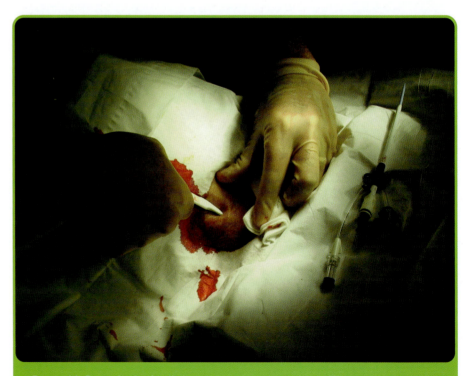

Figure 11. Bury the knife all the way to the white plastic. That will assure a big enough hole for the main line. If you make too little of a hole, then the introducer will tear through the skin and that's no fun!

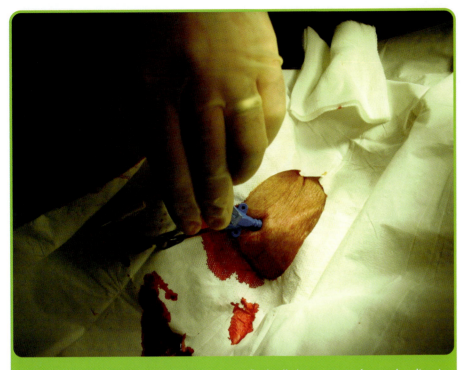

Figure 12. Secure the line, making sure you flush all the ports and sew that line in so it doesn't jump out on you.

SUGGESTED READING

American Society of Anesthesiologists. *Recommendations for infection control for the practice of anesthesiology*, 2nd ed. Park Ridge, IL: ASA; 1998, p 15.

Andrews RT, Bova DA. How much guidewire is too much? Direct measurement of the distance from subclavian and internal jugular vein access sites to the superior vena cava-atrial junction during central venous catheter placement. *Crit Care Med* Jan 2000;28(1):138-142.
Determines that patient height, weight, and measurements from previous chest radiographs are less reliable in predicting a safe wire length than is the access site selected. Concludes that 18 cm should be considered the upper limit of guidewire introduced during central catheter placement in adults.

Aoki H, Mizobe T, Nozuchi S, et al. Vertebral artery pseudoaneurysm: a rare complication of internal jugular vein catheterization. *Anesth Analg* 1992;75:296-298.

Armstrong PJ, Sutherland R, Scott DH. The effect of position and different manoeuvres on internal jugular vein diameter size. *Acta Anaesthesiol Scand* Apr 1994;38:229-231.
Studies different variables and their effect on IJ size; found no correlation between diameter and subject habitus; artery palpation and neck extension reduced its diameter; Trendelenburg increased diameter; abdominal binder and Valsalva increased size.

Badley AD, Steckelberg JM. Infectious rates of central venous pressure catheters: comparison between newly placed catheters & those that have been changed. *Mayo Clin Proc* 1996;71:838.
In a population of ICU patients in whom catheter change was governed by clinical judgment, no differences were noted between the observed rates of infection of new site replacement catheters and guidewire exchange catheters.

Civetta JM, Gabel JC. Internal jugular vein-puncture with a margin of safety. *Anesthesiology* 1972;36:622.

Daily PO, Griepp RB. Percutaneous internal jugular vein cannulation. *Arch Surg* 1970;101:534.

Depierraz B, Essinger A, Morin D, Goy JJ, Buchser E. Isolated phrenic nerve injury after apparently atraumatic puncture of the internal jugular vein. *Intensive Care Med* 1989;15:132-134.
A case report of a missed diagnosis of phrenic nerve paralysis that occurred after an unsuccessful, but apparently atraumatic attempt to puncture the internal jugular vein prior to cardiac surgery.

Dzelzkalns R, Stanely TH. Placement of pulmonary artery catheter before anesthesia for cardiac surgery: a stressful, painful, unnecessary crutch. *J Clin Monit* 1985; 1:197.

A threefold argument against the placement of preinduction PA catheters. Information provided by a PA catheter may be misleading since it is an indirect measurement that depends on many variables; correction of hemodynamic abnormalities detected by a PA catheter does not improve induction of anesthesia or outcome after cardiac surgery; and inserting a PA catheter produces cardiovascular stimulation that can lead to myocardial ischemia.

Eckhardt WF, Iaconetti DJ, Kwon JS, et al. Inadvertent carotid artery cannulation during pulmonary artery catheter insertion. *J Cardiothorac Vasc Anesth* 1996;283-290.

A case report describing this complication of central venous cannulation.

Fabian JA, Jesudian MC. A simple method of improving the safety of percutaneous cannulation of the internal jugular vein. *Anesth Analg* 1985;64:1032.

Gilbert TB, Seneff MG, Becker RB. Facilitation of internal jugular venous cannulation using an audio-guided Doppler ultrasound vascular access device: results from a prospective, dual-center, randomized, crossover clinical study. *Crit Care Med* 1995;23:60-55.

Concludes that the use of an audio-guided Doppler ultrasound vascular access device was associated with increased success of cannulation and a decreased frequency of significant complications in a population of high-risk patients with obesity or coagulopathy.

Gratz I, Afshar M, Kidwell P, Weiman DS, Shariff HM. Doppler-guided cannulation of the internal jugular vein: a prospective, randomized trial. *J Clin Monit* May 1994;10(3):185-188.

Concludes that the Doppler-guided cannulation technique can reduce the number of attempts required for successful IJ cannulation.

Gravenstein N, Blackshear RH. In vitro evaluation of relative perforating potential of central venous catheters: comparison of materials, selected models, number of lumens, and angles of incidence to simulated membrane. *J Clin Monit* 1991;7:1.

Studies several variables including lumen number, material, and length to determine the potential for atrial or caval perforation by central venous catheter insertion.

Ho AM, Chung DC, Tay BA, Yu LM, Yeo P. Diluted venous blood appears arterial: implications for central venous cannulation. *Anesth Analg* Dec 2000;91(6):1356.

Discusses identification of inadvertent arterial puncture, and that this sign is removed if one puts saline in the aspirating syringe because dusky venous blood turns bright red on dilution.

Jain U, Shah KB, Belusko RJ, et al, Subclavian artery laceration and acute hemothorax on attempted internal jugular vein cannulation. *J Cardiothorac Vasc Anesth* 1991;608-610.

A case report describing this complication of central venous cannulation.

Kapadia CB, Heard SO, Yeston NS. Delayed recognition of vascular complications caused by central venous catheters. *J Clin Monit* 1988;4:267.

Three patients are described in whom vascular complications occurred after placement of central venous catheters. Inappropriate catheter length and site of cannulation, catheter movement, and unsuitable catheter material can lead to complications. Guidelines for cannulation of central veins are defined, and recommendations for chest roentgenography, which could result in early recognition of catheter misplacement, are provided.

Khalil KG, Parker FB. Thoracic duct injury: a complication of jugular vein catheterization. *JAMA*, 1972;221:908.

A case report.

Klipper WS, Waite HD, Tomlinson CO. Endotracheal cuff perforation complicating subclavian venipuncture. *JAMA* 1974;228:693.

A case report.

Kua JS, Tan IK. Airway obstruction following internal jugular vein cannulation. *Anaesthesia* 1997;52:776-780.

A case report of a patient that developed airway obstruction leading to cardiac arrest after removal of an internal jugular central venous catheter.

Lobato EB, Sulek CA. Cross-sectional area of the right and left internal jugular veins. *J Cardiothoracic Vasc Anesth* Apr 999;13(2):136.

States that hepatic compression and positive inspiratory hold effectively dilate the RIJV when the Trendelenburg position is not possible; may facilitate cannulation, possibly by making the vein less collapsible due to increased intravascular pressure.

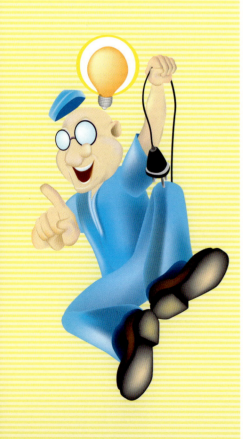

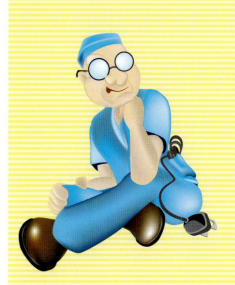

Mennim P, Coyle CF, Taylor JD. Venous air embolism associated with removal of central venous catheter. *BMJ* Jul 18 1992;305:171-172.

Royster RL, Johnston WE. Arrhythmias during venous cannulation prior to pulmonary artery catheter insertion. *Anesth Analg* 1985;64:1214.

Sanford TJ. Internal jugular vein cannulation versus subclavian vein cannulation. an anesthesiologist's view: the right internal jugular vein. *J Clin Monit* 1985;1:58.

Seeberger M, Wu X, Skarvan K. Does short term central venous catheterization of the internal jugular vein cause the thrombi of pathologic relevance? *Anesthesiology* 1998;89:A1203.

Seldinger SI. Catheter replacement of the needle in percutaneous arteriography. *Acta Radiol* 1953;39:368.

Shield CF, Richardson JD, Buckley CJ, et al. Pseudoaneurysm of the brachiocephalic arteries: a complication of percutaneous internal jugular vein catheterization. *Surgery* 1975;78:190-193.

Streisand JB, Clark NJ, Pace NL. Placement of pulmonary arterial catheter before anesthesia for cardiac surgery: safe, intelligent, and appropriate use of invasive hemodynamic monitoring. *J Clin Monit* 1985;1:193.
An argument that preinduction placement of the PA catheter provides valuable, objective information for the cardiac anesthesiologist without incurring significant risk to the patient.

Whittet HB, Boscoe MJ. Isolated palsy of the hypoglossal nerve after central venous catheterization. *Br Med J* 7 April 1994;288(6423):1042.
A case report of this rare complication.

INTRODUCTION

A Swan-Ganz catheter, more precisely, a flow-directed pulmonary artery catheter, lays out a lot of cardiac information for you. From its proximal port, the Swan gives you a central venous pressure reading; from its distal port, it gives you pulmonary artery and pulmonary artery occlusion pressure readings when wedged. Swans can give you cardiac output, mixed venous oxygen saturation, or continuous versions of both cardiac output and mixed venous oxygen saturation.

Swans have their champions ("You can't manage an ICU patient *without* one.") and their detractors ("Swans are not only *not* helpful, they themselves are *dangerous*."). The debate has raged for years and shows no signs of abating. Throw *this* curveball into the game: Transesophageal echocardiography is now doing a lot of what Swans used to do.

So, the role of Swan-Ganz catheters is open to debate. But, love them or hate them, you do need to know how to place and troubleshoot them.

INDICATIONS

- Assessing hemodynamics, you can assess function and filling pressures.
- Monitoring volume status in a patient where CVP alone will not suffice.
- Monitoring effect of inotropic support in a patient when arterial line alone will not suffice.
- Management of the critically ill patient, especially one whose urine output defies traditional remedies, or one whose hemodynamics defies routine maneuvers.

RELATIVE CONTRAINDICATIONS

- Status postpneumonectomy. If the Swan floats to the arterial stump on the side of the pneumonectomy, it can tear or erode the stump causing a massive bleed. The use of fluoroscopy is recommended to assist in placement of the Swan in this condition to ensure that the catheter goes to the appropriate side.
- Small size. Typically, you don't float Swans in kiddies. However, small pedi Swans are available, but rarely used.
- Clots in the right heart. You may dislodge them with the Swan!
- Pulmonary hypertension. Difficulty with wedging, increased risk of PA rupture, propensity to have coiling of the catheter in RV.
- Left bundle branch block. Theoretical risk of causing complete heart block by inducing a right bundle branch block with the Swan. (Rare. Less than 1%

chance of this occurring according to many studies.) If you do have a patient with LBBB, have transcutaneous pacing capability nearby. It is not recommended to have the pacer pads attached to patient ahead of time, but have everything readily available and working.
- Surgery in the right heart. Swan could get damaged or in the way.
- Heart transplant: *be careful* to pull back Swan before removing heart!

EQUIPMENT

- Introducer in place (see Chapter 1).
- Introducer can be, well, just about anywhere.
- For most anesthetic purposes, the introducer will be in the right IJ, but the introducer can be on the left IJ, either EJ (though EJ passage can be problematic), either subclavian vein, either femoral vein, or even antecubital. If the blood can float to the heart, then you can float the Swan to the heart. The catheter is, after all, flow-directed. RIJ is preferred because it is the shortest and less circuitous route to the right heart.
- Pulmonary artery catheter sleeve (named the "Swandom" or "Condom" by those of an irreverent nature).
- Pulmonary artery catheter itself. These come in a lot of flavors, from the plain vanilla, just a Swan, to the more exotic kinds—continuous mixed venous oxygen saturation, continuous cardiac output, pacing Swans, paceport Swans.

Whoever "Ganz" is, he must be ticked. No one talks about "floating a Ganz," it's always, "floating a Swan." Must be sort of like the **second** guy to step on the moon. Who was that, anyway?

Low-level anesthetic functionary, idly speculating during a cardiac case. Somewhere, sometime.

Let's be Supersafe and Put in a Swan

A Jehovah's Witness patient was scheduled for an open cholecystectomy. The patient had a cardiac history, so, to be supersafe, a Swan-Ganz catheter was planned.

The Swan: the ultimate cardiac thing.

With the Swan in, nothing can go wrong, because, well, Swans are for, you know, cardiac safety, you'll be able to tell anything with it!

Forget the fact that the surgeon was fast.

Forget the fact that the fluid shifts were going to be small.

Forget the fact that the patient would be extubated post-op and require no ICU management.

Let's put in a Swan because, because that's what you do with cardiac patients.

Swan: PA rupture.

Bleed: Jehovah's Witness, can't transfuse.

Call thoracic surgery, they say, and rightfully so, "Thanks for calling us now!"

Patient died.

So much for being supersafe.

- They do not yet have a Swan that can walk your dog and cook a pizza, but that very thing is currently in Stage III trials.
- Transducers hooked up to the Swan.
- Sterile setup—don't forget to gown up lest you brush the Swan against your forearm.
- An extra pair of eyes watching the patient as you do your thing. Even if you're not an exhibitionist, you will want someone to keep an eye on you and your patient.
- Good venous access in case you need to rescue the patient from your evil doings.
- In rare cases, a C-arm to help guide the Swan when you're having a terrible time and just can't get it to go.
- Pacing capability (for example, external Zoll pads), if you are floating a Swan in a patient with a preexisting left bundle branch block.

BEWARE THE SWAN THAT COMES TO YOU FROM A MEDICAL ICU

- Not to harp on this, but do be wary of a Swan that comes to you from afar.
- See how far the Swan has been floated, we've seen it at 30 (Swan is in the right ventricle, causing ectopy) and at 70 (oh damn, if you inflate the balloon here, you may rupture the pulmonary artery).
- Not uncommonly, kinks, introducers not sewn in and hanging out of the skin, or uncapped introducers (potential route for air embolism) may be encountered in a foreign Swan. Inspect, inspect, inspect, and have a high index of suspicion anytime you're handed a Swan.

PHILOSOPHY OF SWANS

- If called to do Swans on critically ill patients, ask yourself whether they need to be intubated first.
- People don't die of lack of a Swan, but they do die of respiratory insufficiency and hypoxemia.
- TEE does do a lot of what Swans do, but you can't keep a TEE in all the time. So, for ICU care, even if you used a TEE during a case, consider putting in a Swan to help out.
- Floating a Swan is fraught with hazard (rhythm disturbances, the ever-present specter of PA rupture), so make sure you are in the zone and paying attention.

- Know your helpers and make sure you are on the same wavelength when you are asking for that balloon to be inflated. If they inflate at the wrong time, you can rupture that PA and then you've had it.
- The more complicated the Swan, the more crap is attached to it, and the more likely the thing is to pull back or pull out.
- The more complicated the Swan, the more attention you have to pay to it, (troubleshooting the continuous cardiac output machine, calibrating the mixed venous oxygen saturation). This can distract you from your *main* job which is to take care of the patient.
- Swan numbers are not the be-all, end-all. Put them in the overall context (blood gas, hematocrit, blood pressure, clinical picture).

SWAN HISTORY AND PHYSICAL

- Know the road map of the patient's circulation.
- Most people can take a Swan with no problem, but a few will present special problems.
- Adult patients who had cardiac surgery as children may present special problems: baffles, rerouting, blind alleys, all kinds of weirdness. Check with their cardiologists to make sure the vessel you stick will admit a Swan into the pulmonary artery circulation.
- Superior vena cava syndrome: Floating a Swan from above may not work because the road is blocked.
- VSD or ASD. Your Swan may tiptoe across to the other side.
- Know what surgery is planned. A heart transplant, for example, requires that you pull the Swan back before it gets amputated!
- If the surgeon is planning on replacing the tricuspid or pulmonic valve, then you don't want your Swan laying across the middle of the surgical field.
- Also, if the patient has a gigantic septic goombah sitting on the pulmonic valve, you don't want your Swan to dislodge and embolize the mass.
- Multiply stuck or multiple-lines-already-there-patients: Look for scarring, Groshongs, ports, pacers. You don't want to get tied up in a knot with other appliances.

TECHNIQUE

- When placing the cordis introducer, do make sure you're not in the carotid (see Chapter 2).
- Clear the area around you. Don't have IV tubing and other things right next to you when you are extending the Swan: You don't want to hit against something and contaminate it.
- If you have to prepare your own Swan, flush all the lines and cap them off with a stopcock so air won't reentrain into them.
- Once you've flushed the lines, keep the tray flat, so fluid won't flow into a non-sterile area, then float back into the sterile area.
- Make sure your transducers are zeroed and leveled appropriately.
- Glove and gown up, make sure your area is sterile.
- Just before you get going on the Swan, take a good look at the patient and the vital signs. There is an almost unavoidable tendency to get wrapped up in your procedure and to forget about the patient.
- Remember, the Swan can wait, an unstable or apneic patient cannot!
- Key Moment: Locating sheath (condom) and taking out of package before insertion.
- Pull the Swan through the condom (sheath), making sure you have the sheath oriented in the correct direction with the locking mechanism toward the patient (look carefully at picture). Don't expand condom yet as it is difficult to then feed Swan all the way through.
- Once the Swan is through the diaphragm of the sheath, check the balloon. That balloon can and does rupture as it goes through the sheath. Don't feel like a manly man if it does rupture, it happens to everyone!
- Pull the sheath up and out of the way so you can navigate the Swan.
- You will inevitably get very excited your first few times inserting a PAC and just stick the Swan in without protection, the condom. You will then have to pull out and start over, i.e., *Swanus Interruptus*. Remember the Swandom.
- Make sure the transducers are hooked up correctly to the Swan and that you can see proper movement of the numbers when you move the Swan around. A nice way to see if the transducer is zeroed correctly and is functioning is to

place the catheter tip at the level of the patient's chest. The PA and CVP should read close to zero. Then raise the tip about 30 cm above the patient while leaving the rest of the catheter (proximal CVP port in particular) at the level of the chest. The PA should now read about 20 mmHg (equivalent to the 30 cm in height you raised the catheter) and the CVP should still read zero. If your CVP reads 20 and PA is still zero, your transducers are functioning, but they are mislabeled on your screen. Either change the labels, or reverse your connection. If your numbers are way off (for instance, only reads 5 mmHg at 30 cm above pt), go ahead and zero, and flush all ports again and reattempt.

- Lay the Swan out so the curve of the Swan will go in the right direction. For the most common approach, the right IJ, the Swan should form a curve going off to the left, that way the Swan will curl through the heart and out the pulmonary artery.
- For other approaches, try to visualize where the heart lies, how the PA goes, and how best to get the damned Swan to go to the right place.
- Put the Swan into the introducer and advance it to 20 cm. That will put the tip, the balloon-tipped end, out of the introducer and near, or in, the right atrium. Watch your monitor for a CVP trace.
- Inflate the balloon with the specially designated syringe, using not more than the 1.5 cc's they allow you to inject.
- Overinflating the balloon can rupture the balloon and overinflating the balloon when it's in the pulmonary artery can rupture the artery.
- Back to balloon inflation: Be sure you close the loop every time you inflate the balloon—you say, "inflate the balloon," then listen for your assistant to say, "balloon inflated" before you do anything. When you say, "deflate the balloon," listen for your assistant to say, "balloon deflated" before you do anything. No kidding, this is important. If everyone is jabbering, the radio is blasting, and no one's paying attention, one of these exchanges can get lost and *kaboom!* PA rupture and patient death!
- Once the balloon's inflated, advance the catheter, watching the trace the entire time.
- When the trace goes from CVP to RV, say, "RV."

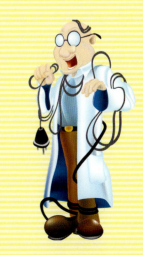

Breakfast and a Swan

A member of the ICU called me to a patient's bedside.

"I'm having trouble with this Swan, it won't wedge, and I can't get the numbers to zero right, and the cardiac output doesn't make sense."

The patient was sitting up in a chair, eating a hearty breakfast, looking wonderful. Greeting me, the patient asked how *I* was doing!

"Here," I said, then I pulled the Swan out and threw it away. "Anyone who's eating breakfast, sitting up in a chair, and asking after *my* health and well-being does not need a Swan anymore."

Laziness with a Capital L

In our Brave New World of off-pump CABGs, beating-heart valve surgery, and percutaneous everything, the burning need for a Swan just doesn't blaze as brightly. And with the TEE going into everybody, who needs it anyway?

One day our ICU attending approached me.

"Did you do that double valve yesterday, with the guy with the rotten ejection fraction and the renal insufficiency?"

That put my teeth on edge. No one asks you, "Did you do…?", but that something awful happened, and now they're going to pin it on you.

"Uh," I looked around, hoping there might be a large crack in the linoleum flooring that might allow me to escape, "yes, I did."

The ICU attending pressed, "Did it occur to you that we might, just might, need a Swan to manage him in the unit?"

"Uh," no linoleum escape route had yet opened up.

"You did him with the TEE yesterday, didn't you?"

"Uh."

And then you figured we'd just get by with a CVP, even though we didn't have a TEE?"

"Um."

"Do you think you guys in the OR might be getting a little bit lazy? You manage everything with the TEE but then, to hell with us in the ICU? Is that what you guys are thinking? This guy has two valves done, two! And his heart and kidneys are bad to start out with. And now you just blow us off and leave us without a Swan. And you want me to keep this guy humming?"

"Er, uh…"

- If you're feeling goofy, say, "LV," just to see if anyone's paying attention. Trust me, you'll get some surprised looks, and you will develop a reputation for being the life of the party. All joking aside, this *can* happen in a large VSD for instance. Learn what an RV trace should look like so that you can suspect something unusual when the trace doesn't fit.

- Once in the RV, keep your eyes peeled for ectopy or for heart block (rare, but dangerous if the patient has a preexisting left bundle branch block). Also be especially aware of sustained ectopy (V tach or V fib) in patients with acute ischemia, particularly right ventricular infarct or ischemia.

- Keep advancing until you get the PA trace.

- Advance until you get a wedge trace, but *don't be a nut for getting a wedge*. If you get to 55 cm, and you don't have a wedge, but you have a good PA trace, then stop there and give it a rest. If you don't get a wedge, you still have a lot of other information. If you push and push to get a wedge, one day you'll get a PA rupture. If you still don't have a PA trace by 50, boy! you better start over!

- Let the balloon down. (Keeping the balloon up will cause a lung infarction, leaving a telltale triangle of pulmonic death on the CXR and embarrassing you in front of your peers.). At this time, your wedge trace should change to a PA trace. If it remains wedged, withdraw catheter (making sure balloon is deflated) until you see a PA trace once again. Reinflate and see if you get a wedge trace.

- Slide the sheath over the Swan and secure it in place. We hope you remembered your Swandom.

- Pat yourself on the back, but don't break your arm doing it.

FANCY FOOTWORK WHEN THE SWAN WON'T GO

- Check the usual stuff first.
- Pull the Swan out and make sure the balloon still inflates.
- Pull the Swan out and make sure it's curling the right way.
- Make sure the transducers are well connected and in the appropriate scales.
- Put the patient's head up and tilt him right side down—that way, the balloon will float up and out of the right ventricle.

- Inject cold water through the Swan to give it some nature. Be aware, this cold-water injectate could cause ectopy.

- If patients are awake, have them take deep breaths to try to suck the Swan into the PA.

- Open the IVs to fill the heart up a little more.

- Try going real slow, letting the balloon catch a wave like an Oahu surfer catching a 35-foot, fast-left, reef break during a winter storm at the North Shore's very own Banzai Pipeline.

- If real slow doesn't work, go with the old standby of all procedures, try something different. Go fast, and maybe you'll get lucky.

- If by chance the chest is open, have the surgeons guide the catheter with their fingers.

- If all else fails (and sometimes it does), get a new Swan. Once they're in the patient long enough, they get warm, soft, and mushy. A new Swan may float out more easily.

- Get a C-arm. Advance under X-ray guidance.

- You can use our friend the TEE to guide the Swan as well.

GLITCH-O-RAMA

- The ultimate disaster is the PA rupture, usually caused by a vigorous hunt to get a wedge (pulmonary artery occlusion pressure).

- Best treatment: prevention and knowledge.

- If obtaining a wedge becomes an impossible and failing quest, then you can always use the PA diastolic to estimate the wedge. This number is usually quite close to a real wedge pressure when there is no pulmonary HTN. Also, without a wedge, you still have other valuable information including cardiac output and mixed venous saturation, so the Swan is not totally useless without a wedge.

- Also, if you don't know your traces well, you run the risk of a rupture by not identifying a wedged catheter. For instance, in the presence of *mitral regurgitation*, it can be difficult to identify a wedged catheter and one might continue to advance a wedged catheter and risk rupture. Mitral regurgitation makes it very difficult to notice a wedge tracing because of the potentially large V systolic waves when wedged. These V systolic waves make the trace closely resemble a PA trace.

- To help identify a wedge tracing, we recommend that you superimpose the arterial and PA pressure traces. PA and arterial tracings will peak in unison. When you wedge a catheter in the presence of large systolic V waves (as in mitral regurgitation), you will clearly notice a right shift of the PA tracing, such that the peak of the PA (or shall we say, "wedge") tracing is offset to the right of the arterial peak and not in unison anymore. You will now know that you are wedged, and that advancing the catheter further is dangerous.

- PA rupture causes massive bleeding into the trachea, awake patients will cough and bring up blood, intubated patients will suddenly fill their endotracheal tube with blood.

- What to do? *Pray.* This can be—and often is—fatal.

- Keep the PA balloon inflated in an attempt to tamponade off the bleed.

- Lay the patient on the side of the bleeding lung to avoid soiling the good lung with blood.

- Get thoracic surgical help.

- You'll need to isolate the lung (see Chapter 30) so both sides don't fill with blood.

- Once you *have* isolated the lung, put the bleeding lung on the up side to hydrostatically decrease the perfusion pressure of the patient's bleeding PA.

- Pray more.

- Other problems with the Swan: kinking or tying in a knot. Send to special procedure for removal under direct vision if this happens.

- Another problem is ectopy: If ectopy is causing a lot of trouble, pull the Swan out of the RV, or rapidly advance the catheter into the PA. A Swan tip in the RV is quite irritating and will cause PVCs more than 70% of the time, so they are to be expected. Just don't leave the catheter tip in the RV. Advance to PA, or pull out if sustained or troublesome arrhythmias occur. Prophylactic antiarrhythmics are of no use.

- Don't kill the patient to get a number.

WHAT DO YOU DO WITH THE DIGITS? SHE AIN'T GONNA CALL YOU!

Interpretation of the numbers from a Swan can be tricky. If you understand the basic concept of Swan Physiology, it will make the numbers you get of some benefit in the management of your patient. Otherwise, the only good a Swan will do is make you look important around your friends and coworkers (they probably won't know you really don't know what you're doing).

Where do we begin? The truth in as little words as possible: The meat, baby.

Transmural pressure

What a concept. So you get a wedge pressure of 18 mmHg. Great. What do you do? Well, as anything else in medicine, you need to put that number in the context of what's going on around it, *literally.* If the heart were not in a closed space (i.e., the chest), one could interpret that number as an absolute value. In real life, you must consider the pressure outside the heart and think about transmural pressure gradient. For instance, if the patient has an abdominal compartment syndrome or cardiac tamponade, the pressure exerted around the outside of the heart may be 15 mmHg. In that case, the transmural pressure (pressure inside-pressure outside, 18-15) is only 3; the wedge is really 3. The number on your monitor is 18, but the heart is *dry.* The heart can't fill adequately enough with a transmural pressure of 3. The pressure of 18 is generated greatly by the transmitted pressure from outside the heart.

Imagine a small balloon that you are trying to fill with water while you squeeze that balloon in your hand. It will take a lot more pressure to fill that balloon than it would if you were not constricting it with your hand. If you release that balloon from your grip, it would hardly have any water in it at all and the pressure inside would be negligible. Same with the heart. If you want to figure out the volume inside the heart chamber by using pressure as an indicator (what the wedge is intended to do), you must consider the transmural pressure gradient. That is why it is recommended to measure the wedge pressure at end-expiration when the pressure inside the chest cavity is closest to atmospheric. Thereby, at this point in the respiratory cycle, the wedge pressure most truly represents the transmural pressure (18-0 is 18; your wedge, not 18-15, or 18-6).

Parking at CVP and Filling the Sheath with Fluid

At times, you will not have the Swan pulled all the way out. For example, in a heart transplant, to keep the Swan from getting sliced in two by the surgeon, you pull the Swan back to 20 cm. That is, the Swan is parked at the CVP level. When this occurs, the distal port of the Swan is just outside the introducer, but the proximal port is back in the sheath!

If you infuse through the proximal port, you will infuse, not into the patient, but into the sheath.

Not good.

You will fill the sleeve of the sheath with fluid. This is untidy, downright contamination-producing, and will produce unwanted hemodynamic effects. That is, that epi you have running wide open has little or no effect when it's all going into the sheath.

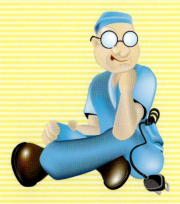

Starling curve

Damn that nasty term. Really, it is quite simple. As you fill a compliant compartment (compliant compartment is one whose volume changes under varying pressures) such as a heart with fluid, it will expand. As it expands, its pressure will increase based on how compliant it is. If it is very compliant (like a thin balloon) the pressure will not go up very much as the volume increases. Less compliant means more pressure increase for volume increase (a thick rubber tire). Based on studying many human hearts with PA catheters placed in them, we have come to approximate the volume of ejected blood (cardiac output) in a *normal* heart for a given wedge pressure, aka Starling curve. This is why you might hear, "A wedge of 25? That patient is too full!" That statement could be true, but once again, don't make the mistake of taking a number as an absolute value. Not every heart is *normal*. If you work at Jackson Memorial Hospital, for instance, that is quite the contrary. So, what to do?

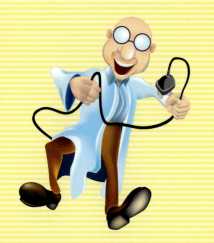

You have a patient you don't know much about as far as cardiac status (probably why you are putting in the Swan in the first place). Maybe the patient has a very hypertrophic and, thereby, noncompliant, ventricle. Maybe they have a dilated cardiomyopathy. What is their ideal wedge pressure to ensure that the heart is adequately full? Figure it out. Here's how: Let's say I have a wedge of 20. Look at your other numbers, particularly BP and cardiac output. Likely your BP is on the low end and so is your cardiac output (otherwise you probably would not have placed the Swan with stable hemodynamics). It's time to make your own Starling curve.

Give fluid to increase the wedge a little (22-24). Did CO go up? How about BP? If they increased a clinically noticeable amount, all bets are that you had more room in that ventricle to fill up and the heart is happier (it's on an increasing portion of the Starling curve). If they did not change at all, it is highly likely that you are on the plateau portion of the Starling curve and filling pressure is not your problem; it may be contractility. If they went down, well you have overshot the curve and the heart is too full, causing valvular dysfunction and decreased forward flow. The take-home point here is that you can't look at the absolute value. One person's heart may need a wedge of 20 to work well, another may need a 10. It all depends on the compliance of the heart. In a 65-year-old man in the U.S. of A., it is highly unlikely that the heart is normal and so an absolute number is useless. You can probably bet that he had long-standing HTN. Maybe alcoholic cardiomyopathy. Get it? *Now you are a pro.*

CONVERTING TO THE ONE TRUE FAITH

- Don't try to convert Swan lovers into Swan haters. It'll never happen.
- Don't try to convert Swan haters into Swan lovers. It'll never happen.

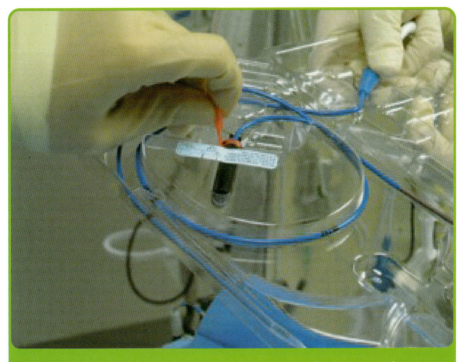

Figure 1. When pulling the Swan out make sure everything is covered . . . you don't want that tip touching stuff out of the sterile field.

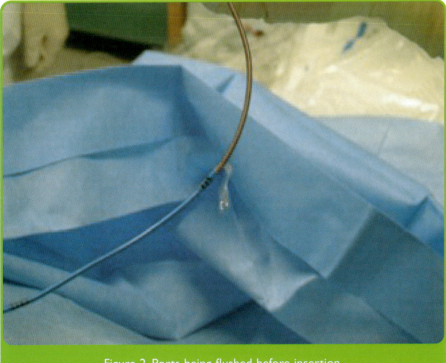

Figure 2. Ports being flushed before insertion.

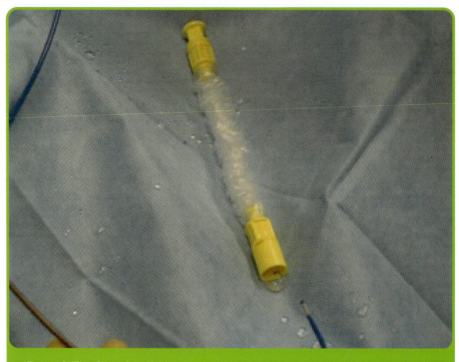

Figure 3. The Swandom!! Also notice that this is a test . . . the Swan is going to enter into the wrong end! Don't do that.

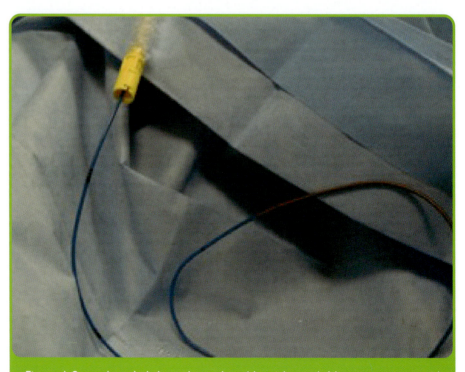

Figure 4. Swan threaded through condom (the right way). Now you can expand the sheath.

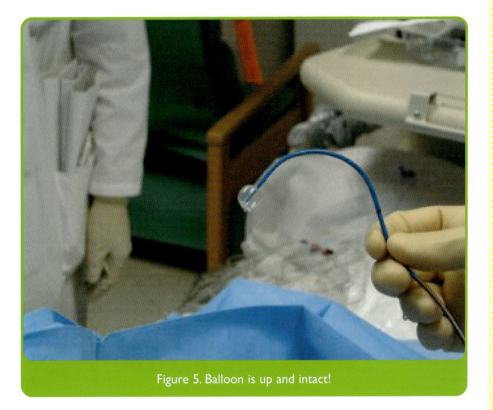

Figure 5. Balloon is up and intact!

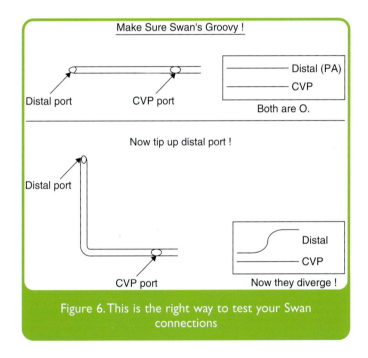

Figure 6. This is the right way to test your Swan connections

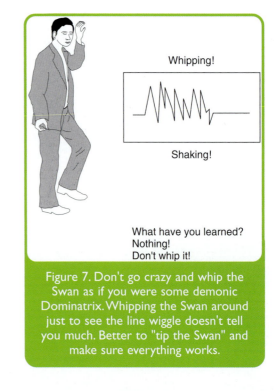

Figure 7. Don't go crazy and whip the Swan as if you were some demonic Dominatrix. Whipping the Swan around just to see the line wiggle doesn't tell you much. Better to "tip the Swan" and make sure everything works.

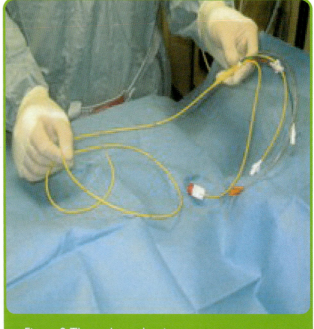

Figure 8. The catheter has its own curvature . . . try to align it so it goes in the "right direction" inside the patient.

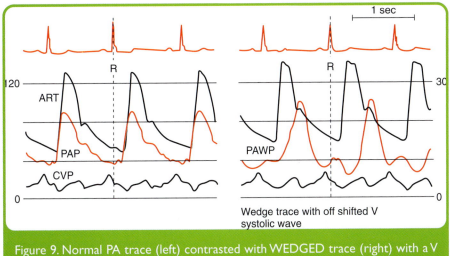

1 sec

Figure 9. Normal PA trace (left) contrasted with WEDGED trace (right) with a V systolic wave. Notice how easy is to be fooled by the similar appearance but the trick is on wave superimposition: The V systolic wave is shifted to the right compared to the a-line trace!

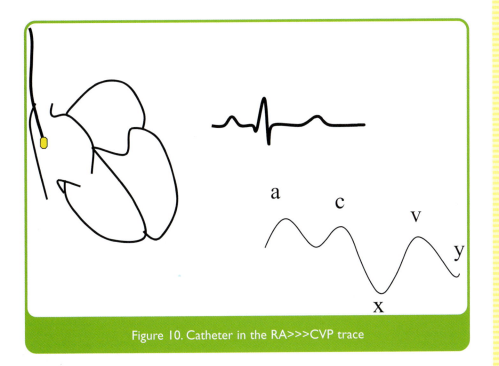

Figure 10. Catheter in the RA>>>CVP trace

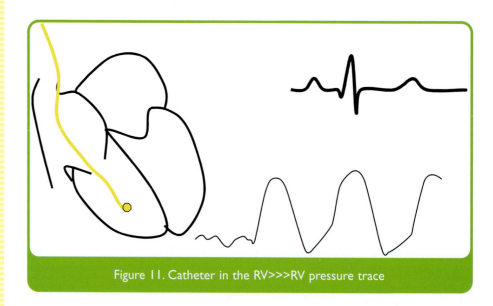

Figure 11. Catheter in the RV>>>RV pressure trace

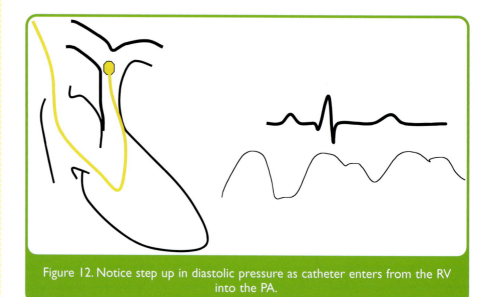

Figure 12. Notice step up in diastolic pressure as catheter enters from the RV into the PA.

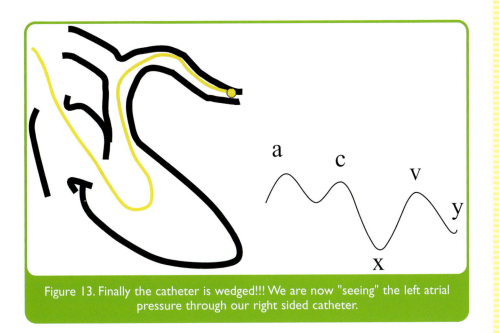

Figure 13. Finally the catheter is wedged!!! We are now "seeing" the left atrial pressure through our right sided catheter.

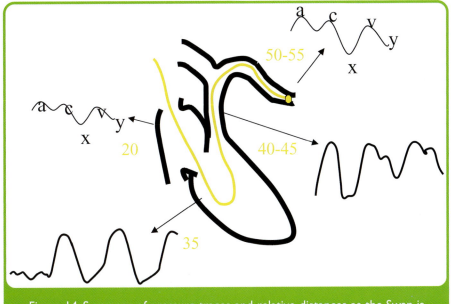

Figure 14. Summary of pressure traces and relative distances as the Swan is floated.

SUGGESTED READING

Connors F Jr, Speroff T, Dawson NV, Thomas C, Harrell FE Jr, Wagner D, Desbiens N, Goldman L, Wu AW, Califf RM, Fulkerson WJ Jr, Vidaillet H, Broste S, Bellamy P, Lynn J, Knaus WA. The effectiveness of right heart catheterization in the initial care of critically ill patients. *JAMA* 1996;276: 889-897.

- *Landmark article that showed an increase in mortality as well as an increase in resource utilization in patients who received a Swan-Ganz catheter. This article stirred a lot of controversy. The editorial that came with this article asked for an FDA moratorium in the use of this device. It made clear that more studies needed to be done to assess the benefits and risks of right heart catheters.*

Iberti TJ, Fischer EP, Leibowitz AB, et al. A multicenter study of physicians' knowledge of the pulmonary artery catheter. *JAMA* 1990;264:2928-2932.

- *Another landmark article that probably explains why the use of the Swan-Ganz has not proven to be of major benefit. Misinterpretation of data is the problem! A third of physicians interviewed could not recognize a wedge trace!*

Keush DJ, Winters S, Thys DM. The patient's position influences the incidence of dysrhythmias during pulmonary artery catheterization. *Anesthesiology* 1989;70:582-584.

- *This paper examines different patient positions during placement of a PAC. It found that placing the patient in a head-up and right-side-down position aids the catheter in exiting the right ventricle into the pulmonary circulation, and decreases ventricular arrhythmias.*

Lopez-Sendon J, Lopez de Sa E, Maqueda IG, et al. Right ventricular infarction as a risk factor for ventricular fibrillation during pulmonary artery catheterization using Swan-Ganz catheters. *Am Heart J* 1990:119:207-209.

- *This paper looks at the incidence of ventricular fibrillation while placing a pulmonary artery catheter in 2,821 patients in the coronary care unit. Of 2,327 patients having acute ischemia, 25 (1.1%) of them developed ventricular fibrillation. That compared with zero out of the 494 patients not having acute ischemia. The most likely subset of patients to have ventricular fibrillation was those diagnosed with right ventricular infarction (4.2%). Clearly, when placing a Swan, ventricular fibrillation is a consideration in persons with a right ventricular infarct.*

Moore RA, Neary MJ, Gallagher JD, Clark DL. Determination of the pulmonary capillary wedge position in patients with giant left atrial V waves. *J Cardiothorac Anesth* 198;1:108-113.

- *The authors examined the temporal relationship between pulmonary artery pressure traces, arterial pressure traces, EKG traces, and found that the PA upstroke and arterial upstroke occurred nearly simultaneously. Resultantly, an easy beat-to-beat method for differentiating pulmonary arterial from pulmonary capillary wedge positions in the presence of giant left atrial V waves is the superimposition of the pulmonary arterial trace on the radial arterial trace. When wedged, there is an immediate rightward shift in the upstroke and peak of the pulmonary arterial pressure trace compared to the arterial trace.*

Salmenpera M, Peltola K, Rosenberg P. Does prophylactic lidocaine control cardiac arrhythmias associated with pulmonary artery catheterization? *Anesthesiology* 198;56:210-212.

- *This study looked at controlling the incidence of arrhythmias by using intravenous prophylactic lidocaine while placing a pulmonary artery catheter. It concludes that lidocaine is of no benefit to be used to prevent arrhythmia during Swan placement.*

Shah KB, Rao TLK, Laughlin S, El-Etr AA. A review of pulmonary artery catheterization in 6,245 patients. *Anesthesiology* 1984;61:271-275.

- *A large study evaluating the safety of pulmonary artery catheters that looked at numerous endpoints. Overall, only 10 patients in the study (0.16%) had serious complications resulting in morbidity, and only one patient (0.016%) died as a result of complication arising from a pulmonary artery catheter (pulmonary artery rupture). As far as arrhythmias go, in 113 patients with pre-existing LBBB, complete heart block occurred in only one patient (0.9%).*

Shah MR, Hasselblad V, Stevenson LW, Binanay C, O'Connor CM, Sopko G, Calif RM. Impact of the pulmonary artery catheter in critically ill patients meta-analysis of randomized clinical trials. *JAMA* 2005;294:1664-1670.

- *This is a recent meta-analysis, with more than 5,000 patients, that showed the neutrality of using the PA catheter: It did not increase mortality, but it also did not confer any benefit. It discusses the lack of evidence-based interventions when using the information the PA catheter provides.*

Wall MH, MacGregor DA, Kennedy DJ, et al. Pulmonary artery catheter placement for elective coronary artery bypass grafting: before or after anesthetic induction? *Anesth Analg* 2002;94:1409-1415.

- *This paper looks at various endpoints to determine whether or not placing a PAC prior to anesthetic induction in an elective CABG has any efficacy. It concludes that there are absolutely no advantages to preinduction PAC placement. In fact, the investigators found that it took longer and actually required more needle sticks to place the catheter while the patient was awake.*

The Surgeon's Bailiwick: The Subclavian

Karim Abouelenin and
Benjamin Yu

I have always depended on the kindness of strangers.

Tennessee Williams
A Streetcar Named Desire, 1947

INTRODUCTION

When it comes to placing subclavian lines, anesthesiologists often depend on the kindness of strangers: the surgeons. "We do IJs, they do subclavians," is a common refrain.

Change that mind-set. There are plenty of occasions you'll want to or need to place a subclavian; you can't just punt it to the surgeons each time. You need a lot of procedural arrows in your quiver and a subclavian belongs in that "quiver."

In a few ways, subclavians are easier than IJs, and in a few ways, they're more nerve-wracking. Like anything else, practice makes perfect and you just have to know what you're doing.

WHY SUBCLAVIAN?

- There are a lot of times when a subclavian comes in quite handy—for example, you're going to do a carotid and the patient has no peripheral access. You don't want to stick the IJ on the side of the surgery. You don't want to stick the other side for fear you nail *that* carotid. Hey, do the subclavian.
- The anatomy can be easier with subclavian lines. In patients with short, obese necks, the anatomical landmarks for an IJ may be difficult to discern. Or, you may have a hard time palpating the carotid. Hmm . . . where could I place the line? Oh, wait . . . I know . . . the subclavian!
- Patients tend to tolerate subclavians better than IJs, so if the line will be in for a while, the subclavian is not a bad idea.
- If you're in the ICU and a long-term patient needs line after line after line, then the occasional subclavian allows the IJs to rest in between lines.
- In a code, you're better off going subclavian. You can't always feel a carotid pulse up in IJ-land during cardiopulmonary arrest, so go subclavian instead.

INDICATIONS

These are generally the same as for the IJ:
- Delivery of volume
- Volume assessment (CVP)
- IV access in a patient with poor or no peripheral access
- Delivery of certain medications or fluids that require central access (e.g., TPN, inotropes, K+)
- Central access for the placement of other devices:

- Swan-Ganz catheter for volume assessment (see Chapter 3)
- Catheters for hemodialysis
- Temporary pacemaker wires

CONTRAINDICATIONS

- Superior vena cava syndrome/thrombosis
- Infection at the site of entry
- Injury to the clavicle that might distort anatomy
- Coagulopathy (relative)
- COPD (relative)
- High PEEP (relative)

EQUIPMENT

- Venous access kit (CVP, Swan introducer)
- Flush syringes (and normal saline for flushing)
- Drapes, gowns, gloves, hats, and mask
- Bed that you can put in Trendelenburg
- Monitor and oxygen

CONSIDERATIONS

- Remember all the usual concerns when you see an existing line from elsewhere.
- If you see fluid being delivered by an infusion pump, disconnect and make sure the line is not in the artery. (An infusion pump can overcome arterial pressure and pump stuff into the arterial system.)
- If someone comes down with high glucose containing IV fluids going in a central line, don't just discontinue that fluid! The patient may develop dangerous

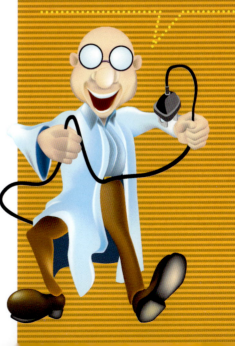

That's Funny Why Should the PLunger Do That?

Proof positive that no good deed goes unpunished.

An ICU nurse bemoaned and wailed a lack of venous access on a patient. I, in passing, heard this tale of unrequited venous access and offered to help.

Into the subclavian I went. At one point while floundering around, I noticed the plunger jumped back a little of its own accord.

"Odd," I thought.

Eventually got the line.

While I waited for the chest X-ray, I retreated to such dining facilities as the hospital afforded, in order to keep my ever-widening girth from ever approaching or even nearing "ideal body weight."

"Code blue! ICU Six!"

Damn, I was just there, what on earth could it be?

Abandoning a well-balanced meal of Twinkies, ice cream sandwiches, and Mountain Dew, I dashed back to the scene of the crime.

You guessed it. Tension pneumothorax.

The plunger had gone back with a positive pressure breath from the ventilator. While I was gorging, the patient was developing a tension pneumothorax.

Proving that God looks after drunks and fools, one of my colleagues heard the code, decompressed the chest, and saved the day, saved the patient, and saved my butt.

hypoglycemia. Make sure you replace that sugar immediately (either peripherally or in the new central line).

- If you're planning to place a PA catheter or pacing wires, the *left* subclavian is preferable to the right (a gentler angle to approach the right heart). This is the opposite of if you're doing the IJ (you want the right IJ for a more straight shot to the right atrium).

- If you're spooked about dropping the lung (as everyone is), then pick your first few subclavians wisely. Do subclavians on cases where the patients will end up with a chest tube anyway—for example, a heart case or a lung case. If you botch it and drop the lung, they're just getting their chest tubes a little early.

- Remember how close the first rib is to the clavicle. If you place your line too medial, you might get the wire in but, when you try to get your line in, the line gets squished between the clavicle and first rib. This'll make you very unhappy and make you utter words that are not sanctioned by any religious or ecumenical body.

- If you're really spooked about a bleed (patient on Plavix, coagulopathic), then keep this scary reminder in your hip pocket: If you do hit the subclavian artery, you can't compress it, no matter how hard you squish down on the clavicle (we've tried). Think about going somewhere where you can compress the mis-stuck artery, namely the IJ or the femoral.

- If you palpate and you feel a bounding pulse right where you are thinking of sticking the subclavian, think again. The subclavian artery, like every artery, can become dilated, tortuous, and can go where it's *not* supposed to. If a little voice inside you says, "Hmm, I don't know, it sure feels like there is an artery right underneath my fingers," *believe that little voice.* Go elsewhere.

SUBCLAVIAN HISTORY AND PHYSICAL

- While obtaining a quick, directed history, you should snoop around for things that would gum up the works—history of radiation to the chest wall, history of clotted subclavian veins after, for example, central lines from an earlier illness, dialysis catheters, Infuse-a-Ports, or history of trauma or injury to their clavicle (car accident, playing football).

- The physical is simple enough: Palpate the clavicle! Patients who forgot about the time when "I fell out of a tree and broke my collarbone when I was five" might now have a distorted subclavian area.

- There are also congenital disorders that might affect the clavicle such as craniocleidodystosis.

PREPARATION

- Make yourself comfortable and give yourself a nice workspace—good lighting, a dedicated Mayo stand for your kit, a bed that can get into the Trendelenburg position.

- As with every other procedure, pay attention to your patient. Are you putting this line in because the patient is in big trouble, can't breathe, volume overloaded, on the brink? Remember your ABCs? Airway comes first: Hold off on the stupid subclavian, secure the airway, assure adequate respiratory exchange, and *then* put the line in.

- Put a roll down the middle of the patient's back to throw the shoulders back and give yourself a straight shot into the subclavian versus going up and over the shoulder. In a pinch, a 1-L bag of LR or saline does nicely.

- If patients are on the ventilator, put them on 100% oxygen, use small tidal volumes, and decrease the PEEP (if feasible) to hedge your bet against a pneumothorax.

- Pull the shoulder down (5 cm caudal from the neutral position).

- Review the anatomy and landmarks. If you're just starting out, marking it all with a skin marker can help you visualize the anatomy.

- Place the patient in Trendelenburg position *before* you gown and glove.

- Don't forget your sterile setup and technique (gown, gloves, hat, mask, drape).

TECHNIQUE

- Perform sterile preparation and drape the patient fully.

- After sterile preparation and draping, inject your local anesthetic to form a 1-cm skin wheal at the insertion site.

- While you're waiting for the local anesthetic to take effect, prepare your catheter: you may flush the ports by injecting normal saline into the appropriate lumens—until you see it flow from the distal end of the catheter—and then clamp each port off. Make sure to leave the distal port unclamped and uncapped in preparation for the guidewire.

- The insertion site should be approximately 1 cm below the midclavicular point of the lower border of the clavicle.

- Use the long needle. Don't bother with a finder.

- Don't use the catheter either. While it's preferable for the IJ, it will get kinked and besquoozled under the clavicle.

- Aiming for the suprasternal notch, the clavicle should cross over your trajectory.

- If you hit the clavicle, walk off it by pushing down on the needle with your fingers.

- Stay parallel to the ground. The idea is to be low, aiming away, out of the chest to avoid sticking the lung.

- You should hit the vein beneath the inner third of the clavicle, near the clavicular head of the sternocleidomastoid.

- Sometimes you'll miss it going in, then get it coming back—what happens is, you compressed and went through it, then aspirated blood when you come back.

- When you get blood, stop!

- One nice thing about the subclavian (versus the internal jugular) is that you don't need to hold the needle in just the exact place. The needle is sort of held between the clavicle above and the first rib below. (With the IJ, nothing holds the needle fast and you have to really hold that needle still—as still as can be—to keep from coming out of the vein).

- Make sure the blood you're aspirating is venous.

- Disconnect the needle from the hub of the syringe and look for *squirtationus arteriosicus*. Some kits come with a short length of tubing that you can use to transduce the needle to verify that the pressures are venous and not arterial.

- Advance the wire. It should go in smoothly, without any hang ups. While advancing the wire, watch for ectopy.

- Nick the skin. When you nick the skin, lay that blade flat on the wire so you feel the vvvvvvvvvvvvvrrrrrrrrrrrrrrrffffffffffffff-ppptt of the wire against the blade, otherwise, you might make the hole (X) here, when the wire is .... (X) here.

- Advance the dilator over the guidewire using the Seldinger technique. Of note, the dilator is tricky, sometimes, to get under the clavicle. Holding the dilator closer to the skin and using a twisting motion helps, sometimes.

- Advance the catheter using the distal port (brown, in most cases) to thread your wire. Again, holding the catheter near the skin helps if you're having difficulty advancing.

- If you haven't already done so, flush each of your ports after first aspirating blood.

- Finally, sew or staple the line in and then take the patient out of Trendelenburg.

- Order a CXR (then read it).

- Revel in the glory of another spectacular procedure completed.

COMPLICATIONS

- Arterial puncture (3%-5%)
- Pneumothorax (1.5%-3%)
- Hemothorax (0.5%)
- Catheter or guidewire embolism

GLITCH CITY

- Hitting the subclavian artery. Big bummer, as there is no real way to put pressure on it. Sometimes you might even have to go all the way to surgical repair and, given the position of the hole, the artery is damned inaccessible. Best treatment: prevention. Don't go deep and don't aim high, that's where the artery lies.

- Dropping the lung. Hey, it happens.

- If you have to decompress the lung in a hurry, remember, you can place a 14-g catheter in the second intercostal space at the midclavicular line. This is just a temporizing measure; get a surgeon to put a chest tube in for you.

- Singer sewing machine in motion. Don't be in a hurry, jabbing and going back and forth like a needle-wielding maniac. Go in slow, come out slow. You really do get this one a lot on the way out.

Craniocleidodystosis . . . What's That?

Little historical tidbit, there is a condition called "craniocleido dysostosis," where there is a congenital absence of the clavicle. These people can scrunch their shoulders so tightly together they can touch their shoulders together anteriorly. During the Civil War, boys with this condition were used to swab out the insides of large (presumably unloaded) cannons. Who said medicine isn't fun?

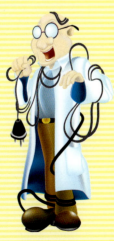

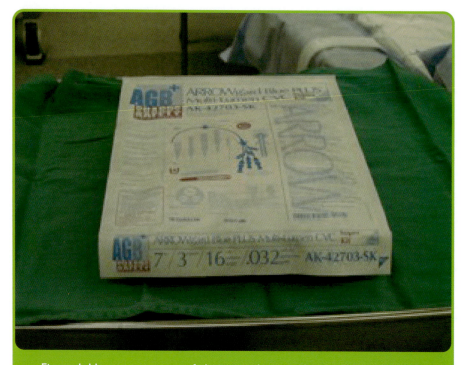

Figure 1. Use your weapon of choice: triple o quadruple CVP's (simple or double lumens are for whimps and the reality is that you usually need extra ports), introducers, rapid infusion catheters, etc.

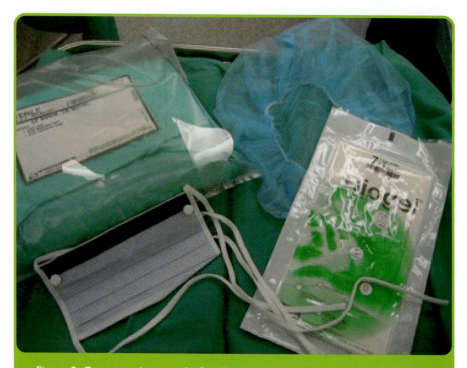

Figure 2. Get everything ready: Sterile set up>>>gown, gloves, mask, hat, the works, as per CDC recommendations.

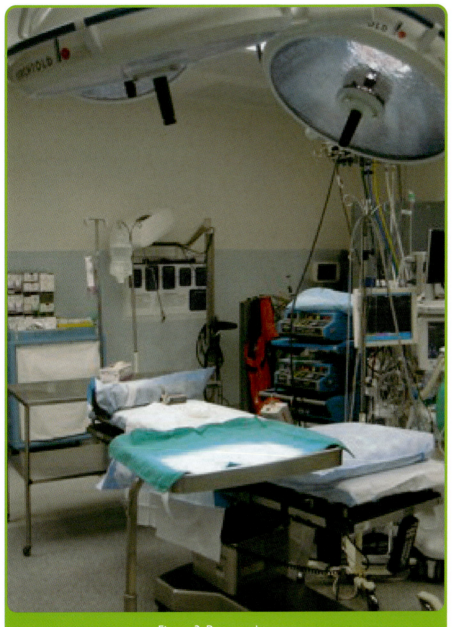

Figure 3. Prepare the area

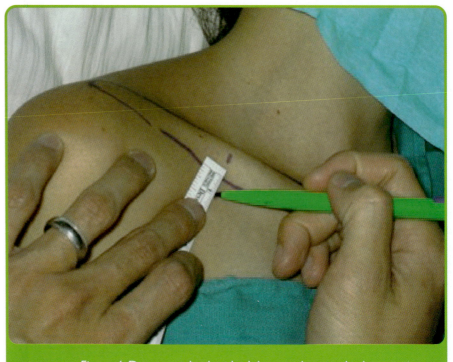

Figure 4. Draw your landmarks. Ink never hurt anybody.

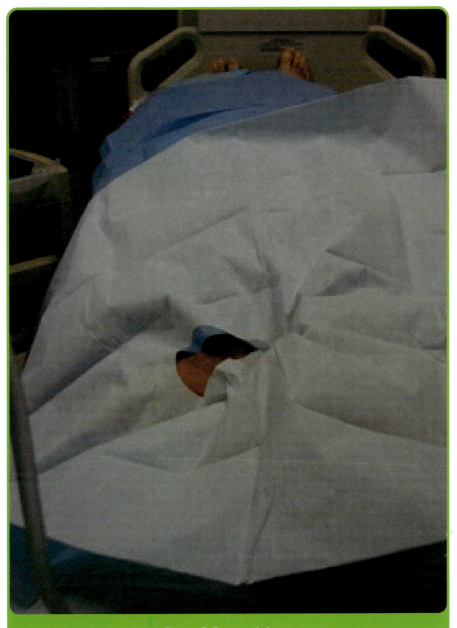

Figure 5. Prep and drape

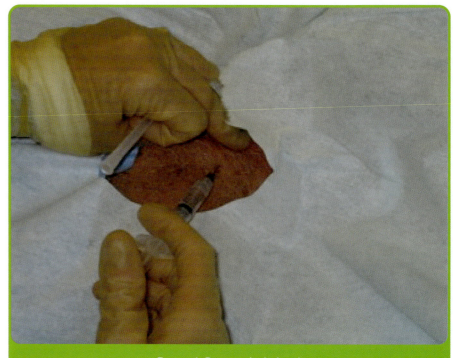

Figure 6. Put in a little local

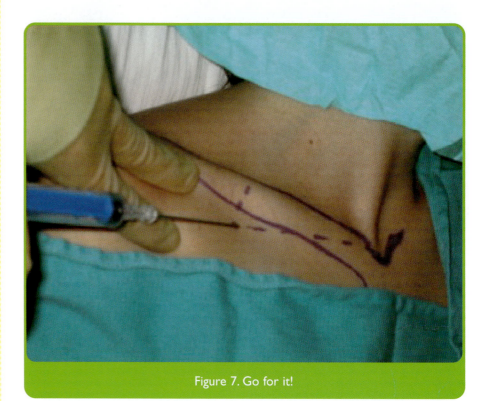

Figure 7. Go for it!

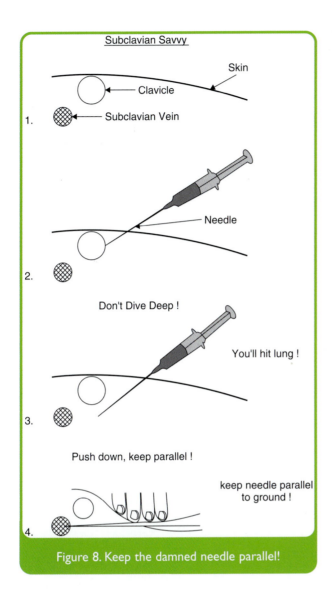

Subclavian Savvy

1. Skin / Clavicle / Subclavian Vein

2. Needle

3. Don't Dive Deep !
You'll hit lung !

4. Push down, keep parallel !
keep needle parallel to ground !

Figure 8. Keep the damned needle parallel!

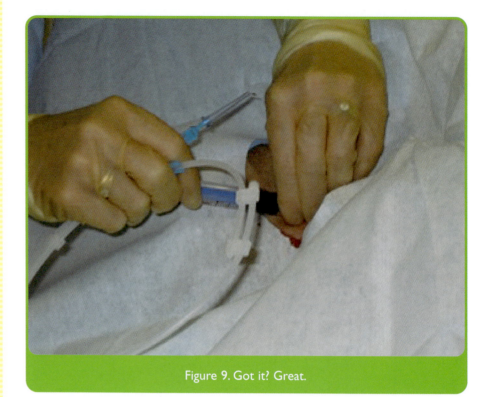

Figure 9. Got it? Great.

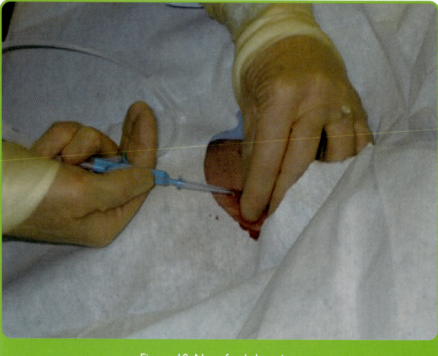

Figure 10. Now feed the wire.

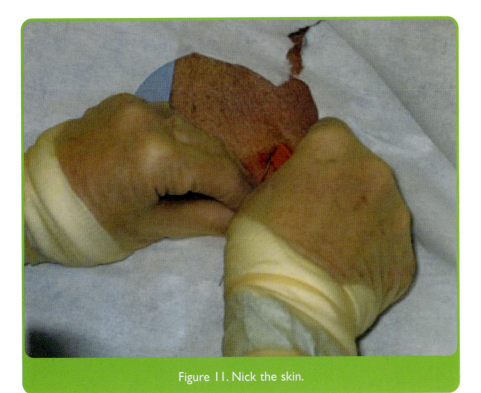

Figure 11. Nick the skin.

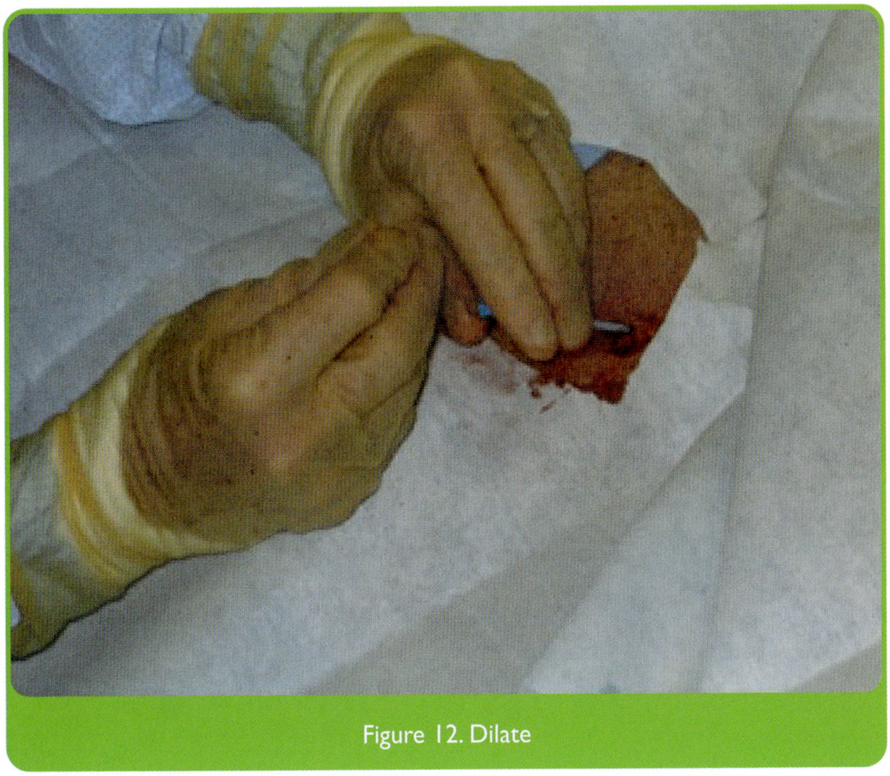

Figure 12. Dilate

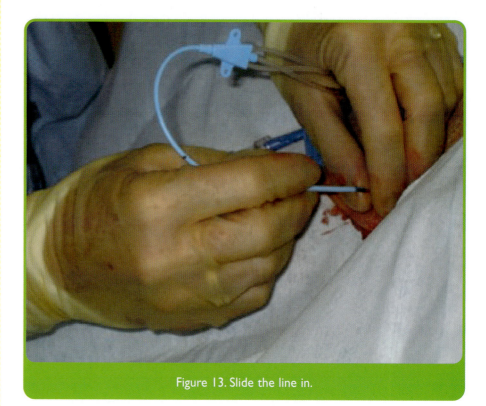

Figure 13. Slide the line in.

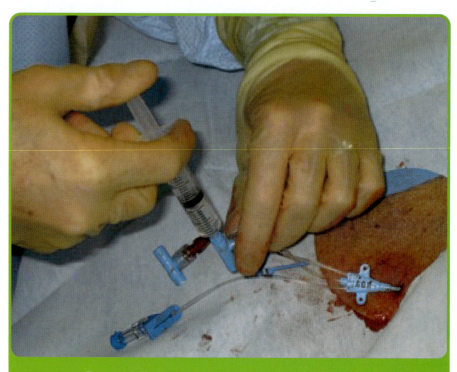

Figure 14. Flush the ports and pat yourself on the back.

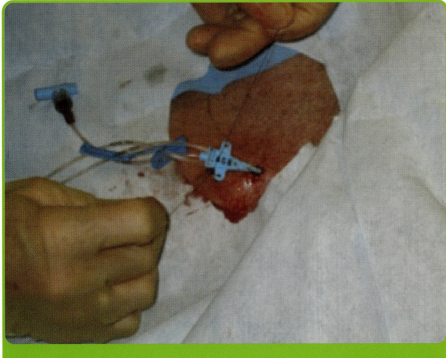

Figure 15. Sew that baby in like you mean it!

SUGGESTED READING

Andrews RT, Bova DA, Venbrux AC. How much guidewire is too much? Direct measurement of the distance from subclavian and internal jugular vein access sites to the superior vena cava-atrial junction during central venous catheter placement. *Crit Care Med* 2000;28(1):138–142.
- *A study looking into how much guidewire is appropriate for placement of central venous catheters. (Hint: 18 cm seems to be the magic number.)*

Deshpande KS, Hatem C, Ulrich HL, et al. *Crit Care Med* 2005;33(1):13–20.
- *The incidence of infectious complications of central venous catheters at the subclavian, internal jugular, and femoral sites in an intensive care unit population, An observational study showing no statistical difference in infection rates of central venous catheters placed in any of the three locations.*

Von Goedecke A, Kellor C, Moriggl B, et al. An anatomic landmark to simplify subclavian vein cannulation: the "deltoid tuberosity." *Anesth Analg* 2005; 100(3):623–628.

- *Another paper regarding anatomy as it pertains to placing the subclavian line. The gold mine here is its bibliography (also applies to the Kitigawa bibliography. As a matter of fact, you'll find a lot of the same papers in both bibliographies.)*

Kitigawa N, Oda M, et al. Proper shoulder position for subclavian venipuncture. *Anesthesiology* 2004;101(6):1306–1312.
- *A well-illustrated, recent article on positioning for placement of subclavian lines.*

McGee DC, Gould MK. Current concepts: preventing complications of central venous catheterization. *N Engl J Med* 2003;348:1123–1133.
- *A great review article detailing the various complications of central venous catheters and how to prevent them.*

Thompson EC, Calver LE. Safe subclavian vein cannulation. *Am Surg* 2005;71(2):180–183.
- *A surgeon's perspective.*

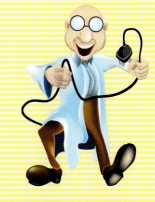

CHAPTER 5

The Bastard Stepchild: The Femoral

Craig Nelson and Jennifer Vaughn

> Truth...never comes into the world but like a bastard, to the ignominy of him that brought it forth.
>
> *John Milton*
> The Doctrine and Discipline of Divorce, 1643

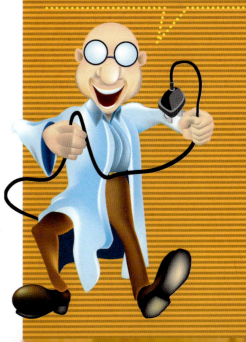

INTRODUCTION

And the truth is: A femoral line is not such a dirty bastard as everyone says.

We just plain don't put in that many femoral lines, but that should not keep you from learning how. Once you've done a few, (like anything else), you get comfortable with it. And once comfortable with it, you're more likely to do it, and then you get better at it, more comfortable with it. Round and round you go, getting better and more comfortable.

The opposite of a vicious circle:

A good circle.

Femoral lines, contrary to prevailing myth, do not get infected any more than other central lines. Yeah verily, we speak the truth.

Another tack on femoral lines? They're great just-in-case lines. You can put them in at the start of a potentially bad case, and you can always pull them out at the end of the case if your worst fears went unrealized.

What if you hit the artery by mistake? In the neck? That's an issue because if you hit the carotid, you could end up with a cerebrovascular problem or an airway problem. In the subclavian arena, an arterial stick can pose a can't-control-the-bleeding problem. In the femoral region? Hey, an arterial stick is not such a catastrophe. It's easy to get to, easy to fix, and you won't lose an airway while doing it.

Pretty handy for a "bastard" line.

INDICATIONS

- Volume access (emergent or otherwise).
- Inotropic access, CVP monitoring, you can even float a Swan from a femoral introducer!
- Hypertonic fluids (TPN, for example).

CONTRAINDICATIONS

- Infection at the site.
- Penetrating abdominal trauma (your femoral infusion will spill into the abdomen).
- Occlusion of the inferior vena cava from tumor (consider this the lower variant of superior vena cava syndrome).
- Prior groin surgery is a relative contraindication.

EQUIPMENT

- Sterile prep and drape stuff.
- Central line kit.
- Helper to pull the abdomen out of the way should the patient require that.

BEWARE THE FLOOR FEMORAL LINE

- No, actually, you don't have to. When someone comes with a femoral line, it's usually from the cardiac cath lab. And, we almost hate to say it, they are pretty good at this. Better than we are, truth to tell.

PHILOSOPHY OF FEMORAL LINES

- Doing a neuro case? Need good access? Want to be able to get at and troubleshoot a central line? Hey, a femoral line works just right. You don't cut off venous drainage from the head, you won't have to crawl up and under the drapes, bumping the patient and infuriating the looking- through-the-microscope neurosurgeons.
- Surgeons working high in the chest? Hey, the *northern route* into the heart might get cut off. How will you resuscitate? Try the *southern route* via the femoral approach.
- If you really sit down and *think* about how you'll get stuff into the patient's heart, you may be surprised at how often a femoral line makes sense.

FEMORAL LINE: HISTORY AND PHYSICAL

- Look for badness in the groin, both the usual stuff (infection, hematoma) and the unusual (inguinal lymphadenopathy compressing and distorting the anatomy).

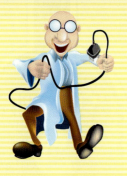

- If the IVC is likely to be interrupted (renal cell cancer, for example, blocking passage), then don't use the femoral approach.

TECHNIQUE

- Prep, drape, get good lighting.
- If the patient's abdomen protrudes, have a helper pull the pannus back and give you a straight shot.
- The landmarks, from lateral to medial, are NAVEL: nerve, artery, vein, empty space, lymphatics.
- For the irreverent, the landmarks, from lateral to medial, are NAVY: nerve, artery, vein, Yahoo! The "Yahoo!" implies some degree of happiness affiliated with the pudendal region, and has nothing to do with the Internet search engine.
- Localize the area.
- This hurts and is more than a little scary, so if you can do this once they're under general anesthesia, then do that.
- Feel the pulse, go medial, and advance at a 45-degree angle to the skin. No need for a finder here.
- Use the long needle, the catheter will get kinked and scrunkled.
- Aspirate while advancing.
- Once you get blood flow, disconnect the needle and watch for arterial spurting (if it spurts, hold pressure).
- If you're in the vein, advance the wire.
- Once the wire's in, make a nick in the skin, laying the flat blade against the wire and feeling for that vvvvvvvvvvvvr-rrrrrrrrrrrrrffffffffffffffffpppt of the wire essence. Remove the needle.
- Introduce the dilator over the wire, but not too much (a few centimeters) to avoid tearing a gaping hole in the vein.
- Advance the line.
- Aspirate and flush.
- Sew in place.
- It's now just a jump to the left, then a step to the right. Let's do the Time Warp again (see *Rocky Horror Picture Show*).

GLITCH-O-RAMA

- The femoral is deep. In the bigger patients, it's real deep, and it can be a source of genuine frustration to find the femoral vein.
- Dropping a lung by this approach would require some damned aggressive needle-work. If you do drop a lung with the femoral approach, consider a new career.
- If the patient is going to ambulate soon after the case, a femoral line is clumsy and probably not a good idea in general. Bedrest is best.
- If you're going femoral, don't put a dinky short line in. The thing will pull out.
- If you're right-handed, go for the right femoral; the mechanics are just easier.
- If you are having a terrible time of it, consider a Site-Rite echo device to help you *find* the vessel.

Now for some *really* far-out glitches

Imagine yourself in the midst of a pediatric femoral central line placement, and instead of aspirating blood, you aspirate a clear, yellow fluid. Or maybe you detect some feculent material in your syringe. Bowel and bladder are just a peritoneal reflection away from the groin, so be careful (especially in the kiddies).

Next imagine a patient who is a tad on the coagulopathic side, so you go the femoral route to avoid a potential bleeding problem in a more clinically important region. That femoral stick can ooze (or trickle or gush) its way into a retroperitoneal hematoma.

Finally, imagine your patient already has a femoral arterial line and needs a venous line (or vice versa). If you place the complementary catheter on the same side as the existing line, it is possible for an A-V fistula to develop.

We can stop being overly dramatic now and close by saying that femoral venous lines, albeit bastards, can be useful in the instances described above. It is therefore completely worth the time and energy spent sticking the groin to learn this technique.

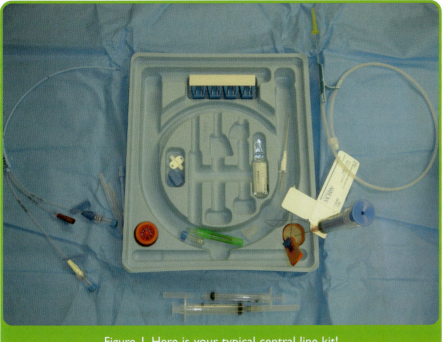

Figure 1. Here is your typical central line kit!

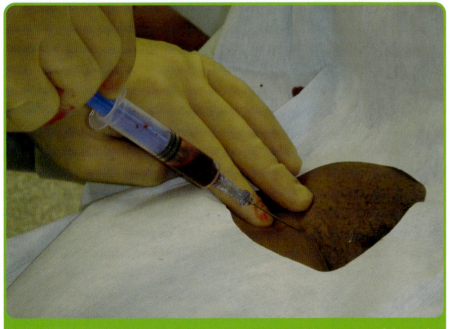

Figure 2. Voila! Non-pulsatile blood coming your way. Note position of the stick in relation to the inguinal ligament. Also note the depth and angle of the needle.

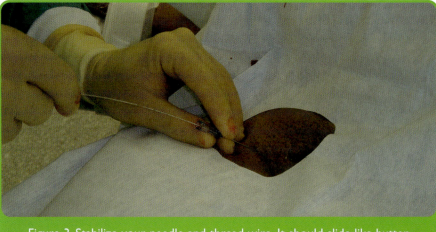

Figure 3. Stabilize your needle and thread wire. It should slide like butter.

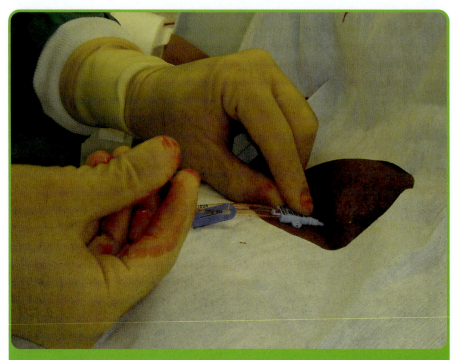

Figure 4. Line is in after threading it over the wire. Never, ever, loose sight of the wire! Please secure the line with stiches.

SUGGESTED READING

Deshpande KS, Hatem C, Ulrich HL, et al. The incidence of infectious complications of central venous catheters at the subclavian, internal jugular, and femoral sites in an intensive care unit population. *Crit Care Med* 2005;33:13-20.

• *The authors performed a prospective, observational study to assess the comparative risk of infection at subclavian, internal jugular, and femoral central venous catheter (CVC) sites in an ICU setting. In 657 patients (831 total catheters) there was an overall "low" rate of CVC infection and colonization with no clinical or statistical difference between the three sites. This study was optimized in comparison to the Merrer study via more experienced operators, uniform protocols for sterile technique and data reporting, and standardized catheter care by trained nurses at a single institution.*

Friedman B, Kanter G, Titus D. Femoral venous catheters: a safe alternative for delivering parenteral alimentation. *Nutr Clin Pract*, 1994;9:69-72.

- *The authors in this study determine that femoral venous catheterization is a safe alternative route of access for the delivery of TPN.*

Merrer J, De Jonghe B, Golliot R, et al. Complications of femoral and subclavian venous catheterization in critically ill patients. A randomized controlled trial. *JAMA* 2001;286:700-707.

- *The authors compared mechanical, infectious, and thrombotic complications of femoral and subclavian venous catheterization in a randomized controlled trial involving 289 ICU patients. Femoral venous catheterization was found to be associated with a greater risk of both thrombotic and minor infectious complications than subclavian catheterization in the ICU setting.*

Sato S, Ueno E, Toyooka H. Central venous access via the distal femoral vein using ultrasound guidance. *Anesthesiology* 1998;88:838-839.

- *The authors describe a new technique for inserting central venous catheters at a site distal to that of traditional femoral venous catheterization.*

Williams JF, Seneff MG, Friedman BC, et al. Use of femoral venous catheters in critically ill adults: prospective study. *Crit Care Med* 1991;19:550-553.

- *This study predates the Deshpande group study, and also concludes that the rate of major infectious complications associated with femoral venous catheters in the ICU setting is acceptably low.*

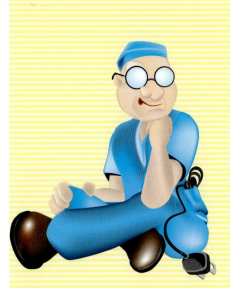

PART 2

ARTERIAL LAND

The Beat-to-Beat Faucet: The Radial A-Line

**Roger Marks and
Ana Lipska**

A man is as old as his arteries.

*Thomas Sydenham, 1624-1689
Date of quotation unknown*

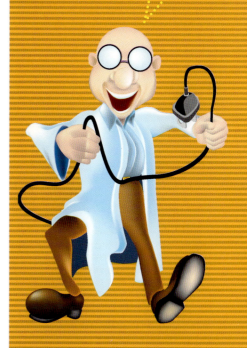

INTRODUCTION

The radial arterial line is the bread and butter of a big case. If you're spooked about blood pressure swings (up or down), if the wait-for-the-Dinamap-to-cycle is just too horrific to contemplate, and if you're going to need any blood gases, then by all means get yourself an arterial line. The radial artery is, far and away, the most common place to get your line.

INDICATIONS

- Beat-to-beat blood pressure measurement.
- Faucet into the arterial system for drawing blood gases.
- Indicator of cerebral insufficiency during a mediastinoscopy (an art line on the right, if cut off during a mediastinoscopy, indicates that the innominate artery is being squished by the scope).

CONTRAINDICATIONS

- Arterial insufficiency in the hand.
- Raynaud's syndrome (a variant of the first contraindication).
- No radial artery (for example, after a radial artery harvesting for bypass). If you *can* stick a radial artery after it's been taken out, call us right away. We've got to see this!

EQUIPMENT

- Something to lock and hold the wrist in extension (not too much, for fear of a median nerve stretch, but enough to get your line and keep the trace).
- Tape.
- Local.
- Cannula (usually a 20-g for an adult, 22 or 24 for the little guys).
- Transducer and pressure tubing.
- You can use an art line kit, or you can just use a regular cannula, tastes vary.

A NOTE ON INFECTION

- If you study the actual mechanism of infection, you find that most infections come from skin flora working their way down the cannula.
- In a low-flow system (in other words, a vein), the bugs take up residence and happily infect most intravenous lines pretty quickly (a few days).
- In a high-flow system (in other words, an artery), the bugs can't take up residence so easily, and an art line is much less likely to get infected quickly.
- So, some would say you can keep an arterial line in until you see ferns blooming visibly out of the site. While this may be a *bit* exaggerated, it makes the point.

RADIAL ARTERY: HISTORY AND PHYSICAL

- You'd be amazed the weird scars and stuff you see in people's wrists.
- Ask whether they've had previous carpal tunnel surgery. If they've had any kind of nerve work or nerve damage, you may not want to stick that side. Any pain in that spot may get tagged to your art line, whether or not you are the guilty party.
- Severe arthritics present the problem of how to get their wrists in the right position.
- Don't forget to ask about Raynaud's! That's not a routine part of our H and P, but you'd hate to find out later that they have it. You are major padoinkled at that point.

TECHNIQUE

- Zero the transducer before you begin so that when you connect the tubing, the monitor will give you a number right away—a correct number!
- Choose the radial artery that is palpated best.

The Resident-Explanatory Impulse

Through some bizarre quirk in our evolutionary makeup, residents feel compelled to explain a lot while placing arterial lines. They feel that by saying what happened, that will somehow make everything better.

"I hit it, but I couldn't thread it."

Yes, and, what do you want me to do? Give you half-credit?

"I thought I was in, but now there's no trace and I can't draw back blood. Where do you think it is?"

Hmm. There's no arterial trace whatsoever and you cannot draw back blood. That's a real brain-buster. Let me think. Maybe you're in the artery, but it's a magic artery with no trace and no blood. Or maybe you're in the artery, but we've been transported to some alternative galaxy by some wormhole in the space-time continuum.

What Kind of ICU is This?

I walked into the ICU, looking for my next patient, a real train wreck. He had been in, well, a train wreck, of all things! He was scheduled for an AKA on the right. All the king's horses and all the king's men had not been able to put his leg back together again.

There he was—spot 7, lucky 7.

Flail chest, vent-dependent, chest tubes, pan-wrapped/casted/pinned.

I looked up at the monitors. No A-line trace.

Odd.

Looked around, no A-line anywhere.

Odder still.

"Does this guy have an A-line somewhere," I asked the ICU nurse.

"No."

"Really," I said, "he doesn't have one? You would think . . ."

"So would I," the ICU nurse said, "so would I. The surgeon doesn't want to put one in. Says it's dangerous."

- Extend the wrist and flatten out the hypothenar eminence so you have a straight shot into the radial artery.
- Do yourself a favor and sit down. If you stand and crouch, you'll end up in Laminectomy Village one day.
- Prep the area.
- Put a little local in.
- Don't bother poking a hole with an 18-g needle like some people do. That just makes an extra hole, and if you miss and have to go elsewhere, you haven't done yourself any favors.
- There are two fundamental techniques, each with its defenders: the *through-and-through* technique and the *go-right-in* technique.
- Through and through: Nail the artery and keep on going, then pull out the needle. Now pull back the catheter until you get flow, then advance the catheter into the artery.
- Go-right-in: Don't nail the artery all the way through. Once you get blood flow, advance an itty-bitty bit (making sure the catheter is in the artery, not just the needle tip), then slide the catheter up.
- Blood should keep flowing, and the catheter should slide easily with either technique. If the blood doesn't flow, then you are no longer in.
- Hold the artery to keep the blood from gooshing all over the place (this makes you lose style points) when you pull out the needle.
- Hook up the art line to the catheter.
- If you miss, apply pressure for several minutes to prevent hematoma.
- A hematoma will make subsequent sticks impossible.
- Make sure your connection is a Luer-Loc. That will lock the line in place on your catheter. A non-Luer is not locked in place and makes fallout at the worst possible time!
- Make sure you have a good trace.
- Secure the line, some say sew it in place, some say do it with a Tegaderm and tape . . . lots of tape.
- You should be able to move your patient to the stretcher by pulling him by the A-line!
- Loop the art line around the patient's thumb (not *your* thumb—that would be a mistake).
- A portable ultrasound device can be used to place the line under direct vision.

HOW ABOUT KIDDIES AGAIN?

Indications
- Major surgery where blood loss and fluids shifts may result in BP instability or, where constant, accurate BP measurement is necessary.
- Repeat blood gas measurements are required.

Sites
- Radial is the preferred.
- Good collaterals are the norm in the hand from the ulnar artery.
- Left side preferred for cardiac surgery.
- Dorsalis pedia and posterior tibial are not much help if the aorta is to be clamped (liver transplant, cardiac surgery).
- Axillary is technically tricky in children, but collaterals are good and it is usually above the clamp.
- Femoral is the last resort.
- Associated with poor perfusion in newborns.
- Sepsis more common.
- Forget the brachial artery. It is an end artery. Though, read on. The next chapter will address this very concern!

Technique
- Asepsis.
- Palpate vessel (transillumination with cold, bright light helpful).
- Nick the skin with an 18-g needle as this will prevent kinking the cannula.
- 24 g for younger than 12 months.
- 22 g up to 10 years old.
- 20 g for those older.
- Use the bevel of the needle pointing down as this will prevent puncture of the back wall of the vessel.
- Advance the cannula when you see blood flashback.
- If advancement is not possible, try a fine guidewire. This may be a necessity in some of the new, improved safety cannulae.
- Secure with Luer-Lok fittings because disconnection may result in fatal hemorrhage.
- Secure with plenty of tape joint immobilization.
- Do not flush excessively (1 mL maximum in infants). Do not use the pressure bag-flushing mechanism in

infants, (use a 10-mL syringe instead). We don't want retrograde cerebral embolus in small babies, or anyone, for that matter.

- Use normal saline with 1 unit heparin/mL in the continuous flush device.

Once again, that's it for our little kiddie diversion.

COMPLICATIONS

- Hematoma.
- Infection.
- Ischemia: One of the most feared complications, but it is an unusual event. The Allen test is not a good screening test.
- Embolization: including air to the *brain*, yes, the brain, as overzealous flushing can push bubbles all the way up.
- Overall, a pretty safe procedure!

GLITCHY GOOMY

- No kidding, sit down and try to relax the rest of yourself when you do an arterial line. An art line requires very fine movement of the little muscles of your hand. If you're bent over and your lower back is crying out, you can't devote enough of your motor cortex to the subject at hand.
- These lines hurt. If the patient is screaming bloody murder, put a little more local in. You work in a hospital, not in the Spanish Inquisition torture chamber.
- When the arm gets tucked, make sure the art line trace doesn't disappear. If the hand that was extended now gets flexed, you can lose your trace.
- In the best of all possible worlds, keep the art line where you can see it.
- If you lose the trace, first make sure that it's not *the real thing* (i.e., death). Still

have a CO_2 trace? Still have a pulse oximeter reading? Still have an EKG? Good. Now, troubleshoot.

- Believe the worst first, always. Only *after* you have proven it's not the worst should you go to technical glitches as a cause of a lost trace.
- Lost trace that is not fatal? Look for a stopcock bumped and cutting you off.
- Look for a disconnected line. Note: Blood will now pour out of the patient which is *not* a good thing.
- Trace looking damped? Make sure there is not a loose connection somewhere.
- You can flush, get a good trace, later it gets damped, flush, get a good trace, later it gets damped, flush . . . . You can do this forever! Such a cycle usually means something is loose and not working well, and you're about to lose your trace altogether . . . sooner than later.
- Trace looking damped? Make sure your flush bag is under pressure. An unpumped-up bag is a common cause of a damped trace.
- Crummy trace no matter what you do? Don't limp through a case with a rotten art line. Put another one in, or ask the surgeons to put one in for you. If you need it, you need it. Don't cower behind the drapes, bemoaning a lost art line and just hoping the case will end soon. That is the very case disaster will strike. (Evil genies watch over us and take advantage of us when we really need a line, but lose that same line.)
- Placed the line and now the hand looks dusky? Few options here. Call a vascular surgeon no matter what. You can inject a little nitroglycerin down the line or else inject a little papaverin (watch for hypotension), then pull the line out. As you pull, aspirate in case there is a clot on the end, maybe you'll get lucky and pull the clot out.

A Blast from the Past

A lot of times, we're really only spooked about induction. An imperfect, but reasonable measure for blood pressure just for the induction time, is—a blast from the past—a finger on the pulse! How's that for ancient history?!

If you feel the patient's pulse ahead of time and make a note of the blood pressure at the time, you have calibrated your monitor. Then, during the ups and downs of induction and intubation, you can at least have a notion of the pressure. You may not be able to tell 140 from 130, but you can at least tell *bounding* from *nonexistent*.

This would be useful in the following case: An adult with mental incapacity who won't cooperate for an A-line. You decide to induce, and want to keep a close eye on the blood pressure during induction. If you don't have the new gizmo, go with Old Faithful, the finger on the pulse. As soon as you can postinduce, get the A-line.

Not the Only Place to Draw Blood

Keep in mind that you don't need an arterial line to draw blood. You can get blood out of a central line, for example, if you just want to follow hematocrits or glucose. You don't need *arterial* blood for information that a *vein* can give you.

Also, truth to tell, you could draw blood out of a peripheral IV, but that line would have to be pretty big, plus you might screw up the IV and clot it off. In general, not a groovy idea to rely on a peripheral IV for a lot of blood draws.

And, finally, you could stick a vein for individual draws, but that, in the middle of a case, is too fraught with clumsiness and struggling. You're crawling under the drapes, putting on tourniquets, dealing with needles. Like they say: Fuhgedaboudit!

Zen Arterial Line Placement

If you ever see an open wrist in the trauma center, and you see how teeny the radial artery is, you'll be amazed that we *ever* get an art line in. The thing looks as narrow as a pencil lead.

So to get a radial arterial line, you have to shift into Zen oneness with that artery.

Be the artery.

Set the artery up so you can get a straight shot into it. Tape the wrist so it's hyperextended (not horrifically so—you don't want to stretch the median nerve), and get the thenar eminence out of the way. If that thenar eminence is sticking up in your way, your needle will need to magically go up and over that hill then slip into the radial artery. In effect, that would describe a near-impossible S movement.

There are different ways to stick the artery (through and through, for example). Myself, I'm not a big advocate of putting two holes in that itsy-bitsy artery if I don't have to. Better to come at the artery in a shallow, shallow, along-the-same-axis-that-the-artery-is-describing angle.

Picture a plane trying to fly into a tunnel: To get into that tunnel, the plane should approach and be describing the tunnel as it flies in . . . that way, the plane can get well into the tunnel. You, too, want to get well into the artery. You want to fly a little way in so you don't end up with just the needle tip in the artery while the catheter is not yet in. When that happens, you can have a hell of a time sliding the catheter in.

When you place an A-line, what is the most useful adjuvant equipment? A chair, believe it or not.

Most people crouch over and visit murder upon their lumbar vertebrae as they place an arterial line. Better to sit down and relax. Not only does this fit into the whole Zen experience, sitting allows you to concentrate your muscles on the task at hand. While sitting, your back, hips, and legs aren't working—all your motor cortex can focus on the fine movement of your fingertips. That's where the action is, after all.

If you miss and you were sitting, you end up with a hematoma.

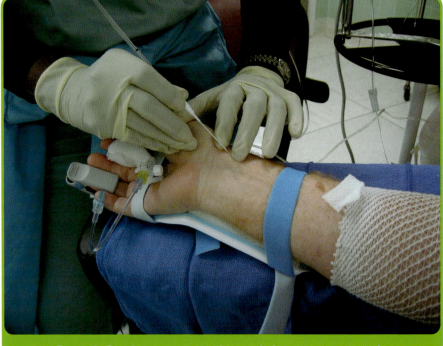

Figure 1. Get the wrist nice and extended, so you get a straight approach to the vessel. You don't want to jump up and over the thenar eminence.

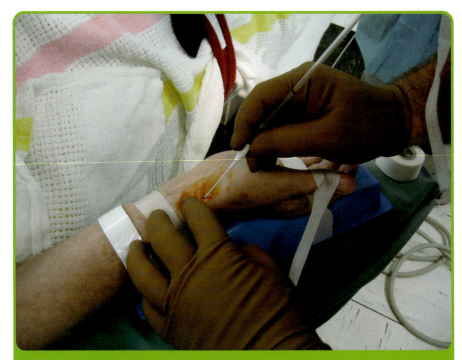

Figure 2. Come in shallow, shallow, shallow. That way you'll get the needle in and will also be able to advance the catheter in that "silly millimeter" that separates success from failure.

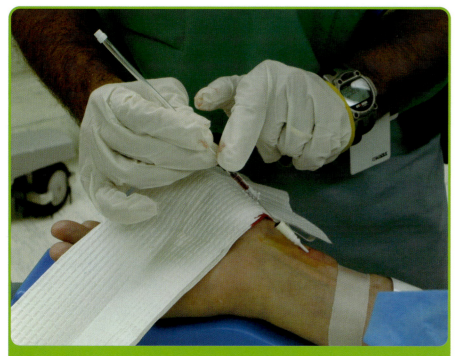

Figure 3. Oh unbridled happiness! The flash, now make sure you advance the catheter into the vessel.

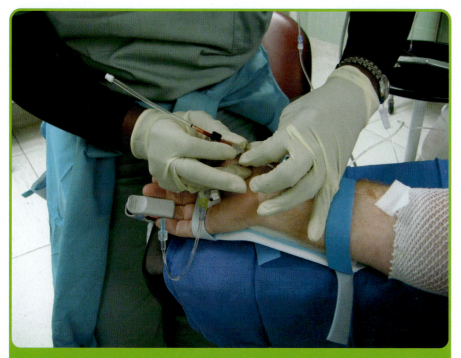

Figure 4. Now slither that baby up there. Unlike a vein (which can roll around), an artery doesn't have to be "held in place".

If you miss and you were standing, you end up with a hematoma, and 10 years from now you yourself end up with a lumbar laminectomy.

Should you use the kit with the little wire?

In theory, the catheter with the slide-up-the-catheter wire will allow you to get the needle in the artery, stop, slide up the wire, then easily slide up the catheter. Oh happiness! No more hitting the artery, but not being able to advance the catheter!

Only problem is, it usually doesn't work out that way. You're better off just getting in a little further, and sliding in the catheter the regular way. I've seen a million episodes of hitting the artery, stopping, and then you can't even slide the wire up.

Damn!

So, the kit looks good in theory, and you can sometimes save the day with that wire, but I'm not too impressed with it.

How about a freestanding wire up a regular catheter?

Again, in theory it works out great—you hit the artery, get flow, but just plain can't slide the damned catheter in. So you slide up a wire and save the day.

Would that it always happened.

Trouble is, just like the catheter with the built-in wire, a lot of times, that wire just won't go.

Non-Zen Arterial Line Placement

OK, what in blue blazes do you do when the A-line gods are arraigned against you and are making your life miserable?

In the wild and wooly world of anesthesia, there is no place so uncomfortable as the I-can't-get-the-line place. The patient hurts, blood's dripping all over the place, you have a mountain of dirty needles amassing all around you, and all the guys are tapping their feet and their wristwatches, and you want to be anywhere but there.

Your Zen composure crumbles, revealing a beet-red, put-a-drunken-sailor-to-shame-swearing monster. No one can hear the sound of one hand clapping as you rant and rave and curse your fate and you denounce the patient's radial artery for failing to yield to your entry efforts.

At this juncture, redirect.

Line directile dysfunction will madden and infuriate you. Feelings of inadequacy will wash over you. Just like any other procedure in anesthesia, you have to prepare yourself mentally to handle line directile dysfunction. Here's how:

The wrong way:

Many a resident, attending, medical student, or out-in-the-real-world anesthesiologist has tried talking a line in.

"I hit it, but I can't thread it!"

"I don't get it, the pulse is right there, how can this not be in?"

"Hmm, I thought it was in, and I even taped it in (sewed it in, tied it down with battleship anchor chains, what difference does it make?), but there's no arterial trace and I can't draw any blood out of it. I wonder if it's in."

"You saw it! That should be in there!"

All of these verbal arguments, though convincing, and more than likely to evince a sympathetic nod from the on-looking nurse/tech/surgeon/dignitary, still don't change one thing.

You're not in.

All the talking in the world won't change that . . . never has and never

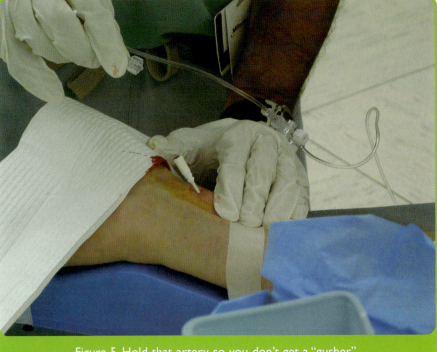

Figure 5. Hold that artery so you don't get a "gusher".

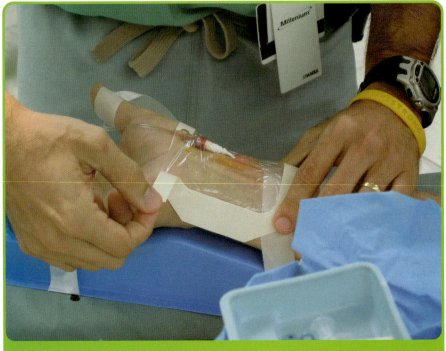

Figure 6. Now secure the vessel and make sure you can see all the connection sites.

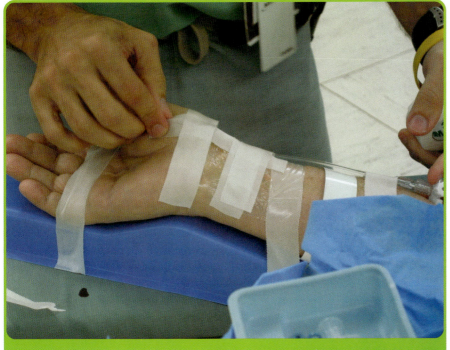

Figure 7. Aaah! A thing of beauty is a joy forever.

SUGGESTED READING

Allen EV. Thromboangiitis obliterans: methods of diagnosis of chronic occlusive arterial disease distal to the wrist with illustrative cases. *Am J Med Sci* 1929; 178:237-244.

- *Original description of the Allen test! It is a historical paper, as the Allen test has not been able to predict who will get hand ischemia with radial A-lines.*

Anderson JS. Arterial cannulation: how to do it. *Brit J Hosp Med* 1997;7: 497-499.

- *Another cool article on arterial cannulation with all the you-need-to-know details of the procedure.*

Barr PO. Percutaneous puncture of the radial artery with multipurpose Teflon catheter for indwelling use. *Acta Physiol Scand* 1961;51:343-345.

- *First description of the radial cannulation with Teflon catheter.*

Bedford RF. Radial arterial function following percutaneous cannulation with 18- and 20-gauge catheters. *Anesthesiology* 1977;47:37-39.

- *This study showed that the incidence of postcannulation radial artery occlusion can be decreased significantly by using 20-g cannulas instead of 18-g cannulas. Also small radial arteries (less than 2 mm in diameter) are more likely to occlude, and remain thrombosed longer than large radial arteries (more than 2.25 mm in diameter.*

Franklin C. The technique of radial artery cannulation. *J Crit Ill* 1995;10:424-432.

- *Good article which describes the correct technique step by step, and everything you should know about the radial artery cannulation. Gives tips for maximizing results while minimizing the risk of complications.*

Levin PD. Use of ultrasound guidance in the insertion of radial artery catheters. *Crit Care Med* 2003;31:481-484.

- *Nifty trick when you cannot find the artery. Radial artery catheters can be inserted under ultrasound guidance using a portable ultrasound device with the same benefits as ultrasound-guided central vein catheter insertion; higher success rate with fewer attempts.*

Lovenstein E. Prevention of cerebral embolization from flushing radial-artery cannulas. *New Engl J Med* 1971;25:1414-1415.

- *This study shows that the volume of flush solution that can produce embolization of air or clot from the radial artery is very small (3-12 mL). We must pay special attention to avoid any air bubbles in the flushing system.*

Oh TE. Radial artery cannulation. *Anaesth Intensive Care* 1975;1:12-17.

- *This article gives a list of precautions to minimize the risk of complications such as use of a modified Allen test, aseptic technique (to better feel the pulse, gloves were not recommended in 1975), etc. Another historical paper.*

will. Plato and Voltaire and Abraham Lincoln could all come back from the great beyond and plead your case with all the eloquence that humankind has ever mustered, but all that *talking* still doesn't translate into any *arterial lines*.

So shut your trap and move on.

The right way:

Go to a different site.

Mentally, if you're always thinking of Plan B ("If I don't get the radial on this side, I'll get it on the other; if that doesn't work, I'll go femoral"), then there's not so much pressure on you while you're doing Plan A. Believe it or not, this really works. It keeps you from going out of your gourd while you hammer and hammer at that poor radial artery, making a Texas Chainsaw Massacre of the patient, and a gibbering idiot out of yourself.

From a time-sensitive standpoint, try this to keep things moving if you're having trouble: If one radial line is just not happening, ask the circulator or holding area nurse to tee up the other side. Have them set the patient's other wrist on an armboard with a roll. Get everything taped and in place so when you go to the other side, you go right to the stick, rather than having to start all over. That minute or two saved makes life a lot easier.

In the computer-speak of the day, you are multitasking, rather than just doing one thing at a time. (Also, if you blow it on the other side, you have just successfully engaged in multiscrewing upping.)

Slogoff S. On the safety of radial artery cannulation. *Anesthesiology* 1983;59:42-47.
- *Large prospective study of the risk of radial artery cannulation showed that the risk of partial or complete occlusion of the radial artery after cannulation was more than 25%, but without any important clinical thrombosis. The Allen test was not useful in predicting ischemia.*

Valentine RJ. Hand ischemia after radial artery cannulation. *Am Coll Surg* 2005; 201:18-22.
- *This paper focused on eight patients with radial cannula-induced arterial thrombosis. It confirms that hand ischemia is a very rare complication after radial artery cannulation. Causes of radial artery thrombosis are multifactorial, but ischemia symptoms can be attributed to digital embolization or in situ thrombosis. Successful surgical revascularization does not prevent digital gangrene in most patients. Big limitation of the study is that it is retrospective.*

Wilkins RG. Radial artery cannulation and ischemic damage: a review. *Anaesthesia* 1985;40:896-899.
- *Puts everything together, gives good overview of prior studies on radial cannulation.*

EEEEK! Do We Dare? The Brachial A-line

Mike Barron and Geoffrey Sanders

Enter these enchanted woods, you who dare.

George Meredith
The Woods of Westermain, 1828

INTRODUCTION

That damned radial artery seems as thin as a pencil-lead at times, and it just doesn't yield to our A-line attempts like it ought to. And the radial artery has a nagging habit, after cardiopulmonary bypass, of damping out, no matter what we do.

Where to next?

Femoral. Yes, you can.

Brachial?

Wait! Doesn't every book say the brachial artery is an end-artery? If I stick the brachial artery, will I not be stepping into an enchanted woods of vascular insufficiency, arms falling off, and *Plaintiff's Attorneys R Us*?

Well, no.

Look at the Cleveland Clinic. They do a zillion hearts a year and they put brachial lines in all the time. Half the people in Cleveland don't walk around with one arm missing from a brachial artery mishap, do they?

Go ahead. Enter those enchanted woods. Put in a brachial art line.

If you dare.

INDICATIONS

- Same as for other arterial lines, beat–to-beat blood pressure measurement.
- Faucet for drawing arterial blood gases.
- Little more reliable in the post-cardiopulmonary bypass period for giving accurate blood pressures than a radial arterial line.

CONTRAINDICATIONS

- Vascular insufficiency.
- Raynaud's phenomenon. (Why risk it?)
- If you're chicken about brachial arterial lines and you don't care if Cleveland Clinic puts them in all the time.

EQUIPMENT

- Don't bother with a short line like you do for a radial art line.
- Use a 20-g, 12-cm kit. Since the brachial area will move around a little, a short line could come out. Put in a long line.
- All the usual sterile prep stuff.

BEWARE NUTHIN'

- You will rarely get one of these from elsewhere because everyone else is scared to put in a brachial a-line.

PHILOSOPHY

- If the radial just ain't happening, and you're not chicken, go brachial.

- If you were having so much trouble with the radial line anyway, then that radial line will probably go to caca later, so go ahead, and get a better line now.
- The brachial artery is bigger so, surprise! surprise! it's easier to hit. Oh, happy days!

TECHNIQUE

- Lay that arm out flat as a pancake.
- Palpate the brachial artery, just medial to the midline in the antecubital fossa.
- Place local.
- Use the hollow bore needle (à la Seldinger).
- Get flow.
- Pass the wire.
- Remove the needle.
- Slide the catheter up the wire.
- Keep the wire in until you are ready to hook up the line. (The catheter is so long, you can't so easily reach up and squish the artery and prevent *exsanguinaticus iatrogenicus*).
- Pull the wire and hook up the line.
- Make sure you have a good trace.
- Sew this baby in place. (It's not so easy to tape this down because it is a radial line, so go with the extra security. Plus, this line has two tabs on the side you can sew into.)
- Place a dressing.
- Go have an unfiltered Camel.

So you want to put a brachial A-line in, but are getting resistance from someone in the OR with concerns about its safety, efficacy, or standard of care. Just mention Michael Bazaral from the Cleveland Clinic and tell them to update their scope of knowledge.

You're looking at two large hematomas from failed radial A-line attempts and the femorals are off-limits by specific case. You can be a hero and get the case started on time by becoming proficient in this alternate A-line site: the brachial artery.

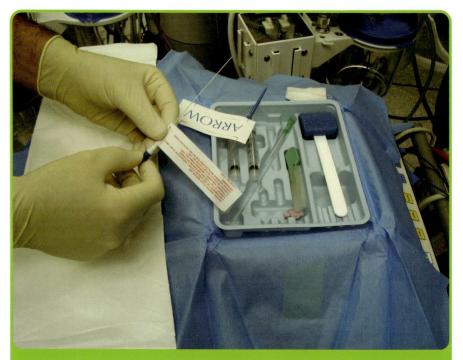

Figure 1. Here is the a-line tray. Notice that we are using a 12 cm long catheter.

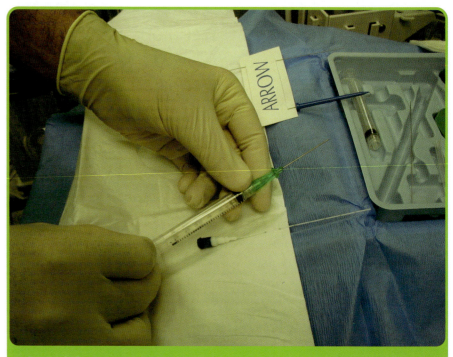

Figure 2. Easier to find the vessel with an angiocath and a syringe and thread it in or you can use a thin wall needle directly.

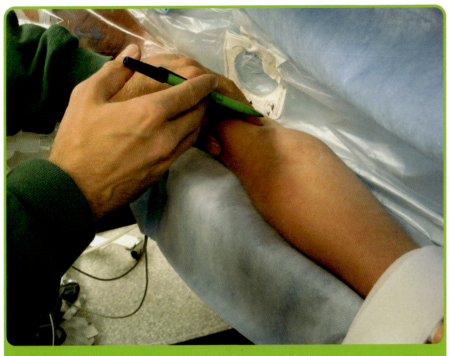

Figure 3. Locate your target!! Better said:feel your target.

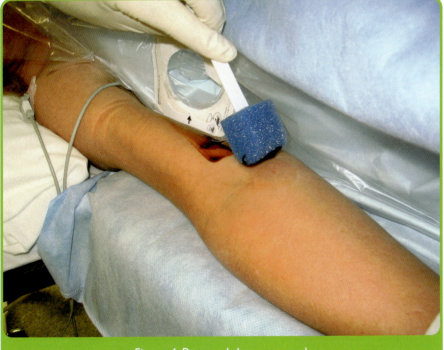

Figure 4. Prep and drape as usual.

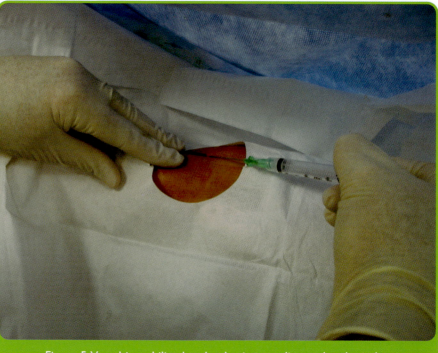

Figure 5. Vessel is stabilized and pulse is pounding under the index and middle fingers of your left hand. Go for that puppy!

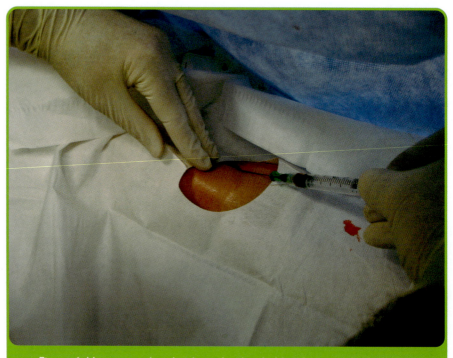

Figure 6. How rewarding: bright red pulsatile blood coming back to you.

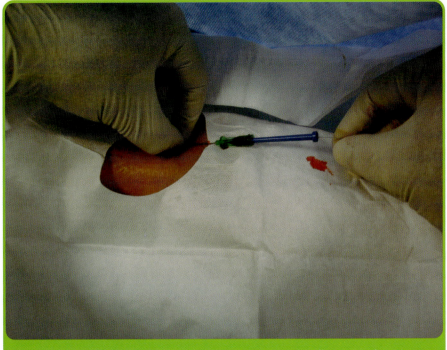

Figure 7. You are in the vessel, thread the wire in, pull angio cath out.

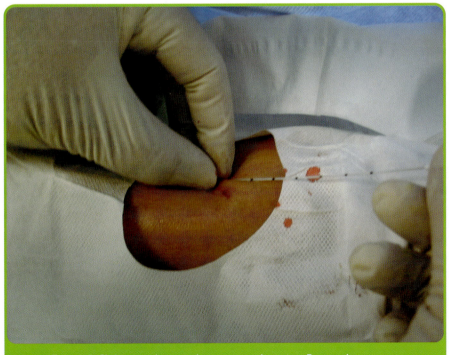

Figure 8. Slide your long catheter over the wire. Remember not to lose sight of the wire at all times.

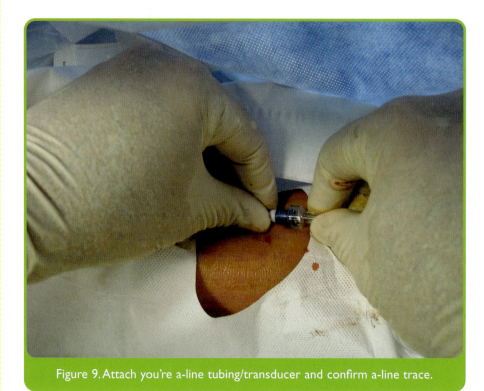

Figure 9. Attach you're a-line tubing/transducer and confirm a-line trace.

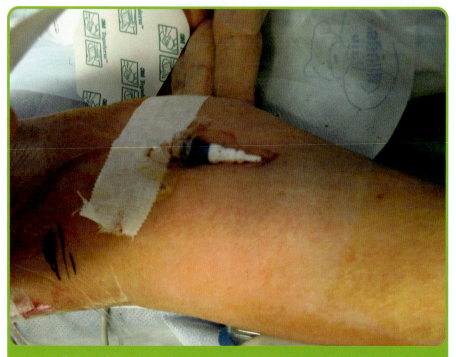

Figure 10. Brachial a-line working!. Make sure it is well secured.

SUGGESTED READING

Barnes RW, Foster EJ, Jansen GA. Safety of brachial arterial catheterization as monitors in the intensive care unit: prospective evaluation with the Doppler ultrasonic velocity detector. *Anesthesiology* 1976;44: 260-264.

- *Another article to explore the safety of brachial artery cannulation. This study is unique in that the perfusion of the upper limb was studied postcannulation in a patient population undergoing open heart surgery via Doppler studies. Results point toward confidence in the safety of this procedure.*

Bazaral MG, Welch M, Golding LAR, Badwar K. Comparison of brachial and radial arterial pressure monitoring in patients undergoing coronary artery bypass surgery. *Anesthesiology* 1990;73:38-45.

- *Excellent study showing not only that brachial A-lines are a possible option for safely monitoring patients blood pressure in a critical case, but a brachial A-line might offer a more accurate means to this monitoring. In addition, this study was done by the well-respected Michael Bazaral who reportedly commonly placed brachial A-lines in the also well-known institution known as the Cleveland Clinic.*

Gravlee GP, Wong AB, Adkins TG, Case LD, Pauca AL. A comparison of radial, brachial, and aortic pressures after cardiopulmonary bypass. *J Cardiothorac Anesth* 1989;(3):1: 20-26.

- *This is another article that compares the accuracy of blood pressure measurement post CPB in various areas compared to the aorta. Results of this study point toward the idea that cannulation of the brachial artery may offer a slightly more accurate measuring area than the traditional radial.*

Jerald O, White RD, Abenstein JP, et al. Comparison of axillary artery pressure with aortic pressure after cardiopulmonary bypass using a long radial artery catheter. *J Cardiothorac Vasc Anesth* 1993;(7):3: 312-315.

- *A somewhat relevant discussion exploring the idea that post CPB, the monitoring of blood pressure more proximal to the aorta provides more accurate monitoring. This idea could suggest that brachial artery cannulation could be superior in some ways to radial artery blood pressure monitoring.*

Moran KT, Halpin DP, Zide RS, et al. Long-term brachial arterial catheterization: ischemic complications. *J Vasc Surg* 1988;8:76-78.

- *This study discusses and potentially refutes claims that cannulation of the brachial artery can cause frequent ischemic complications.*

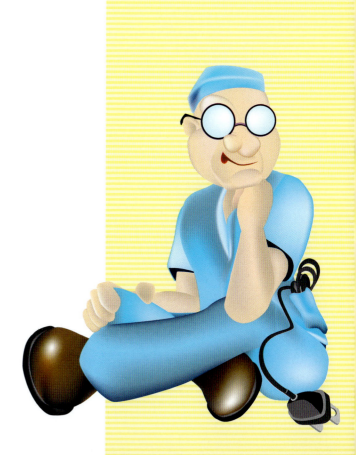

An Ever-Present Friend in Time of Need: The Femoral

Craig Nelson and Kiley Reynolds

INTRODUCTION

Femoral arterial catheterization is an ever-present friend in time of need. When the arms won't yield an art line, go femoral. In cases of severe vasculopathy, it is the only frontier yet to be confronted before the word "cutdown" has to be muttered.

And one fine day you may have to stick your femoral friend to get an arterial line.

Though largely seen as the domain of the cardiologists (who, by means of femoral arterial access, have bankrupted cardiac surgery and cardiac anesthesia), we, too should know how to get this crucial line.

The femoral artery is a big hogger, so it should admit even blundering attempts at cannulation. And some days the arms just don't cooperate to allow us access to arterial flow, so we have to go femoral.

The femoral artery is a friend in need and a friend indeed.

INDICATIONS

- Beat-to-beat blood pressure measurement.
- Automated cuff dysfunction: arrhythmias, severe hypotension, morbid obesity.
- Multiple arterial blood gases measurements.
- Easy access if you anticipate the need for an intraaortic balloon pump later (better to already have access to the femoral artery, then you can just place a wire and go for the gusto).
- A few specialized cases where you need to know the blood pressure above and below (the aortic arch aneurysm where you will be doing partial cardiopulmonary bypass).

CONTRAINDICATIONS

- Surgery above that may involve the aorta or interfere with aortic pressures due to compression.
- Recent femoral artery surgery (fem-pop, fem-fem crossover, aortobiiliac . . . pick your poison).
- Simultaneously existing central venous catheter in same location due to risk of AV fistula formation.
- Infection or anatomic abnormality at the site.
- Aorto-occlusive disease (how accurate will the blood pressure be?).

TECHNIQUE

- Direct arterial puncture and cannulation
- Guidewire-assisted cannulation
- Direct visualization through surgical exploration

EQUIPMENT

- Heparinized versus normal saline (no difference in thrombosis at or distal to cannulation site) pressure bag, pressure monitoring kit—primed and zeroed.
- Access kits for femoral artery (Arrow makes a nice kit) (20 g, 12 cm kit) versus central line kit (16-g, 16-cm single-lumen central line kit). You want a long catheter with a soft tip. If you use a shorter, stiffer line, you could poke through the back of the femoral artery. Also, femoral lines require larger gauge catheters (16-18) to minimize catheter whip.
- Sterile prep, drape, and gloves (used appropriately).
- Helping hands to pull the abdomen back.

PHILOSOPHY OF FEMORAL ART LINES

- Don't get hung up if you can't get an arterial line in the arm. Just go femoral. Beating your head against the wall will not make an arterial line go in. Going to a new spot often will.

A man that hath friends must show himself friendly; and there is a friend that sticketh closer than a brother.

Proverbs 18:24

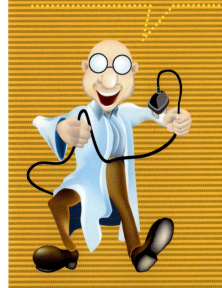

Beware the Cardiac Cath Emergency

- When patients come flying down to the OR from the cath lab, they will often have their groin lines still in.

- If you hear of patients coming down from the cath lab, be sure and remind them *not* to pull out the groin lines, because those lines might save you in the rush-rush of a cath lab disaster.

- Make sure you know which line is which! Often there will be a bandage over them, and it won't be evident which is the venous and which is the arterial.

- Take the bandage off, and take a good look.

- When time is of the essence (trust us, it will be), use those groin lines for your IV and your A-line. Don't bother to put in your own until later when the crisis is past.

- In the panic, people in the cath lab sometimes won't sew in those lines, so make sure they don't get pulled out.

- In the middle of a case, if your radial arterial line poops out, ask the surgeons (the groin will often be in the field by now) to help you and get a femoral line.

- These sticks do hurt, and the vessel can be deep. If you can do these under general anesthesia, then do the patient a favor.

PROCEDURE

- If you are right-handed, go for the right femoral. If left-handed, go for the left femoral. The angle of approach is more natural.

- If ambidextrous, go for the aorta.

- *Just kidding*! Just wanted to see if you're paying attention.

- Prep and drape the area.

- Use liberal local anesthetic if the patient isn't under general anesthesia.

- Don't bother with a finder.

- Use the long needle, not the catheter (the catheter will get kinked).

- Have your helper pull the abdomen out of the way so you have a straight shot.

- Palpate the artery, remembering the lateral to medial mnemonic, NAVEL to the navel (nerve, artery, vein, empty, lymphatics).

- Start below the inguinal crease (higher might have you sticking intestines, which this book does not recommend). Also, above the inguinal ligament, the artery is named the "external iliac." Laceration of the artery above the ligament creates a potential space that can hold a massive amount of blood undetected till cardiovascular changes occur . . . a little late. The external iliac artery is hard to compress due to the posterior projection of the artery.

- The artery can be deep so this could be a little vexing.

- Hope that today is your lucky day.

- When you get flow, make sure the blood is bright (it better be) and pulsatile (it better be that, too, or else something is most egregiously wrong).

- Pass the wire. If the wire doesn't pass easily, don't force it. Forcing wire just bends the wire, traumatizes tissue, and dislodges arterial plaques heading for the toes. Readjust needle and aspirate for blood. Repass the wire.

- Once the wire passes easily, pull out the needle.

- Make a nick in the skin, this can be a teeny one, because you can wiggley-jiggley a 16 g through the skin without a big production in the knife department.

- Advance the catheter.

- Aspirate and flush.

- Secure.

- Give the line a nice curve around and coming back up toward the head of the bed so your line won't kink off during the case. This is essential. Take your time because this is the last time you might see this line till the end of the case. Catastrophic bleeds can occur from a free-flowing 16-g arterial catheter.

MAINTENANCE

- Correlate invasive with noninvasive blood pressure.

- Send an ABG, which gives you a baseline.

- Flush the line at least every hour. This may be the most effective way to troubleshoot an overdamped line occurring during the case.

- Make sure the pressure bag has, and is, keeping pressure.

- Keep the transducer at the level of the heart. In specialized cases, such as the sitting crani, you may opt to leave the transducer at the level of the head because this will most closely approximate cerebral perfusion pressures.

- Eyeball your site, if this is possible during the case. This will keep Murphy and his law in check.

COMPLICATION

- Hemorrhage. Usually from disconnect. Never let this happen, this is user error. The potential space for blood collection in the thigh is immense and can go unnoticed. Diligence is the only answer. High-risk patients (coagulopathic, multiple sticks) require good followup and checkout.

- Infection. Rules are that the longer an indwelling catheter is in place, the more likely an infection will occur. How long should a catheter be left in place? Simple answer: the least amount of time as possible. There is no predetermined time that a catheter must be changed except if infection is evident or, in the cases of infection of unknown origin, where all indwelling lines are changed.

- Pain. Local incision pain versus a neuropathy from nerve damage due to traumatic cannulation.
- Thrombosis. Cold extremities are an emergency. Cool extremities are a concern and the catheter should be removed and evaluation performed.
- Spasm. Loss of tracing with intact distal pulses. Hard to discriminate from thrombosis. Time for a new site.
- Accidental drug injection. Enough said. Know your lines. Label your lines.

WHEN THE LINE GODS CONSPIRE AGAINST YOU

- Use an ultrasound location device if you are having a hard time.
- The femoral pulse can feel so big that you can get lost as to where it's really artery and where it's transmitted pulse.
- If you get dark blood, then you may be in the vein. You're too medial. If in doubt, get an ABG. Better yet, a transducer; if the pressure correlates with the noninvasive pressure, think oxygen and look at the patient (maybe sedated the patient a little too much, or the patient may have become disconnected from the ventilator).
- If the patient goes Yipe! you may have hit the nerve. You're too lateral.
- The vessel can be so deep that you almost have the needle going straight in, then it's hard to have the wire take the corner and advance well. When this happens, try to flatten your angle of approach.
- A cut-down is an alternative. A pain in the ass, but it is, after all, an alternative.
- Try putting a pillow under the patient's knees, which alters how the vessels lay and might give you a better shot.
- If you get intestinal fluid back through the needle, call a general surgeon.
- Watch for hematomas. If you stick through the back wall (or if the cardiologist stuck through the back wall in the cath lab), patients can lose a gallon of blood in their thighs or in their retroperitoneum.

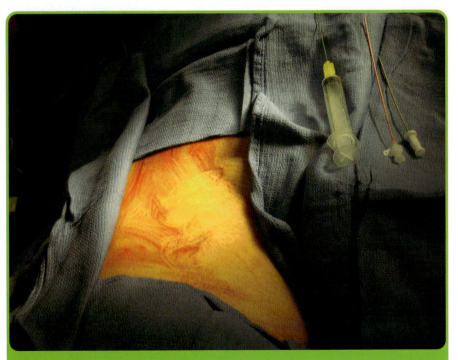

Figure 1. Prep and drape the area. Have equipment ready!

AAG! What Did You Inject?

A cath lab emergency came flying down to the OR on winged feet.

In the rush to get going, someone grabbed a groin line and injected etomidate to induce the patient. The patient lost consciousness, and we got going.

Inspection revealed the etomidate had gone in the arterial line, leading to a panicky search for "What the hell happens when you give etomidate through an arterial line"?

Lucky for us, etomidate (unlike pentathol), causes no harm when injected arterially.

We are *much* more careful about inspecting groin lines now.

What Did You Say That Hematocrit Was?

Yes, people do bleed from the cath site, and it can go undetected for a long time.

I went to an ICU for an intubation. They told me the patient was scheduled for bypass operation the next day, she had been cathed today, and she wasn't looking too good.

Upon arrival, I noticed precious little difference between the sheet of the patient's bed and her skin. After intubation, a hematocrit was sent out with the first blood gas.

Um, did you say, the hemato*crit* was 5? Are you sure that's not the hemo*globin*?

We, uh, went to the OR a little earlier than expected.

Beware the Radial Art Line Post Bypass

Great thinkers have wrestled with great questions for great lengths of time:

Why are we here?

Where did we come from?

What happens after we transfer to the Celestial Care Unit?

Why does the stupid radial arterial line register a lower pressure postbypass?

If you are doing a heart case, and everything else looks good after coming off bypass, but the radial art line is giving you a pressure of 60, have the surgeon feel the aorta and give you an estimate of the blood pressure. If the surgeon says, "It's way higher," then do yourself a favor ... have them put in a femoral line for you. Femoral lines equate more consistently with aortic pressures. Make sure this gradient doesn't exist prebypass; this signifies occlusive disease, and will require higher pressures to maintain perfusion in the upper extremities and, possibly, above the neck.

You don't want to be treating low blood pressure, cranking up all your inotropes and vasopressors, when all you're doing is treating an inaccurate reading. A femoral line is a lot less damaging than driving the patient's blood pressure up to 500!

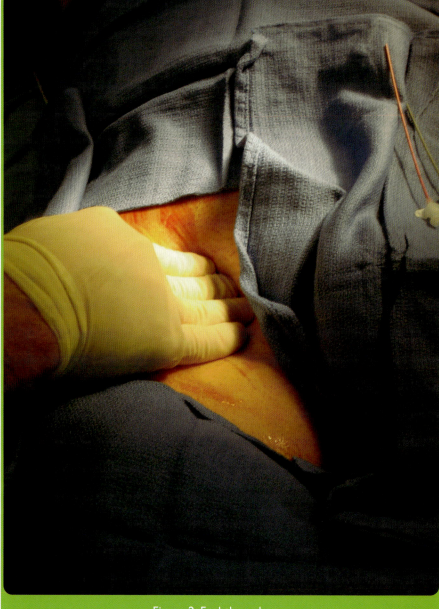

Figure 2. Feel the pulse....

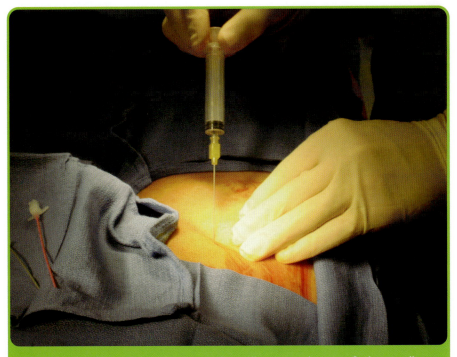

Figure 3. Go for it. Use the thin wall needle; no need to use finder needle.

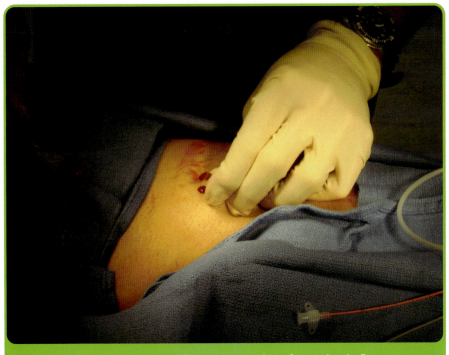

Figure 4. You found it! Disconnect and confirm pulsatile flow.

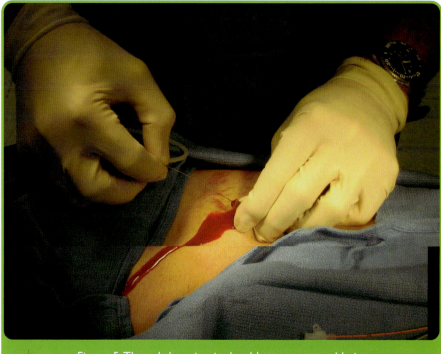

Figure 5. Thread the wire; it should go smoooooothly in.

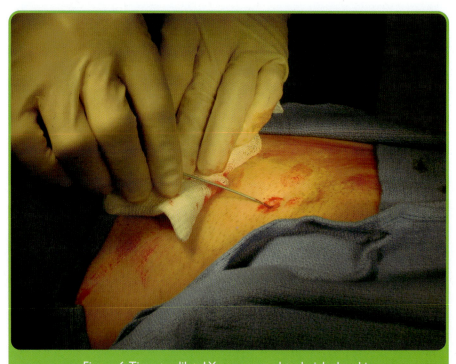

Figure 6. Time to dilate! You may need to knick the skin with the scalpel to let the dilator through the skin.

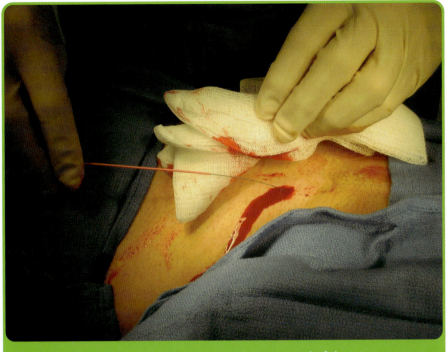

Figure 7. Thread catheter; never loose control of the wire.

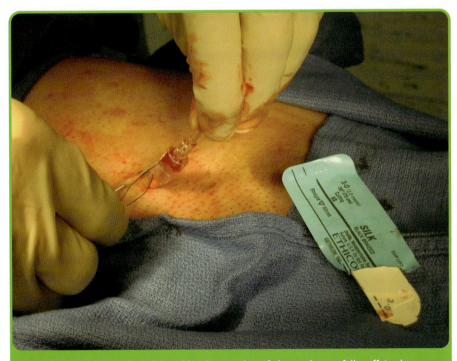

Figure 8. Secure catheter. You know that if the catheter falls off, is the resident's fault!

SUGGESTED READING

Barr PO. Percutaneous puncture of the radial artery with a multipurpose. Teflon catheter for indwelling use. *Acta Physiol Scand* 1961;51:343-345.
- *The Seldinger technique has revolutionized the world of indwelling catheters. Not a need-to-know article, but it is for those of us that want consultant-style verbiage, and knowledge of the system we are using.*

Bazaral MG, Welch M, Golding LAR, Badhwar K. Comparison of brachial and radial arterial arterial pressure monitoring in patient undergoing coronary artery bypass grafting. *Anesthesiology* 1990:73:38-45.
- *Minor reference with great implications for those involved with cardiothoracic surgeries.*

Bowdle TA. Complications of invasive monitoring. *Anesthes Clin North Am* Sep 2002;20(3):571-588.
- *Covered mostly in the basics, but more in depth and in detail if the thirst for knowledge is great.*

Cutler TD, Weidemann HP. Complications of hemodynamic monitoring. *Clin Chest Med* Jun 1999;20(2):249-267.
- *More broad complications involving all of hemodynamic monitoring.*

Fowler GC. Arterial puncture. In: Pfenninger JL, Fowler GC. *Procedures for Primary Care Physicians*, 1st ed. St. Louis: Mosby; 1994, p 340-347.
- *Bare bones of arterial lines; the basics are never to be overlooked. Best article for newbies.*

Fowler GC: Percutaneous arterial line placement. In: Pfenninger JL, Fowler GC. *Procedures for Primary Care Physicians*, 1st ed. St Louis: Mosby; 1994, p 293-299.
- *Fowler does it again; pretty much the same as his above reference.*

Frezza EE, Mezghebe H. Indications and complications of arterial catheter use in surgical or medical intensive care units: analysis of 4932 patients. *Am Surg* 1998;4(2):127-131.
- *Know why to put the line in, and what harm you may cause. Clinical-based medicine at its best.*

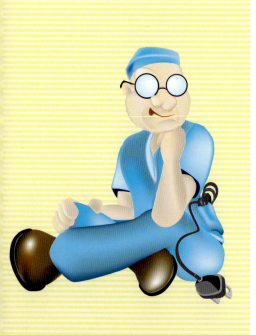

PART 3

INTO THIN AIR

The Mask of Zorro: Mask Ventilation

Christopher Gallagher and Fernando Gavia

Then wilt thou speak of banqueting delights,

Of masks and revels which sweet youth did make.

Thomas Campion
A Book of Airs, 1601

INTRODUCTION

While you are reveling away your sweet youth, do learn the art of mask ventilation. Intubation gets all the press. Each edition of *Anesthesiology News* has a dozen ads for whizbang intubation gizmos. But don't forget the basics!

You need to *walk* before you *run*, and you need to *mask ventilate* before you *intubate*.

If you mask ventilate well, you will prevent yourself from getting into disasters, and if you mask ventilate well, you will extricate yourself from disasters.

This is a craft worth learning.

INDICATION

- Ventilatory support. Better to ventilate than to mess around with a difficult intubation where everybody has tried to get the tube in and, for that reason, your patient has spent a good amount of time without ventilation. It is amazing how time flies when you are distracted getting the tube in; with mask ventilation, at least, you are providing for gas exchange. Not as elegant as intubating, but your patient is *alive*.

CONTRAINDICATION

- Full stomach or risk of aspiration (not actually so, since you can mask ventilate through cricoid pressure and, after all, if you couldn't intubate, you'd *have* to mask ventilate just making sure you are aware of the unprotected airway and the risk of aspiration).

EQUIPMENT

- In the operating room, an anesthetic circuit with supplied oxygen.
- On the floor, an Ambu bag with supplied oxygen.
- A properly fitting mask.
- Suction nearby in case of vomiting. (Make sure it's on and you can reach it.)
- A black strap to hold the mask on and free up your hands. (Our personal prejudice.)

BEWARE ONE PARTICULAR ASPECT OF THE MASK

- Mask CPAP at home is one thing.
- Mask CPAP in the hospital is quite another.

- If patients are so bad that only a tightly applied mask with high FIO_2 will keep them going, think strongly about intubating them.

PHILOSOPHY OF MASK VENTILATION

- In a code or near-code situation on the floor, mask ventilate the patient while the intubation stuff is getting opened and readied.
- Get the patient's saturation as high as you can before biting the bullet and intubating. You never know who might give you trouble.
- In the OR, you want to develop a smooth mask-ventilation style that puts you under low stress. You are setting up the intubation while you're mask ventilating.
- Do a good job with the mask, and you have all the time in the world when the intubation approaches.
- Do a bad job with the mask, and you'll be listening to the sat drop while you're intubating, you'll get panicky, and you'll screw up.
- You also want to develop a relaxed style of mask ventilation. If you clench your hand into the claw of death, your hand will quickly tire.
- If you are relaxed, you could mask ventilate all day. And one day, you just might have to!
- And if you get good at it, your attending might ask you to mask ventilate the case and do the charting simultaneously.

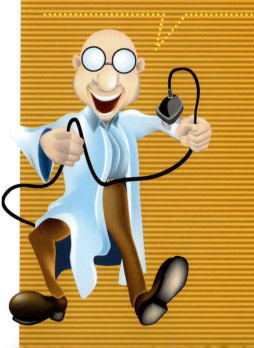

Mask CPAP Stalactites

I was called to an ICU to "evaluate a patient for possible change of respiratory modality." ("Hey, intubate this guy.")

The patient was on mask CPAP and had been for about two days. The oxygen was blowing into his mask at about a thousand liters per second. I got the same feeling I get every single time I see a patient in the hospital on mask CPAP ... why isn't this guy intubated and on a ventilator?

At intubation, he had a dried piece of mucus the size of a cigarette package (I kid thee not), completely occluding all visualization of anything whatsoever resembling a normal structure seen in human beings.

If you see a patient on mask CPAP, think long and hard about what the next best step is.

What's Up with All those Masks, Anyway?

What's up with those stupid masks, anyway? There stand Bruce Wayne and his young ward (what the hell is a "ward"), whatszissname. Now they put on their little masks, some colorful tights that define the precise moment when metrosexuality began, and boom! no one recognizes Batman and Robin. Am I the only one that wondered about that?

And Superman, come on! Didn't even *have* a mask. Just wore those dorky glasses as Clark Kent, then he takes them off. Call it the "antimask" look. And no one pegs him, not clueless Lois. Not dotty Jimmy. Nobody.

Lone Ranger? Same deal. Come to think of it, his clothes were pretty tight, he wore gloves (probably to protect his nails), and he'd built up his upper body to a pretty buffed state. Maybe metrosexuality actually began in the Wild West of yesteryear.

High ho, Silver, away!

MASK HISTORY AND PHYSICAL

- Read old records to see if the patients were hard to mask ventilate or to intubate.
- Take a good look at their faces and see if they will be tough to mask.
- Beard? Big mustache? These will make mask seals hard to obtain.
- Want a trick when a Santa Claus beard comes along and you think, "No way can I mask this guy!"? Once the patient is induced, place a large Steri-Drape over his face, smash it down and flatten all the facial hair, then poke a hole in the area of the mouth. Voila! Perfect seal for a mask!
- Obese? Masking may be hard; plus, obese people are at greater risk for aspiration.
- On a weird bed? Those orthopedic jungle gyms can make access tough and masking impossible.
- Unstable neck from injury or arthritis? When you mask, you always pull back a little. This could be catastrophe when the cervical spine is at risk.
- No teeth ... yeah! easy intubation, but guess what ... expect a difficult mask seal. Try getting some gauze under their cheeks.

TECHNIQUE

- To keep your hands free, put a black face strap on the mask. No kidding, this makes your life a lot easier.
- Make sure the oxygen is on. (Don't laugh, it happens.)
- Hold the mask with your left hand.
- Use your right hand to squeeze the bag.
- With your thumb, index, and middle finger forming a *C* of pressure, hold the mask on tightly.
- Don't squish the mask into the patient's eyes.
- Speaking of eyes, make sure your ID, pens, stethoscopes, lucky amulets, "Go Hurricanes" pins, and stuff are not hanging down in the patient's eyes.
- Use your ring finger and pinkie to lift up the patient's chin.
- Make sure you are pulling up on the bone of the chin, not on the soft tissue.
- When you squeeze the bag, "love that air in."

- Don't squish real hard or you'll just pump air into the stomach.
- If air doesn't go in, (chest doesn't rise, no CO_2 on trace, embarrassing flatulent sounds are produced), readjust the head, pulling back.
- If pulling back doesn't work, try this trick: Turn your patient's head to the side a little. (You'll be amazed, this really does open up the airway a lot of times.)
- If the patient can tolerate it, place an oral airway.
- To place the oral airway, use a tongue depressor: Depress the tongue and push the oral airway in while making sure it actually opens up the airway, but doesn't just jam the tongue up and make things worse.
- If you're still having trouble, consider a nasal airway.
- Caution: The nasal airway can help you, but it can also stir up bleeding and hurt you!
- If you place the nasal airway, goop it up well with K-Y or some other lubricant, place it gently, and slide it in. Don't force it or you'll get bleeding.
- To make ventilation easier, especially in obese patients, put the table in reverse Trendelenburg, which takes weight off the diaphragm, and makes *your* life much easier.
- If you're having a tough go of it, use two hands to hold the jaw up and have a second person squeeze the bag.
- In an anesthetic induction, ventilation will often be tough until the relaxant hits. This creates a kind of Catch-22. "Hmm, he's hard to ventilate, should I now give him relaxant and make it easier to ventilate, or do I give him relaxant, burn my bridges, and now he's still hard to ventilate, and we're driving toward Disaster Junction?" We say, "give the relaxant."

PEDIATRIC TECHNIQUE: MASK INDUCTION

- This is a common form of induction in pediatrics.
- You can do it in adults, though this is much less common.
- A wild, thrashing, hold-on-for-dear-life mask induction is always a possibility, but why make your life miserable? Sedate the kid ahead of time (PO midazolam, for example) and everybody wins.

- Keep the kid comfortable. You can, for example, put the kid in your lap.
- Place the mask on the child and turn on a nonpungent potent anesthetic with or without nitrous oxide plus oxygen.
- Increase the potent agent incrementally.
- Children will often get a little wild in Phase II.
- Once the child is breathing easily and calmed down, place your IV.

MASK GLITCHES

- Taking masking lightly. "We can always intubate, after all." Guess what, that is not a given!
- Not doing a real assessment of how hard it might be to mask ventilate. This is especially common on orthopedic beds where, all of a sudden, you just can't get at the patient.
- Beards. Big ones, big problems!
- Hairpieces. With this new fashion statement (which we don't understand), big, attached hairpieces will push the patient's head forward, making it hard to achieve extension and good positioning for mask ventilation.
- Obesity. If patients are really huge, you better just intubate them awake because it is damned near impossible to mask ventilate them. God forbid you induce anesthesia and miss the intubation—you will then try fruitlessly to mask ventilate, they will desaturate quickly, and you're done for.
- Vomiting. Put the patient's head down, turn it to the side, suction like mad.

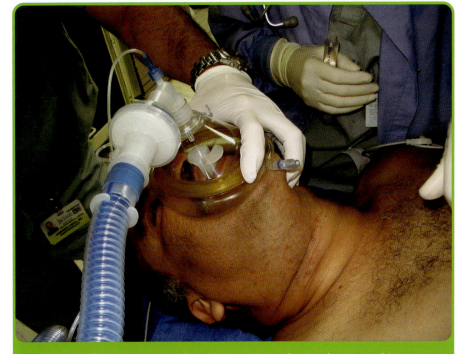

Figure 1. This was supposed to be a routine induction but turned into an unexpected failed intubation. You'll see how important good mask ventilation is when things go sour! Here, the case starts and mask ventilation proceeds.

Is it Really Worth it to Strap Up and Preoxygenate?

To keep your hands free, preoxygenate by holding the mask in place with a face strap. This will allow you to push your own drugs for induction. By using a face mask, you also allow good preoxygenation while you do other preparations—put on monitors, strap down the patient's arms, look over your stuff one last time—suction, vital signs, equipment. An efficient takeoff is much appreciated by one and all, and using a face mask to preoxygenate while you do other stuff, is an efficient use of time.

But wait, is it that big of a deal to preoxygenate?

Yes, yes, a thousand times yes. Consider every case a scuba dive into the unknown. Before any scuba dive, you fill your tanks up with air. Similarly, before every anesthetic induction, you fill the *tanks* with oxygen. Those tanks are the patient's lungs. Furthermore, if you preoxygenate for a full three or four minutes, you saturate the patient's FRC with oxygen, giving you little reserve oxygen tanks to draw on. That complete preoxygenation can provide you an additional 90 seconds before you desaturate.

How valuable is 90 seconds in a catastrophe airway Armageddon?

A lot of time. That extra time can allow you to get help, get in an LMA, try something new, even cut the neck if you absolutely have to!

Trouble doesn't ring a bell, that's why it's trouble.

People do not come down with tattoos on their forehead that say, "I will be the surprise you never wanted to see, a perfectly normal person who turns out to be impossible to intubate and impossible to ventilate."

Go on the assumption that anyone and everyone can be The Big Bad Surprise, and preoxygenate them completely. You will never regret preoxygenating. You may damned well regret *not* preoxygenating.

How Do You Preoxygenate the Claustrophobic Patient Who can't Stand the Mask?

Well golly Moses, if you really have to preoxygenate, what do you do when patients absolutely cannot tolerate the mask? Do you just say, "The hell with it, I'll not preoxygenate and hope nothing goes wrong?"

Holy desaturation Batman!

Here's a trick that really really works, as they say on late-night TV commercials. Take the mask off, and have the patients put the elbow of the circuit in their mouths. They breathe in oxygen like a straw. No one gets claustrophobia through a straw. Then you induce, and as soon as they are unconscious, you put the mask on the circuit and away you go.

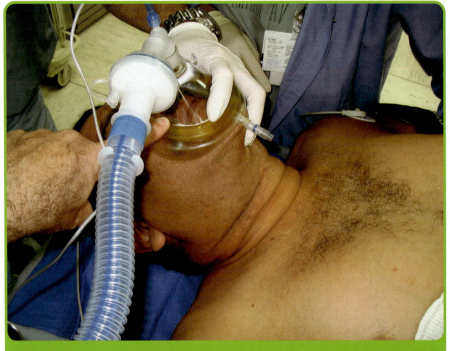

Figure 2. Note on the right side how ventilation can "escape." A helping hand (here, my finger), presses down on the right to help "seal the deal."

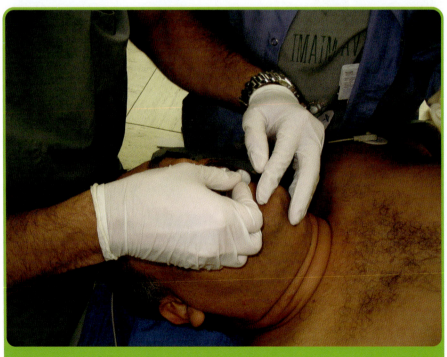

Figure 3. In goes the oral airway, that's usually helpful.

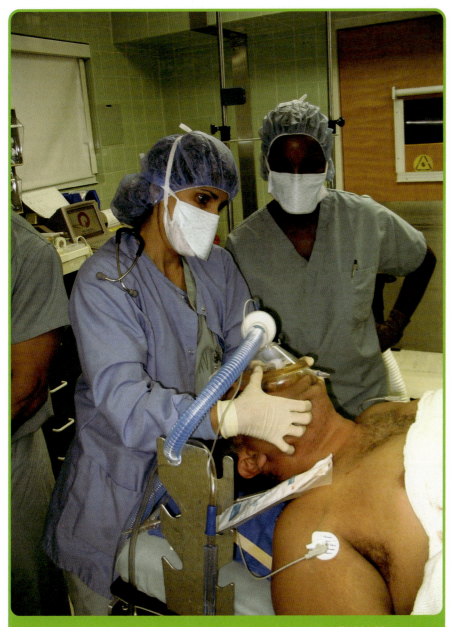

Figure 4. Two-handed mask ventilation—the more skilled holds the mask, then the helper squeezes the bag.

Another Look at Reverse-Trendelenburg

A little bit of reverse Trendelenburg makes the medicine go down.

Look at anyone anywhere that in any way is having trouble breathing. They sit upright.

Whether it's epiglottitis, CHF, asthma, mediastinal mass, pneumothorax, you name it, there is one universal behavior that patients seek to improve their breathing mechanics. They sit up. They do everything they can to get weight off their diaphragm.

Take their cue.

If, as you induce, you tilt the patients just a little bit upright, you will take a titch of weight off their diaphragms, making them just a tad bit less likely to desaturate and just a skosh easier to ventilate. All these titches, tad bits, and skoshes may add up to the difference between good and bad, life and death, and we kid thee not!

A little easier to ventilate and a little less likely to desaturate means things stay cool and calm during induction and mask ventilation. If, in contrast, the patients are a little more difficult to ventilate and a little more likely to de-saturate, you quickly head down the road to ruin during mask-ventilation time. You start to panic, you squeeze the bag harder, you fill their stomachs with air, they desaturate (and now, pos-sibly, vomit and aspirate), you get more panicky, aaaaaaaaaaaaaaaaaaaaaaaaaah!

That little tip up may make all the dif-ference!

The Oxyhemoglobin Curve Revisited

It's worth taking a look at the oxyhemoglobin dissociation curve at this time. We always think of that curve in its scary direction—once the sat goes to about 90%, the sat plunges like a roller coaster. But keep in mind, that same curve works *for* you as well as against you.

If patients desaturate badly, and you readjust things and just get a little more oxygen into them (for example, just a few little puffs of air after readjusting the mask), then that sat will jump up pretty fast too. You'll be hip deep in caca, then you finesse a few breaths, and you at least get up into the survivable-for a-minute-anyway high eighties on the pulse ox.

The Hardest are the Easiest

One truism about mask ventilation: The hardest people to mask are the easiest to intubate. Look at the edentulous patient. Their faces fall away from their mouths, and it can be difficult to gather enough face into the mask to effectively ventilate. Fortunately, their edentulousosity (?) makes them quite easy to intubate, so when you're getting frustrated as hell trying to mask them, place the tube.

One exception: facial hair.

If we ran the earth, every guy, plus every bearded lady in the circus, would get clean-shaven before undergoing anesthesia. Beards, even short stubbly ones, make it hard to get a good mask seal. No matter how hard you mash down, a little air sneaks out the side. If you are facing a lot of additional airway/oxygenation problems at the same time (obesity, full stomach, poor lungs), this not-so-trivial problem of a beard becomes disastrous in no time flat.

Yet another exception: The patient after a rhinoplasty.

After you extubate, you can get in airway trouble and have to mask ventilate. If some plastic surgeon just finished carving the perfect nose (say, oh, Michael Jackson's), and you smash the mask down on this aesthetic creation, you may undo the beauty.

To keep the mask off the nose, yet still ventilate, just turn the mask around and seal it over the mouth. Yes indeed, you can ventilate this way and spare the nose your brutality.

Thus you can serve the cause of oxygenation and beautification at the same time.

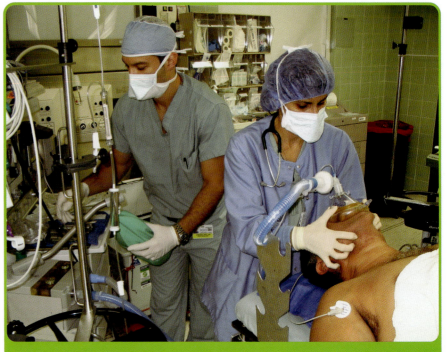

Figure 5. All efforts are focused on masking. Attempts at intubation failed, and rather than "pursue failure," you go for the all-important ventilation. You never HAVE to intubate, but you always HAVE to ventilate.

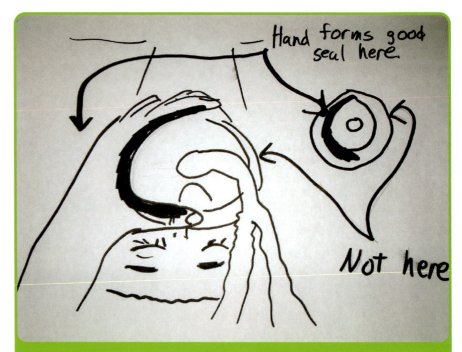

Figure 6. This drawing "from the top" shows how your hand creates a "C-shaped" seal on the mask. A little extra help pushing down at "3 o'clock" on the mask can help a lot.

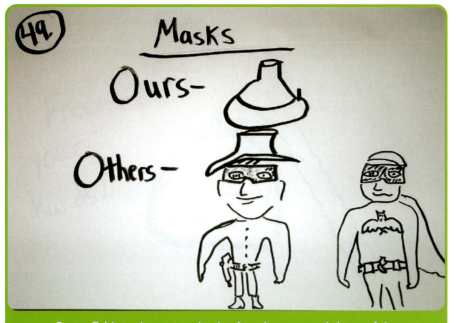

Figure 7. Note the various kinds of masks, ours, and those of the superhero variety.

SUGGESTED READING

Diaz JH. A new transparent disposable plastic mask for children and adults. *Anesthesiology* 1993;78:1195-1196.
• *Describes the use of the mask rotated 180 for patients with acromegaly.*

Durkan W, Fleming N. Potential eye damage from reusable masks. *Anesthesiology* 1987;67:444.
• *Cleaning chemicals used for reusable masks can cause eye injury.*

Edmondson WC, Rushton A. The upside down facemask again. *Anaesthesia* 1992;47:361.
• *Describes the use of the mask rotated 180 for children with certain facial deformities.*

Glauber DT. Facial paralysis after general anesthesia. *Anesthesiology* 1986;65:516-517.
• *Yes, pressure from a mask or mask strap can cause a pressure injury to the underlying nerves.*

Hauswald M, Sklar DR, Tandberg D, et al. Cervical spine movement during airway management. Cinefluoroscopic appraisal in human cadavers. *Am J Emerg Med* 1991;9:535-538.
• *Shows that cervical spine movement is more pronounced during mask ventilation than during tracheal intubation.*

Lanier WL. Improving anesthesia mask fit in edentulous patients. *Anesth Analg* 1987;66:1053.
• *Describes the use of a triangular-shaped mask in edentulous patients.*

McGowan P, Skinner A. Preoxygenation— the importance of a good face mask seal. *Br J Anaesth* 1995:75:777-778.
• *Shows that air dilution occurred with failure to obtain a tight mask seal during spontaneous respiration.*

Mortimer AJ. An airtight seal between facemask and beard. *Anaesthesia* 1986;41:670-671.

Seavell CR, Priestley GS. Solving a hairy problem. *Anaesthesia* 1995;50:271.

Smurthwaite GJ, Ford P. Skin necrosis following continuous positive pressure with a face mask. *Anaesthesia* 1993;48:147-148.
• *Report of skin necrosis after prolonged mask application in the presence of hypotension.*

Breaking Laryngo-Spasm, the Ultimate Test of Mask Ventilation

Most of the focus on mask ventilation is at the beginning of the case. The patient gets induced, you take over, mask ventilation happens. At the end of the case, the patient's breathing on his own, you pull out the tube, go to the PACU, fill out a grossly overweighted billing slip, and head to the yacht club.

Piece of cake.

Only one zinger in this deal: Sometimes when you pull the tube out, the patient goes into laryngospasm and your yacht sinks! Now you're having to mask ventilate *with attitude* because everything is going to hell. The patient is desaturating, his chest is moving up and down, generating negative pressure pulmonary edema, and you are in a world of hurt.

What to do, Boy Wonder?

As with everything else in medicine, an ounce of prevention is worth a pound of personal injury lawyer subpoenas. Do your damndest to extubate the patient when laryngospasm won't happen. That means either a deep extubation or a real live awake extubation. By "awake," we mean this: The patient's *brain* is awake as well as his *airway*. If just your airway is awake, then you cough, buck, and flail around. Remember, your *airway alone* has only one way to protect itself . . . slam the vocal cords shut. When your *brain* is awake (the patient responds to commands such as "Open your eyes"), you have a lot of ways to protect your airway.

So extubate the patient only after you've established Brain Awakeness.

So you blew it and now he's in laryngospasm. Now what?

Apply the mask and get the mother of all seals, you need to ventilate this patient pronto. Don't be shy about asking for help, laryngospasm is scary as hell and can get ugly fast. Especially when you do the next maneuver both your hands may be tied up, so have someone else hold positive pressure on the bag.

Drive your fingers behind the upward-going ramus of the jaw, and pull like there is no tomorrow. If I had a dime for every time I've run in a room and done this maneuver and unlaryngospasmed a patient, I would be driving drop-top big-finned pink Cadillac today, rather than the '73 Pinto that I do drive.

This maneuver does not, in my humble opinion, break laryngospasm. This maneuver hurts so bad (try it on yourself), that it pole vaults patients from being only airway awake to being brain awake. It's giving pain to counteract anesthesia. It's like giving two amps of Narcan push.

They wake up.

They take a big breath in.

Laryngospasm gone.

If that doesn't work, you can always give a low dose of SUX (10-20 mg), which usually weakens patients just a little, and allows you to give positive pressure mask ventilation through the now-parting vocal cords.

When someone goes into laryngospasm and you apply positive pressure by mask (using all the tips I gave before), you don't really break laryngospasm by the column of air. You just have the column of air there, waiting to jump in when the vocal cords finally open. It's like amassing your troops outside the gates of Troy, ready to rush in as soon as your guys open the gate.

Snow JC, Kripke BJ, Norton ML, et al. Corneal injuries during general anesthesia. *Anesth Analg* 1975;54:465-467.
- *Key point: Don't put the face mask over an open eye.*

Stoneham MD. The nasopharyngeal airway: assessment of position by fiberoptic laryngoscopy. *Anaesthesia* 1993;48:575-580.
- *Correct position of airway should have the pharyngeal end below the base of tongue, but above the epiglottis.*

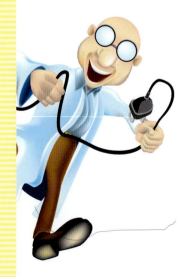

The Zirconium Jewel of Sort-of-Intubation: The LMA

Michael Lewis

INTRODUCTION

"What indeed hath God wrought?" might have been on the minds of American anesthesiologists when they first saw the Laryngeal Mask Airway (LMA). It was first described by Dr. Archie Brain in 1983 in the UK. It was designed to bridge the gap between basic airway management adjuncts such as the face mask and the more complicated technique of endotracheal intubation. Later in the 1980s, it was brought into the USA. Since its inception, the LMA has been used on more than 30,000,000 patients in both the USA and UK.

It now has a coveted seat in the difficult-airway algorithm. In many hospitals, a routine elective case means inserting an LMA. They are forever on standby for that can't-intubate, can't-ventilate nightmare scenario. The LMA is now often part of the drill when it comes to securing a difficult airway.

INDICATIONS

- Airway support for a routine anesthetic (not a full stomach or aspiration risk).
  - Known or unexpected difficult airways. It is a very useful tool in the can't-intubate, can't-ventilate scenario; you'll concede the aspiration risk, but you need *something* to establish effective ventilation.
  - Airway vehicle for doing a fiberoptic intubation (LMA Fastrach).
- Airway establishment during resuscitation in the unconscious patient with absent glossopharyngeal and laryngeal reflexes when tracheal intubation is not possible.

CONTRAINDICATIONS

- Aspiration risk (the LMA does not secure the airway against aspiration).
- Upper airway pathology that could occlude the LMA (big fungating mass in the mouth, say, that could get dislodged if you ram an LMA in there).
- Patients with decreased pulmonary compliance.

EQUIPMENT

- LMA.
- Tongue depressor.
- All the usual airway equipment to intubate, just in case.
- Suction.
- A big syringe (20 cc) to inflate the big LMA cuff.
- If you do the Fastrach, you may want to have fiberoptic equipment ready.

PHILOSOPHY OF LMAs

- You don't have to instrument the airway, avoiding the hemodynamic swings seen with endotracheal intubation.
- When compared to intubation, the LMA is considered easier and faster to place correctly.
- At the end of the case, things can be a lot simpler with an LMA as opposed to all the bucking and straining that you see with an emerging intubated patient.
- Don't let complacency set in! If you can't intubate someone, and you put an LMA in instead, you may be in big trouble later if the patient vomits.
- Practice the skill of intubating with a LMA Fastrach; it's an extremely useful tool and, like any specialized instrument, don't do it the first time in an emergency.
- You can do, and some people do, LMAs in weird positions (lateral, even prone!), but keep in mind, you *may* have to change gears and intubate at some point during the case.

LMA HISTORY AND PHYSICAL

- You *never know* which patient the LMA will not work on, so always keep the "if no go, then intubate" in mind.
- Evaluate aspiration risk.

What hath God wrought?

First words sent by trans-Atlantic telegraph, 1870s

Welcome to My Case

I went into a room to relieve a colleague for lunch. The patient looked like a difficult airway—obese, short chin. I noticed an LMA was in.

He states "Oh yeah, I couldn't intubate this guy no matter how hard I tried. So I put this in."

"Um, uh, why didn't you . . . ?"

"See you. I'll be back after lunch."

So How Secure is Secure?

You are not protected against aspiration if you use an LMA. An endotracheal tube or a tracheostomy tube with intact cuffs is considered secure airways. (You can, of course, aspirate during intubation or after extubation, so it's not as if the endotracheal tube guarantees you'll never aspirate during your anesthetic journey.) Consider an LMA to be *mask ventilation on a stick*. The cuff provides some protection against aspiration, but that cuff does not seal off the trachea from whatever is floating around in the stomach.

How Can You Argue with the Difficult Airway Algorithm?

Look at the American Society of Anesthesiologists' Difficult Airway Algorithm. (That would have to be viewed as a pretty definitive *What If?* guide.) There sits the LMA, an approved rescue technique. This LMA is no red-haired bastard stepchild; this is a welcome member of the airway Tinker Toy family.

- Know the operation: What position the patient will be in, if insufflation will be used (insufflation will increase abdominal pressure, possibly increasing aspiration risk).

- In a curious twist of anatomical fate, the very person *easiest* to intubate (edentulous) is often the *hardest* to LMA-ate (the mouth and face fall away and you can't get a good seating). On the flip side, the very person *hardest* to intubate (narrow mouth) can sometimes prove the *easiest* to LMA-ate (the narrow upper airway holds snug to the LMA and gives you a good seal).

- LMAs can be very forgiving. X-rays have shown them folded back, doing all kinds of weird things, and still they often work!

- Everybody has a secret recipe for placing the LMA. The fact that so many different techniques exist is further testimony to the LMA's resilience. There must not be any single *best* way, since so many different ways work!

TECHNIQUE

- The LMA *can* be placed in the awake patient, using topical anesthesia. In most cases, you will place an LMA in a patient using general anesthesia.

- With all your just-in-case equipment ready (intubating supplies, suction), following induction, pick up the right-sized LMA: normal woman, size 3; normal man, size 4; big man, size 5. Kids, smaller. As with any other instrument, have different sizes ready to go in case you need a bigger or smaller one.

- You can place the LMA any of a number of ways, and I've seen them all work, and all not work.

- Be sure and lubricate the LMA, avoiding mucosal damage. The lubricant should be water-soluble, and placed on the posterior surface of the LMA.

- You can completely deflate, push straight back. Alternatively, you can completely deflate, push straight back, put your finger in the mouth, make sure the tip of the LMA didn't bend backward, then push straight back. Again, you can do all the above using a tongue depressor. If stuck, you can use the laryngoscope, and place the LMA under direct vision.

- Do all the above with the cuff slightly inflated.

- Put the LMA in sideways, then twist and advance.

- Put the LMA in sideways and partially inflated, then twist and advance.

- Put the LMA in all the way backward, then twist all the way around and advance.

- Put the LMA in all the way backward with it slightly inflated, then twist all the way around and advance.

- So you can see that, except for standing on your head and placing it with your feet, you can place the LMA almost any way you want.

- The key, no matter how you place it, is to get it seated well, deep in the mouth, so when you inflate the cuff (use 15–20 cc), the LMA will push out a little bit (about 0.5 cm) and when you deliver an inspiration, you get good ingress of oxygen (chest rises, good CO_2 trace, no noisy leak).

- If all that good stuff doesn't happen, then deflate the cuff, and reposition.

- Be gentle! Don't force the LMA; you'll just cause bleeding that will eventually lead to airway edema, and lots of trouble.

- If it just isn't happening, intubate the patient. You don't want to be sweating for the whole case with a nonoptimal LMA.

- Confirm the adequacy of your LMA placement by checking for equal chest excursion, bilateral breath sounds, minimal air leak, and, most importantly, positive ET CO_2.

- If there's a little leak, but airway passage is still OK, patients get back breathing on their own and air moves fine, you can leave the LMA in.

- Can you use the ventilator with an LMA? If the seal is good, it works out fine. Use tidal volumes or around 8 mL/kg, limit peak inspiratory pressures to 20 cm H_2O.

- Keep in mind when the surgeon starts cutting, your level of anesthesia may not be too deep (the LMA doesn't *require* as much anesthesia as an endotracheal tube), so have a little IV agent around and ready to go if the patient responds.

TECHNIQUE FOR A FASTRACH

- The LMA-Fastrach is a modified version of the standard LMA with a large-bore metal tube, a metal handle, and an epiglottis-elevating bar. The LMA-Fastrach is placed inside the mouth, and the endotracheal tube (ETT) is passed through the device, and blindly inserted into the trachea. It can accept up to a 9.0-mm endotracheal tube, but you can also use a fiberoptic scope to guide you in!

- How do you do it? Be ready for regular intubation as with any LMA.

  - Induce. Have a lubricated LMA ready. Lubrication is the secret!

  - Hold the metal handle of the LMA with your left hand and insert in the mouth (help yourself by opening the mouth with your right hand). Apply steady pressure on the hard palate and push it in . . . it should slide into position.

  - Inflate the cuff.

  - Make sure you can move air in and out, and have decent seal. Give muscle relaxant if you feel that's appropriate.

  - Lubricate the dedicated ETT and insert it through the LMA. If resistance is encountered, try rotating the tube until it slides in.

  - Inflate the ETT cuff. Check for bilateral breath sounds and positive CO_2.

  - Now comes the tricky part: extricating the intubating LMA, but not yanking out the endotracheal tube.

  - Deflate the cuff on the LMA.

  - Place the *pusher* element inside the LMA to hold the endotracheal tube in place, and slither the LMA out.

  - Once you can, grab the endotracheal tube and hold it in place in the mouth as the LMA completes its journey out.

  - Hook up the breathing circuit, and make sure you can adequately ventilate through the endotracheal tube.

  - Voila! Pretty slick, *yes?*

- Alternatively, you can place the fiberoptic through the intubating LMA, loading the ETT tube on the scope.

- The LMA usually gets all the soft tissue out of the way and, as soon as you come out of the opening of the LMA, you should be staring at the cords.

- Slide through the cords with the fiberoptic.

- Advance the endotracheal tube, and make sure it's in good position.

- Inflate the cuff on the endotracheal tube.

- An alternative is to place an endotracheal tube changer down the endotracheal tube as insurance, or, for that matter, put an endotracheal tube changer down the intubating LMA in the first place, position it, then use that to intubate.

LMA GLITCHES

- The main glitch does not know when to throw in the towel. If you just can't get it, to hell with it, intubate the patient.

- Vomiting. In the middle of the case, if they vomit, do the usual stuff when an unprotected airway has emesis—head down, head to side, suction (mouth and LMA), then intubate and secure that airway.

- Bleeding. Don't ram this beast into the patient. That's mucosa in there. Easy does it.

- Fighting to get it in! Just make sure the tip is not bent backward as the LMA went into the mouth . . . insert your finger and straighten the tip and the device will slide in, I am telling you!

With All these Different Ways, How Do *You* Do It?

Here's my personal how-to:

Do all the smart stuff you'd do with any induction: have suction ready, pre-oxygenate all that good stuff. Induce, tilt their heads back so their mouths pop open (a good circulator will sometimes hold the patient's forehead down for you, but that only happens when you are blessed with the world's greatest circulator), then shove that monster in there. Don't force it, don't ram it! Forcing it causes bleeding. Surgeons are allowed to cause bleeding, we are discouraged from same. If it doesn't go, then wiggle a little this way, then that, then wiggle it again. Inflate the cuff (you'll see the tube push out a little when you inflate), then gently "love some oxygen" into the patient. If the chest doesn't rise and embarrassing sounds should start erupting, reposition. Don't ignore those sounds—a big leak will become a big problem.

Pretty, Not in Pink

Anyone who's done fiberoptic intubations knows that you hit the mucosa and all you see is pink. You're doing a fiberoptic with a resident, and you ask, "What do you see?" "Pink."

You have a fiberoptic tower with a TV and you place the fiberoptic, and you see, guess what? Pink. Pink, pink, pink, pink, pink. It drives you crazy!

Along comes the intubating LMA. This puppy allows you to establish ventilation, and then it guides you just about right to the doors of the vocal cords. What a deal! If that LMA is anywhere near where it ought to be, your fiberoptic pops out right near the vocal cords, the cuff of the LMA holds back all the pink stuff, and you have a straight shot. No more pink!

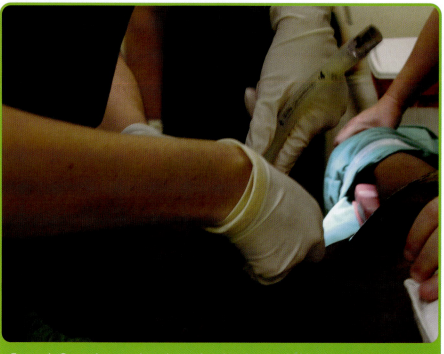

Figure 1. Open the mouth with one hand and insert LMA. Notice how the LMA is held like a pencil. Constant pressure against the hard palate is the way to go!

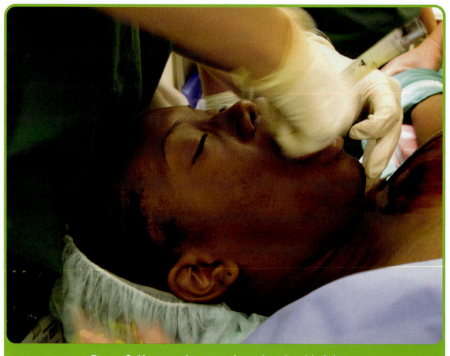

Figure 2. Keep pushing gently and it should glide in.

222

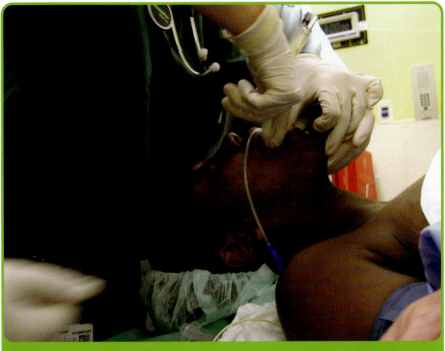

Figure 3. If it gets stuck, straighten the tip with your finger.

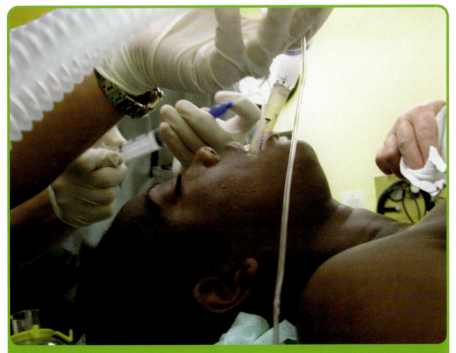

Figure 4. This is how it looks when it is well seated. As you inflate
the cuff the LMA moves slightly out.

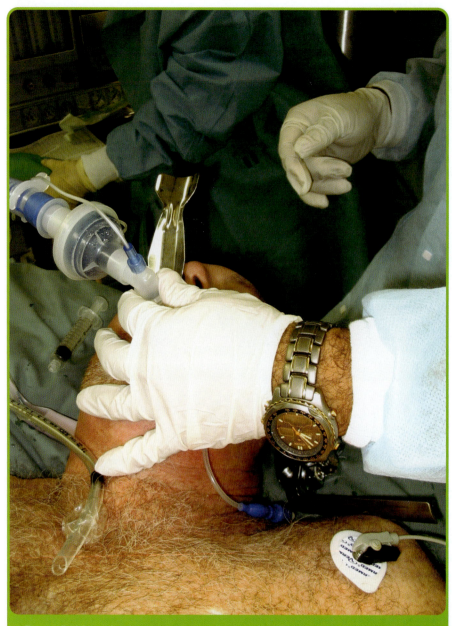

Figure 5. When the insertion is complete and cuff is up, connect to anesthesia circuit and check for adequate seal and good air movement.

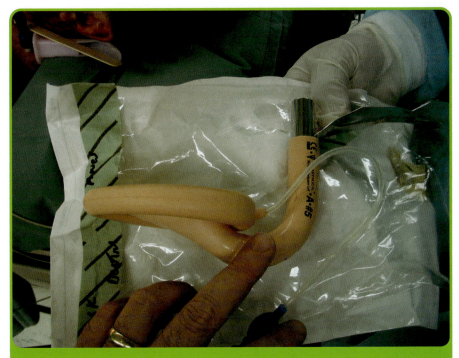

Figure 6. This is the intubation LMA. Notice the metal handle and the C shape body.

SUGGESTED READING

Benumof JL. Laryngeal Mask Airway and the ASA Difficult Airway Algorithm. *Anesthesiology* 1996;84:686.

- *See how far we have come since the 1980s when anesthesiologists were resistant to the use of the LMA. LMA has been shown to be useful in the difficult airway algorithm. It is an important option, and it should be immediately available. Some even consider it a first-treatment choice.*

Ezri T, Szmuk P, Warters RD, Katz J, Hagberg CA. Difficult airway management practice patterns among anesthesiologists practicing in the United States: have we made any progress? *J Clin Anesth* 2003;15:418–422.

- *This article summarizes that younger anesthesiologists with more than 10 years of experiences were found to prefer use of fiberoptic and LMA in difficult airway scenarios. This may be due to increased attendance at airway workshops conferences that emphasize use of these techniques over others.*

Flaishon R, Sotman A, Friedman A, Ben-Abraham R, Rudick V, Weinbroum AA. Laryngeal Mask Airway insertion by anesthetists and non-anesthetists wearing unconventional protective gear: a prospective, randomized, crossover study in humans. *Anesthesiology* 2004;100:267–273.

- *One can use the LMA for mass casualties, and under difficult conditions. The study looked at the speed of insertion of LMA in a population of anesthetists versus other specialists. The conclusion was anesthetists in protective anti-chemical gear (like the kind you'd wear in a terrorist attack) insert LMA at the same speed as they would in a normal surgical attire. They were also two to three times faster than other specialties or novices wearing either attire.*

Griffin SC. Cardiovascular changes with the Laryngeal Mask Airway in cardiac anaesthesia. *Br J Anaesth Jun* 2004;92(6);885–887.

- *This paper shows one advantage of the technique in terms of hemodynamic stability as compared to laryngoscopy and intubation. LMA and the intubating ILMA provide a hands-free airway. Insertion of LMA has no effects on heart rate and mean arterial pressure. ILMA, on the other hand, causes increase in both similar to that seen in direct laryngoscopy. Recovery was prompt, and removal of the tracheal tube/LMA/ILMA was not associated with hemodynamic changes suggesting this is less stressful than airway insertion. No recall discomfort on postoperative day two with these methods. The article shows no need for pharmacological techniques to control the circulation in patients with ischemic heart disease, and cardiovascular stability can be achieved with the LMA.*

Raphael J, Rosenthal-Ganon T, Gozal Y. Emergency airway management with a Laryngeal Mask Airway in a patient placed in the prone position. *J Clin Anesth* 2004; 16:560-561.

- *This paper shows how agile this device is. The placement of LMA has been used for airway management during various elective procedures in prone position, but the patient was supine during the insertion of LMA. In other cases, patients have already been in prone position before the induction of anesthesia. This article discusses the use of LMA in a prone, anesthetized patient undergoing major reconstructive spinal surgery as an emergency measure. The case reviews that loss of airway control in an anesthetized patient placed in prone position is a life-threatening complication. The only reasonable solution for an accidental extubation in this case was to insert an LMA. Turning the patient was too time-consuming, and needed at least four people that at the time of emergency were not available! Besides, these turnings can also cause severe neurologic or infectious complications. The authors believe that the above case is the first reported case of use of an LMA as a means of emergency airway management during surgery in a prone patient.*

Pennant JH, White PF. The Laryngeal Mask Airway. Its uses in anesthesiology. *Anesthesiology* 1993;79:144.

- *This article summarizes that LMA is a useful airway device for most adult and pediatric patients. Advantages: easy, atraumatic to insert, suitable alternative to face mask and tracheal intubation. It facilitates blind and fiberoptic techniques of intubation. This article was published in 1993; the role of LMA in emergency scenarios was not established then.*

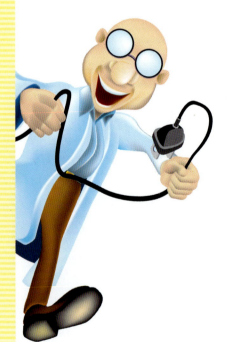

CHAPTER
11

The Vanilla Ice
Cream of
Intubation:
Laryngoscopy

Bryan Robbins and
Christian Diez

INTRODUCTION

The best cartoon ever anywhere showed a man in an ice cream store. His back was to you, the reader. You saw, face-on, a kid standing behind the ice cream counter. Behind the kid was a big sign saying "Today's Flavors."

The flavors listed were:

Vanilla

Wood

Liver

The kid says to the customer, "We're out of vanilla."

When it comes to securing airways, we're *never* out of vanilla. We do direct laryngoscopy to secure the airway almost all the time. That is, we do the vanilla thing, the normal thing, the regular thing.

For the record, the most popular flavor of ice cream, year after year, *is* vanilla.

For the record, the most popular intubation technique, year after year, is direct laryngoscopy. We have lots of cool gizmos and wowie-zowie techniques, but we do plain old laryngoscopy most of the time.

So we need to know this vanilla technique.

INDICATIONS

- Need to secure an airway for general anesthesia. (Most common.)
- Need to secure an airway for ventilatory support in an ICU setting.
- Specifically, you need to support an airway when patients need PEEP, when patients can't handle their secretions, when patients can't adequately support their own ventilation, or when they cannot protect their airways.

CONTRAINDICATIONS

- There's no real *contraindication* to placing a laryngoscope, there's just a time when there's a better alternative.
- Anticipated difficult intubation . . . better to do an awake intubation.
- Anticipated difficult intubation and the upper route is blocked (severe facial trauma, large tumor in the airway) . . . better to do an awake tracheostomy.

EQUIPMENT

- Laryngoscope and a blade (a size-3 Macintosh blade can be used to intubate 80% of patients).
- Extra laryngoscope.
- Extra blades.
- Endotracheal tube.
- Extra endotracheal tubes.
- Syringe to inflate the pilot balloon on the endotracheal tube.

- Unless you are planning to do awake laryngoscopy, you'll need standard induction agents and neuromuscular relaxants tailored to the patient's needs.
- Stethoscope.
- In the OR, an anesthesia circuit to hook the patient up to after intubation.
- In the ICU, a ventilator to hook the patient up to after intubation.
- In case of an emergency, at least an Ambu bag and oxygen supply to ventilate the patient after intubation.
- Suction.
- Monitors: An end-tidal CO_2 monitor is essential, either an automated one as in the OR, or a portable device that should be in any crash cart intubation kit.
- Monitors: oxygen saturation monitor, EKG, blood pressure cuff.
- Something to secure the endotracheal tube in place, most often tape, but you can also use umbilical tape to tie the tube in (if the patient has a beard or if the skin is burned), or you can suture the tube in place (for facial surgery where tape will interfere with the surgery, or you can use a plastic tube holder (as is in vogue in many an ICU).

BEWARE THE ENDOTRACHEAL TUBE FROM ELSEWHERE

- When a patient comes to you intubated, give that endotracheal tube the once over.

It's the opening that has the vocal cords.

Wise counsel from many attendings. Various dates and times in history

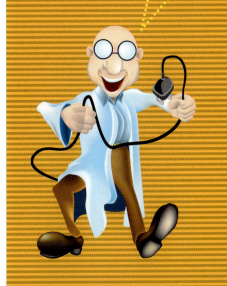

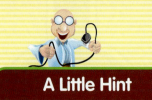

A Little Hint

Never trust another person's airway exam.

A woman came to me, her preop completed by someone else in our preop clinic. No mention of anything in the airway department.

When I examined her airway, she leaned her head back and I saw a very ugly- looking tracheostomy scar.

"What's this?" I asked.

"Oh," she said in an offhand manner, "the last time they couldn't put the tube in and they had to cut my neck open. 'In a real hurry' they told me."

Get the . . . You Know, the Special Thing in the Other Room . . . You Know What

Don't count on other people to magically find stuff for you once you're in trouble. "Quick! Get that special instrument, it's in Room 34 or maybe 35! I think it's in the third drawer down on the left toward the back of the room!" Such a request, delivered with the octave-higher-than-normal-voice-of-the-panic-stricken, is unlikely to get you that silver bullet you're looking for.

- Listen for breath sounds. Make sure the endotracheal tube is actually in the trachea (for the umpteenth time, don't laugh—you'll be amazed what happens out there).

- Listen for breath sounds. Make sure the endotracheal tube is not too far down.

- Listen for a leak. Some endotracheal tubes have worked their way out and the cuff has herniated over the cords. The more the cuff leaks, the more people inflate the cuff, pushing the tube yet *further* out.

- Listen for a leak. Cuffs can and do rupture.

- Look how the endotracheal tube is secured. Tape and holders can pinch off the pilot balloon.

- Look how the endotracheal tube is secured. Sometimes it's not *secure* at all!

- Make sure you can pass a suction catheter down the endotracheal tube. Note especially that if someone has been in an ICU a long time, the lumen of the endotracheal tube can be filled with dried secretions, making a 7.0 tube into more like a 3.0 tube. We've seen it.

PHILOSOPHY OF DIRECT LARYNGOSCOPY

- This ties very much in with the next chapter, Awake Fiberoptic, but it bears repeating. When you induce patients in anesthesia, you are, literally, *betting their lives* (and your medical license) that you can breathe for them.

- Do not take laryngoscopy lightly, ever, ever, ever.

- When you are just beginning, practice on an intubating dummy a lot of times. When you do your first real live patient look for someone edentulous. Your job will be much easier without having to worry about the teeth.

- If you're a student, look for a room that has a lot of cases with healthy patients, that way you'll do a lot of intubations. If you assign yourself to some monster 12-hour case, you'll only get one intubation.

- Trouble does not ring a bell, and people will surprise you with a difficult airway where you never suspected one, so keep your guard up.

- Key to good laryngoscopy is, believe it or not, good mask ventilation. If you mask well, then when you do your laryngoscopy, you have a well-saturated patient and you have time to do a careful look. If you mask poorly, then when you do your laryngoscopy, you have an already desaturating patient and you will have no time, and you'll do a rushed job.

- A rushed laryngoscopy does not bode well, as you will be looking like mad for those cords and may see cords where there aren't any.

- Use both your hands to see what you need to see. Bring your right hand up to push down the larynx, and bring those cords into view. Once you have the view, have helpers push down in the *exact same place* in the *exact same way*. Don't just tell them, "push down," rather, take their hands and guide them. Intubation is a game of millimeters, as opposed to most professional sports, which are games of inches.

- When you are intubating, commandeer anyone else you need to help you. If that means you have someone break scrub, then have them break scrub. Remember, you are securing the airway, the most important thing to the patient's *life*, so you get whomever you need.

- A second pair of hands and eyes is most useful if things go wrong. And it's easier to call across the room than across town for help. If you anticipate a bad airway, ask another anesthesiologist to stick around and help until the airway is secured.

- When the table's turned and someone asks you, by all means, help out.

- When you are the helper and someone needs help visualizing the vocal cords, push down into the throat, incline up toward the intubator, and if that doesn't work, then wiggle the trachea back and forth in an attempt to give them some view of the opening. At times, the epiglottis will swerve to the side when you wiggle the trachea, and you'll be able to see at least a little opening.

- If you think you'll need extra stuff (Eschmann intubating stylet, Bullard scope, intubating LMA, fiberoptic), then get that equipment before you induce. It's a lot easier to get it ahead of time than to shout like crazy and try to round up stuff when you've already screwed the pooch.

LARYNGOSCOPY HISTORY AND PHYSICAL

- Do your usual history, asking if there was ever any trouble getting a breathing tube in.

- Successful oral intubation requires four anatomic traits:
  1. adequate mouth opening
  2. sufficient pharyngeal space
  3. compliant submandibular tissue
  4. adequate atlantooccipital extension
- A few stealth "I-was-hard-to-intubate" clues should catch your ear: "they chipped a tooth last time," "my throat was *really* sore last time." Both these tell you they had a hard time getting the tube in.
- Get an old anesthetic record, and look closely at the intubation note.
- On physical exam, the following features predict a difficult intubation:
  - short chin
  - short thyromental distance (A thyromental distance less than three finger breadths, approximately 7 cm, impairs visualization of the glottis.)
  - big teeth
  - neck immobility
  - thick tongue
- Careful inspection of all points mentioned is crucial during the airway physical exam. Not one part of the exam can stand alone in predicting difficulty, but multiple indications to either an easy or difficult intubation increases the yield of being prepared. However, sufficient pharyngeal space and good thyromental distance were found in one study to be the most helpful when used together.
- Keeping in mind "mask ventilation as a rescue device," examine the patient for anything that would make it difficult or hazardous to mask: obesity, full stomach, big beard.
- If they have a mustache, look that over as well. A short Che Guevara mustache won't cause problems, but a huge, bushy "I say, old chap, I'm Dr. Thiggleby and we'll be on safari together" mustache will be a problem. When you get the view of the cords, the mustache will get right in your line of vision and you'll get all messed up. What to do? Tape the mustache down flat, your view will be fine then.
- Beards—again—not only can be difficult to mask ventilate, but they can be hiding scary things. Some people with beards are trying to hide short chins, prior facial trauma, or other things that can make them a difficult intubation. Inspect!
- Another way to get a good mask seal with a beard? Put Vaseline or K-Y jelly on the beard. This gives you a good seal and allows you to mask well, and *that is all*! Don't even go there!
- Look around for loose or artificial teeth. If they have removable dentures, take them out, and make sure someone keeps an eye on them. (They're expensive.)
- Some people are supersensitive about taking their dentures out ahead of time, and they don't want their relatives (who may be in the holding area with them) seeing them with their teeth out. Let them keep them in until you're in the OR, then take them out there.
- If you're doing a floor intubation in a code, and someone has dentures in, you sometimes may have trouble getting them out. Use a tongue depressor to pry them out; it'll make your intubation a lot easier. If that doesn't work, try dynamite, but clear the room when you light the fuse.

TECHNIQUE

- Check out all your laryngoscopic equipment ahead of time. Batteries fail. Lightbulbs burn out. Just to be sure, have extra stuff handy.
- Check your endotracheal tube and make sure the pilot balloon is OK; there is no need to check the balloon by filling it with air, then emptying it. Just hook up a 10-cc syringe, aspirate until the pilot is empty, and if the plunger snaps back, then the pilot balloon is intact. But remember that the right way is the way your attending wants it done.
- Positioning is the foundation of laryngoscopy and intubating. You cannot intubate a patient who is lying on his belly. We do not intubate patients who are standing up. Patients are positioned supine, with the neck raised and extended. Degree and amount depends on patient body habitus and anatomy.
- Is suction ready, monitors on and working? Make sure all is well before you ride into the valley of the shadow of the arytenoids.
- Induce.
- Mask ventilate (if appropriate).
- Hold the laryngoscope in your left hand.
- Open the mouth with a scissors movement of your right hand. This is very important. The mandible will not break off onto the floor. (OK. Fine. It did once!) Snap that mouth open until you feel it, you will know once you do it.

Proper Care and Feeding of Your Brain

The most important instrument during intubation is your head. If your head is malfunctioning, the intubation can go south in a hurry. And the best way to take care of your head is to *place the laryngoscope in a well-oxygenated patient*. Translation: Do good mask ventilation, then when you place the laryngoscope, you are hearing the high tone from the pulse oximeter, *beep-beep-beep*. You know you have plenty of time, you can look around and get perspective, and you place the tube, no problem. If, in contrast, you do poor mask ventilation, and you are listening to the ominous *boop-boop-boop* that bespeaks impending doom. You know that time is short, you get panicky, and you start seeing vocal cords just because you are so damned desperate to intubate something, anything, and get out of this jam. That leads to badness, 4+ badness, in your intubating technique. So, odd to say, but good *mask ventilation* is a key to *good laryngoscopy*.

Anatomy of the Tongue 101

A little anatomy review: The tongue has two parts, the wiggley, squiggley front part, and the fixed, don't-go-anywhere root part. That front part is the problem. If you don't hook the tongue out of the way, the tongue will slither/slide/slink over your laryngoscope like some malicious octopus. Then you end up with the tongue to the *right* of the laryngoscope blade, and you look and feel the ninny.

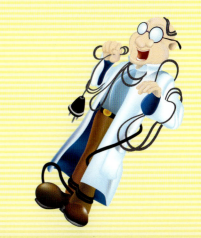

To Stylet or Not to Stylet, That is the Question

Make sure you use a stylet in the endotracheal tube. After all, if you don't need the stylet, it's no big deal if you have it in, but if you do need the stylet, not having it in as a pain. So have the stylet in for every case

No Kidding! Get that Mouth Open

Scissors the mouth, really open, we mean open, open, open. All the action is down at the vocal cords, and the more time you spend around at the entrance to the mouth, the more time you waste.

Check Your Irrational Exuberance When You Get the Tube In

In your thrill and ecstasy at seeing the cords don't pass the endotracheal tube all the way down to the patient's acetabulum. Just get the balloon a couple centimeters past the cords.

- Alternately, you can tilt the patient's head back and let the mouth open of its own accord (don't tilt back if the patient's C-spine is at risk of damage).
- For a beginner, use a curved blade, a Mac 3 for most adults, or Mac 4 for a big adult. That curve will keep you off the teeth.
- Put the blade in the right side of the mouth and go all the way in, all the way in, all the way in. As a beginner, you will tend to just slip the blade in about a zillionth of an angstrom, and will then lift and look for the cords. Unless you are intubating a paramecium, you will not see anything useful. Put that blade all the way in.
- However, if it is a difficult laryngoscopy, a left-molar approach may improve laryngoscopy grade versus midline- or right-molar approach.
- By putting the blade all the way in, you hook the fixed part of the tongue, the base of tongue, and you keep the tongue from slithering over the laryngoscope blade and obscuring your view.
- Once all the way in, lift along the direction of the handle, this will keep you from cranking back and crunching the teeth. Of note, human beings are genetically bred to want to crank back on the laryngoscope. No one knows why, since cranking back doesn't help the view, but it's an urge you'll need to fight.
- Lift along the direction of the handle, and slowly pull back until the epiglottis falls, plop, into your view.
- Once the epiglottis falls into view, push in just a little bit on the laryngoscope; this will engage the tip of the laryngoscope in the vallecula and will allow you to lift the epiglottis. If you don't do that little advancement, then you won't be able to lift the epiglottis.
- Now lift and you should see the cords.
- Mandibular advancement, or BURP maneuver (backward, upward, rightward, pressure of the larynx) will improve the laryngeal view during direct laryngoscopy performed by inexperienced physicians.
- Place the endotracheal tube between those cords.
- Pull the laryngoscope out carefully (you can break teeth coming out just like you can break them going in).
- Inflate the pilot balloon.
- Hook up the breathing circuit and ventilate.

- Make sure you are in by physical exam (chest rises, good breath sounds), and by seeing a good, continuous CO_2 trace.
- Secure the endotracheal tube.
- For a straight blade (the Miller), you will lift the epiglottis directly, rather than lifting it indirectly.
- Don't be too fussy about that lifting of the epiglottis. If you use a Mac like a Miller or a Miller like a Mac, and you still get the endotracheal tube in the right place, you won't get too many complaints.

TECHNIQUE: BULLARD SCOPE

- All kinds of specialty laryngoscopes are out there, each promising to save the day when regular scopes don't do the job.
- One of many is the Bullard scope.
- The Bullard allows you to load the endotracheal tube right into the scope.
- One advantage of the scope is that you can slip it in even when a patient has minimal mouth opening.
- By means of a built-in eyepiece, you can see out the end of the blade.
- Once you see the cords, you can advance the endotracheal tube in.

TECHNIQUE: LIGHT WAND

- Another specialty intubation device is the light wand.
- The patient is induced, and mask ventilation is assured.
- The light wand, with the endotracheal tube loaded on to it, is entered into the pharynx.
- Room lights are dimmed.
- You look for a bright light in the hypopharynx, then you try to advance the wand into the trachea.
- If the light gets dim, you went posterior.
- If the light stays bright, and you can advance it and keep the light bright, then you should be in the trachea.
- This is the coolest thing when you see it, and fans of the light wand absolutely love it.
- Once in, you advance the endotracheal tube and confirm its position.
- Remember, there is no universal tool, some limitations of the light wand's success include obesity.

VIDEO MACINTOSH INTUBATING LARYNGOSCOPE SYSTEM

- Laryngoscope handle with Macintosh blade attached. However, the difference here is a fiberoptic camera at the end of the blade that projects onto a TV similar to a fiberoptic setup.

- Thought to be a great tool for teaching. This way your attending can see if you are really seeing the cords!

- Secondly, some suggest that being able to look at a monitor may afford more coordination to the anesthesiologist and will allow an assistant, who may be giving laryngeal pressure for manipulation, a view also.

- This thing is so cool you'd just die to see it. But it costs a small fortune. Next time you go to a meeting, you'll see a display for it, along with, probably, some little Butterfinger candy bars. Go to a private place when you have to pick the stuck-on Butterfinger essence out of the tops—occlusal surface, if you want to go absolutely DMD nuts about it—of your molars, though.

LARYNGOSCOPIC GLITCHES

- Everyone's heard the horror stories of lost airways, they are almost all preceded by, "I thought I could get it." Have a healthy respect for just how hard an airway can be.

- Remember that obese patients will desaturate quickly, so if you fail to intubate them, you will be in trouble quickly. Now you're trying to mask them, and that's not easy either. Approach the obese patient with a bushel-basket full of caution.

- The Eschmann intubating stylet is a godsend. This tube-changer with a little upward hook at the end will give you that little millimeter or two that you need when someone's airway is a little anterior. We kid thee not, this device has saved our own butts a dozen times, and the butts of many of our friends a lot of times, too. We are serious, we carry one with us **all the time** in the hospital, it is *that* helpful.

- If you don't get a good view, don't try to force the endotracheal tube in. You'll just tear up the airway, cause bleeding and swelling, and make everything worse. If you just plain can't see anything, go to an alternative technique, waking the patient up, or using an intubating LMA.

- During your training, make sure you become adept using both straight and curved blades. Don't get married to the Mac or the Miller. Be a polygamist, married to both. Sometimes, you just can't see with a Mac and the Miller saves you. Other times, the case is reversed. Your best bet is to know them both.

A Grandstanding Maneuver if You Feel Like It

When you're feeling cool, you can pull the stylet out with your teeth. This is admittedly grandstanding and unhygienic, but it generates a lot of oohs and aahs.

Oh, God, Please Do Not Send me to the Damned Radiology Suite

Off to the radiology suite and you have to intubate someone with a bad airway already. You put the scope in and what do you see, a hemangioma at the base of the tongue that you didn't see with the regular airway exam. Fortunately, rather than just ramming the laryngoscope in, the resident slowly advanced it, and thereby avoided smacking into the hemangioma. Thank goodness.

Ooops, though, the resident nicked the lip, and that's all anyone remembered afterward. The resident saved the day, saved the airway, got the intubation, but nicked the lip, so he's still listed as the goat. Oh well.

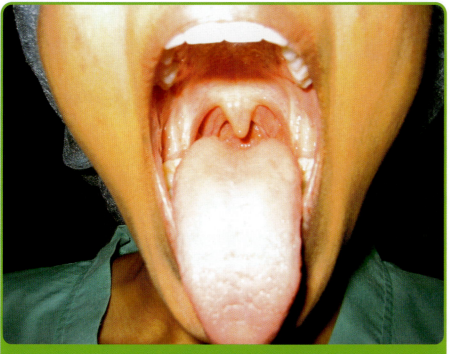

Figure 1. God all fishhooks, you could intubate this person with a drainage pipe.

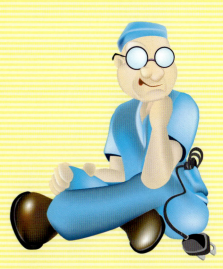

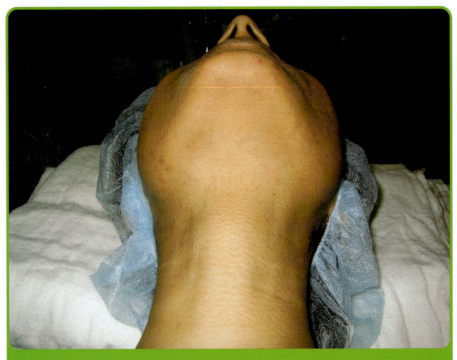

Figure 2. Good neck extension, there's about 50 feet between her chin and her thyrohyoid membrane.

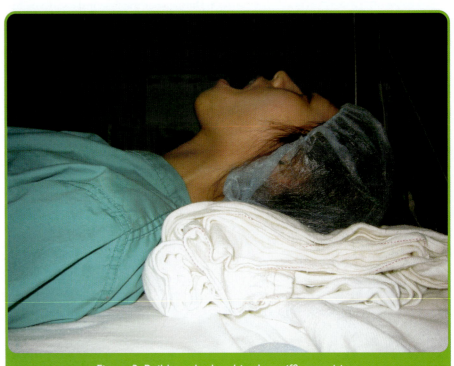

Figure 3. Build up the head in the sniffing position.

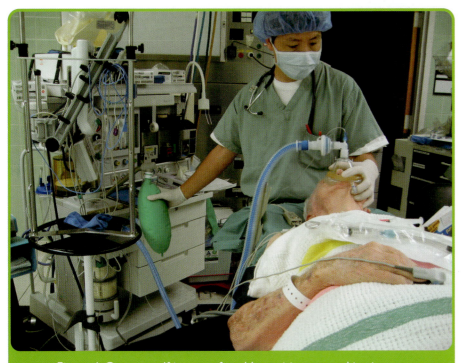

Figure 4. Get yourself in a comfortable position so masking is easy. Get some good Feng Shui going for you.

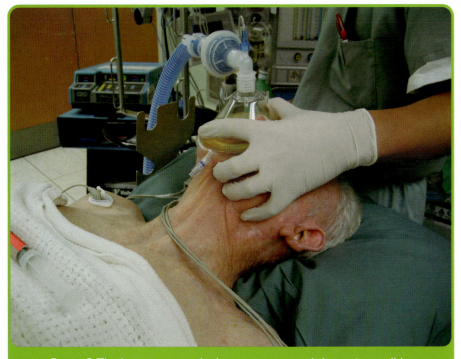

Figure 5. The better you mask, the more saturated the patient will be and the easier it will be to do the intubation. No pressure!

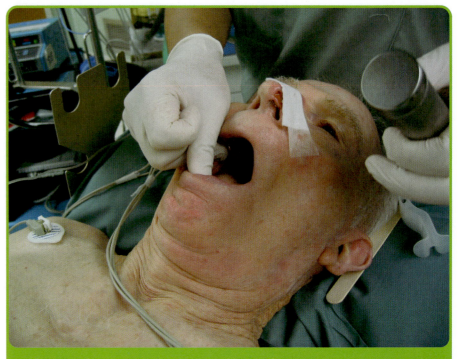

Figure 6. Get that mouth open wide. You don't want to be dancing around the teeth or the front of the mouth. Get past all that.

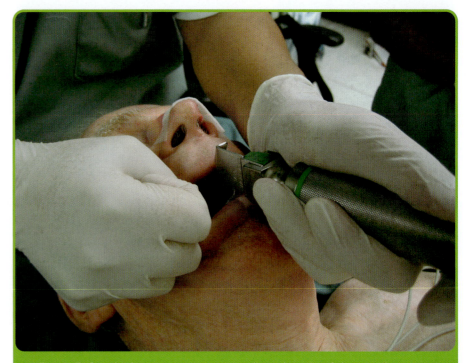

Figure 7. Get the laryngoscope over on the right side of the mouth, getting that pesky, waggly, slithery tongue out of the way.

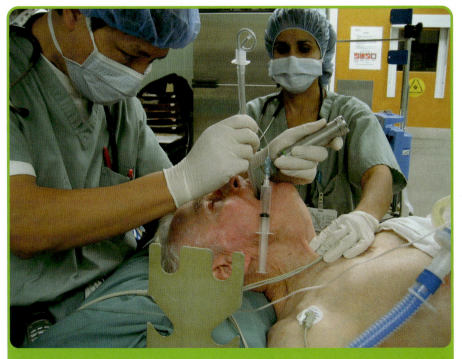

Figure 8. Keep your head far enough back when you place the tube to get some perspective. Don't bury your nose in their mouth.

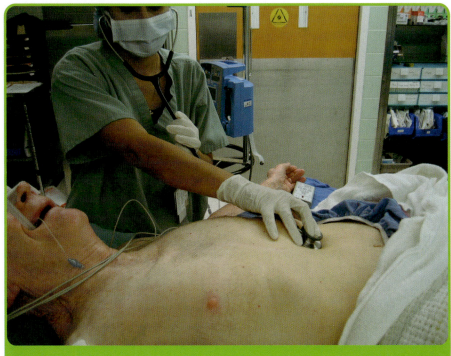

Figure 9. Best first place to listen? The stomach, of course. If you hear bubbly-dee fubble-dee, guess where you are?

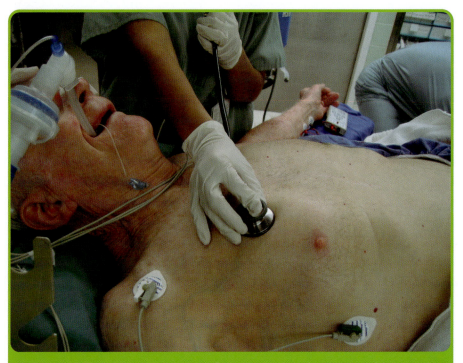

Figure 10. Then listen to the chest. Biggest mistake of newcomers? Irrational exuberance and pushing the tube too far down. You'll hear breath sounds on the right but not the left. (Most often a mainstem goes down the right because it's a straighter shot.)

SUGGESTED READING

Benumof JL, Jonathan C, Saldman L J. *Anesthesia and Perioperative Complications*, 2nd ed. St. Louis: Mosby; 1999, p 6–7.

Frank CM. Predicting difficult intubation. *Anesthesia* 1991;46:1005.

Hagberg CA. Special devices and techniques. *Anesthes Clin North Am* Dec 2002;20(4):907–932.
• *Great article to see every different way to intubate.*

Kaplan MB. A new video laryngoscope—an aid to intubation and teaching. *J Clin Anesth* Dec 2002;14(8):620–626.
• *A cool way to see exactly how you are intubating.*

Shiga T, Wajima Z, Inoue T, Sakamoto A. Predicting difficult intubation in apparently normal patients: a meta-analysis of bedside screening test performance. *Anesthesiology* Aug 2005; 103(2): 429–437.
• *Superb article! This is the basis for knowing who will be easy or difficult to*

Tamura M, Ishikawa T, Kato R, et al. *Anesthesiology* March 2004;100(3):598–601.

Wong SY. Factors influencing time of intubation with a lightwand device in patients without known airway abnormality. *J Clin Anesth* Aug 2004;16(5):326–331.

Get to know the lightwand, Harry Potter.
• 5. *Yamomoto K, Tsubokawa T, Ohmura S, Itoh H. Anesthesiology Jan 2000;92(1):70.*

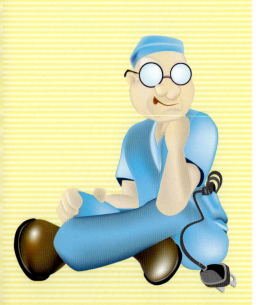

The Crown Jewel of Intubations: Awake Fiberoptic

Christopher Gallagher and Ahmed Zaky

INTRODUCTION

Yea, verily I say these words unto you, all ye who would venture into that land of airway management. For it will come to pass that each and every one of you, great and small, rich and poor, wise and cretinlike, will come across the difficult airway.

And there will be great gnashing of teeth and rending of garments.

And unhappy will be the assembled host.

And spooky and *boop-boop-boop*-ic will be the pulse oximeter.

And so it will come to pass on this day most terrible, that you will raise your hands on high and cry out to a universe devoid of compassion, and you will say, "Whysoever did I not follow the path of righteousness, and do this damnable intubation awake?"

You will note in this chapter that we go to a lot more length than usual to explain every aspect and thought about securing an airway awake. Why? This is **the most important procedure we do**. Who are we kidding? If you can get the tube in, you can fix almost any other problem that comes along.

But if you can't get that tube in, well . . . consider this:

Fiberoptic intubation is considered an invaluable method to secure the airway. In the ASA closed-claim study, adverse respiratory events including inadequate ventilation, esophageal intubation, and difficult tracheal intubation form the largest single class of injury.

Before we leap into how *to use* this slick instrument, let's look at how *it's designed*.

> These things must be done delicately, delicately.
>
> *The Wicked Witch of the West*
> The Wizard of Oz, 1939

DESIGN

The flexible fiberoptic bronchoscope consists of fiberoptic light bundles that transmit light to the airway and an image back to the viewer. The bronchoscope also consists of a channel for suction and passage of other instruments such as brushes and forceps, a controller knob for ante- or retroflexing the instrument, and fine and gross adjustment foci. The outer diameter (OD) of the bronchoscope is of relevance to anesthesia. The outer diameter of the bronchoscope should be at least 2-mm narrower than the lumen of the ETT to prevent excessive increases in airflow resistance and decreased tidal volume.

INDICATIONS

Establishing an airway

- Predicted difficult airway (conscious intubation)
- Unpredicted difficult airway ("cannot intubate, but can ventilate" scenario)
- Unpredicted difficult airway (via LMA, in the "cannot intubate, cannot ventilate" scenario)
- Endotracheal tube change

Verifying an Airway

- Endobronchial intubation for one-lung ventilation
- LMA position
- Single-lumen ETT

Diagnostic

- ETT obstruction
- Endobronchial intubation
- Airway pathology in mechanically ventilated patients
- Biopsy taking
- Bronchoalveolar lavage (BAL)

Therapeutic

- Suctioning secretions obstructing the airway
- Pulmonary toilet
- Hemoptysis tamponade either directly or indirectly by a Fogarty catheter introduced through the bronchoscope to site of bleeding
- Foreign body removal
- Endotracheal intubation and tube change
- In bronchopleural and tracheoesophageal fistulas by introducing sealing material

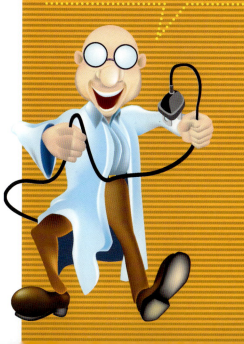

Overcoming Surgeon Opposition

"Oh, no, you're going to do what? God-damn it!"

- Such is the collegial encouragement our surgeons rain down upon us when we do an awake intubation. A few maneuvers on your part can change their swords into plowshares.

Be time efficient. If you dry the patient up early, start topicalizing early, then proceed expeditiously in the OR (spray a little topical, put on the pulse ox, spray a little more, put on the EKG, spray a little topical, place the airway, put on the BP cuff, cycle the cuff as you place the tube into the airway), you can intubate awake in just about the same amount of time it takes to intubate the normal way.

Pay attention to the hemodynamics as you proceed along. Many a surgeon complains (and rightly so) that the patients get stressed to high heaven during an awake intubation, raising concerns of myocardial ischemia and stroke. Take time out during the procedure to tend the hemodynamic garden with judicious use of nitrates, beta-blockers, and antihypertensives.

Let the surgeon watch! Oh yes, oh yes. If you do a few smooth-as-silk intubations where the patients are comfortable and relaxed, you'll be amazed at how surgeons and OR staff will come to rethink awake intubations. Hey, they're not this medieval form of torture after all!

CONTRAINDICATIONS

Flexible fiberoptic bronchoscopy should not be performed in the following six situations:

1. Absence of consent from the patient, which can be from a few different angles . . .
   - Kids who can't cooperate (try talking a two-year-old into an awake intubation).
   - Adults who can't cooperate (mentally incapacitated from congenital or acquired central nervous system pathology).
   - Adults who might be able to cooperate, but are now under the influence of drugs or alcohol and just won't hold still.
2. Lack of trained personnel. Your job is to make sure *you* do not constitute a lack of trained personnel.
3. Refractory hypoxemia. This, of course, is a relative thing. We mean, if there is no other way to secure the airway, then of course you would do a fiberoptic intubation to *cure* the refractory hypoxemia. The lesson here is: If someone is doing horribly, don't putz around and do a *teaching* fiberoptic intubation or delay. Just go for the quickest way to secure the airway immediately (usually direct laryngoscopy).
4. Inability to normalize platelet count and coagulation if biopsy is planned. This is more a consideration for surgeons, of course, since we don't take biopsies too often.
5. Unstable cardiac disease. Again, it's easy to say this, and all textbooks do, but keep in mind: Hypoxemia is not good for cardiac disease, so if a fiberoptic is the best way to secure the airway and relieve that hypoxemia (and the subsequent cardiac ischemia), then do the fiberoptic.
6. Uncontrolled bronchospasm. Here we go again. Yes, an awake fiberoptic in the case of bronchospasm can make the bronchospasm worse. *But*, if someone's going down the tubes and the only way to secure the airway is with a fiberoptic, then do the fiberoptic.

So as you look at these contraindications, you see a lot of "yes, buts" in them. This is, after all, the airway, and that is the *A* of *ABC*—when you're securing the airway, you do what you have to do. Here's a real live contraindication, no ifs, ands, or buts:

- Upper airway so smunched up that a fiberoptic would get lost in a sea of blood and torn-up tissue (need to go with a trach in such a case).

AWAKE INTUBATION: HISTORY AND PHYSICAL

- Ask about difficulties with intubation in the past.
- Examine old anesthetic records looking for the intubation notes.
- Look for subtle clues such as, "Seven attempts, four different practitioners, five different blades, finally got it with a prayer to all major deities and a blind stab."
- Examine the airway for the usual suspects: short chin, thick neck or tongue, big teeth, trach scar (!), immobile neck.
- Look for tight-packed fat in the area under the chin. This is the area you will be attempting to lift with a laryngoscope. If the fat is tight and immobile rather than loose and jowly, you'll have trouble lifting it.
- Any appliances on the head or neck (halo, jaw wired shut, Man in the Iron Mask).
- Obese? Always think of "What will I do if I don't get the tube in the first time?" An obese person, being hard to mask ventilate and quick to desaturate, could paint you into a corner in no time flat.
- Beard? Same question, they could be hard to mask ventilate if you miss the first time.
- On weird orthopedic beds and hard to get to? Again, if you can't get at their airways and then you have problems, do you have a plan B ready?

Now let's set it up and do the damn thing already!

EQUIPMENT

Fiberoptic apparatus

- Clean fiberoptic scope attached to light source and camera if present.
- Test the adjustment focus against the writing on the camera.
- Feel comfortable rotating, anteflexing, and retroflexing the scope before use.
- Attach appropriate size ETT to the scope after removing its connector, but know where it is.

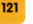

- Lubricate the scope with a silicon-based fluid.

Ancillary airway equipment
- Trumpets
- Source of oxygen
- Source of suction
- Cotton-tipped applicators
- Ambu bag
- Emergency airway cart in case of difficult airway scenario

After finishing with the scope
- Manually clean the scope with a detergent.
- Disinfect it by immersing it in 2% glutaraldehyde for 20 minutes.
- Rinse it with water or 70% alcohol.
- *Mycobacterium tuberculosis* is a ubiquitous organism transmitted by contaminated bronchoscopes.

Medications
- Glycopyrrolate.
- Lidocaine 4% topical solution.
- Lidocaine viscous solution.
- Lidocaine 5% ointment.
- Phenylephrine-soaked cotton tipped applicator.
- Medications entailed by the individual case. For example, labetalol for hypertensive patients, esmolol for patients with coronary artery disease, and albuterol for patients with asthma.

Monitoring
- Pulse oximeter
- Capnograph
- EKG
- Noninvasive blood pressure monitor

TECHNIQUE

Caveat: This is our own personal technique, and there are many others. The single biggest change in recent years has been the advent and widespread use of the intubating LMA, which affords a whole new option in the case of a lost airway.

- Glycopyrrolate the nanosecond we suspect a patient may be difficult. (That way, even if we do an asleep intubation, if we have to back out and wake patiens up, at least their airways will already be dry.) Go away for 20 minutes, at least.
- Explain to patients what we're going to do. No need to freak them out or to turn

them into Airway Anatomy PhDs. We just say, "Before you go to sleep, I'm going to numb up your mouth and look in with a flashlight." Alright, you could criticize us for candy-coating it a little, but that is, in effect, what we do.

- Sedate to taste. (Ourselves? A little midazolam. Some people use dexmedetomidine and swear by it. Whatever you use, don't convert an awake intubation into a 99%-asleep-oh-damn-he-stopped-breathing intubation.)
- Grab our prepackaged airway kits that have all the stuff we like.
- Place an endotracheal tube in a bottle of warm water to make the tube soft and less traumatogenic.
- Place 5% lidocaine ointment on the top of a tongue depressor like an ice cream cone. Place this way way back in the mouth, all the way back to the posterior pharynx. (This is the place where the meanie pediatrician and family practice docs swab your throat for strep.) This is the toughest part to anesthetize, because this is the part where patients will fight you. (How much do you like it when those bastards swab your throat?) So, we start topicalizing this part first, giving it the most time to get numb.
- All other things being equal, we'll go through the mouth, because we don't want a nosebleed. But if we have to go through the nose, then we give some Neosynephrine drops up each nostril. Make sure the patient breathes it way in. Then, like everything else in the airway, give the medicine time to do its thing. Then we spray up the nose with 4% lidocaine using the Mucosal Atomization Device. To goopity-goop up the nostril, we fill a 10-cc syringe with 2% lidocaine jelly (keep these percentages and jellies/ointments straight) and squoozle it into the nostril. (We like a lot getting injected in there so it can completely coat all the little twists and turns in those conchas.)
- We take the smallest possible nasal airway and pass it through that lidocaine-besquoozled nares. We pass this *only to see if something can pass, this is not and no nasal airway should be viewed as a dilator!* Pupils dilate, cervixes dilate—nasal airways don't have a *dilate* function. All they do is *ream*. Passing a bunch of these nasal airways just causes bleeding.
- If the small nasal airway passes, the next thing is that we place into the nose a lidocaine jelly-besotted endotracheal tube. As you pass it, you'll feel a woomph as

Other Forms of Awake Intubation

There are other ways of getting an awake intubation:

Place the LMA awake and go through there. That takes some ambitious topicalizing and we haven't seen it much, but it's possible.

Retrograde wire. You topicalize and sedate as for any awake intubation, then you slide a wire through the cricothyroid membrane, work it up out the mouth or nose, then use that wire as a kind of Seldinger technique for advancing the endotracheal tube. You read about this a lot, but don't see it too often. If you're ever going to practice this, try it on a patient scheduled for a laryngectomy, so if you gum up the works, the whole shebang's coming out anyway.

Awake trach. More on this later. This is reserved for a patient where other awake intubation techniques present a hazard. For example, if a patient has an enormous fungating tumor right on his epiglottis, then any fiberoptic technique, no matter how exquisitely handled, may cause the friable tumor to bleed, crumble, and zoink the airway.

Other Forms of Topicalizing

Myself? I prefer to do everything topical. No needles in the neck unless I have to. But needle-o-philiacs out there do like to do injectable blocks.

Transtracheal (I've talked to patients who've had these and they say it's icky, and their throats hurt for a long time afterward. After going through that crunchy cartilage, I tend to believe them.)

Draw up 2 or 3 cc of 4% lidocaine.

Wipe off the neck.

Stick through the cricoid cartilage, aspirate air, and inject.

Because patients will cough and possibly jump up, have your forearm resting on their chests when you inject. Alternately, use a skinny angio cath and pull the needle out, that way if they jump up, you won't spear anything.

Superior laryngeal.

Inject a cc or two on either side of the hyoid bone, a C-shaped bone hovering above the larynx. To bring the bone to you, push from the left side of the hyoid bone when you inject on the right side, and push from the right side of the bone when you inject on the left side.

There's blocks you can do in the mouth, but even venturing near the mouth with a needle in hand makes me think I went to dental, rather than medical, school.

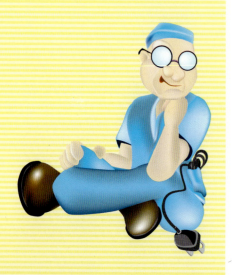

you pop back into the posterior pharynx. At this point, you're golden. (To help patients through the woomph push, we tell them, "This will be unpleasant for about three seconds, now breathe through your mouth." That usually distracts them just enough to allow you to get the endotracheal tube into the posterior pharynx.

- If we go orally or nasally, we place a Mucosal Atomization Device with 4% lidocaine liquid in their mouths and tell them, "pant and breathe deep," and we breathe along with them.

- Topicalization is not a spectator sport! The more you get into it and work with the patient, the better it goes. (When we do it, people think we're nuts, but such is the price one pays.)

- If we go orally, we place the Williams Airway (the pink one . . . we find the Ovassapian Airway wiggles around too much). On top of the airway, we put a fine coat of 5% lidocaine ointment, so wherever the airway touches, there will be yet more local.

- Whichever route you take, have an assistant lift the chin. This keeps everything straight and aligned. If you're going orally, it locks the Williams Airway between the upper and lower teeth. This means when you look with the fiberoptic, you will only have to go ahead and you'll see the cords. (If they don't lift the chin, the airway will go a little off to the side and you won't get a straight shot at the cords. You'll slide into the cheek or some damn thing, and you'll just see the infamous "It's all pink!" view.

- We load the endotracheal tube as close to the cords as we can. Nasally, that means placing the endotracheal tube through the nose into the supra-whoomphic section of the posterior pharynx. If orally, that means we load the endotracheal tube into the Williams Airway.

- Our thinking is this: If we do get the fiberoptic through the cords, we want the shortest possible advancement between us and glory. If the endotracheal tube is a mile back up the fiberoptic, we have to slide the tube all the way down, through the mouth or nose (overcoming Mr. Whoomph in the nose), then go through the cords. And all this time, the patient may be coughing and struggling.

- Better to have the endotracheal tube right near the cords and just go *zip* from up close.

- When you place the fiberoptic, you can either look right through it with your eyeball, or you can look via camera at a

TV screen (the same thing the surgeons do now for all their fiberoptic procedures).

- Adjusting to the camera takes a little, well, adjustment, but it allows all in the room to look along, an obvious advantage in the teaching setting. For laughs, look around the room during one of these, and you'll see everyone using body language to try to finesse the tube in.

- Respect and love your fiberoptic. Remember, those little light elements in there are spun glass, no less, so they can break. (Look at a surgeon's headlight cable, sometimes you'll see little shafts of light shooting out where the fiberoptic glass threads have broken.) Over time, if you crank the living bejeebers out of the fiberoptic, the view will get fuzzier and fuzzier, until you develop a kind of macular degeneration of the fiberoptic. Turn the shaft of the fiberoptic as a unit, don't twist it.

- Hook oxygen up to the suction port of the fiberoptic, that way you will blow spit and blood out of the way (like Moses parting the Red Sea) to clear your vision.

- If you hook up suction to the fiberoptic, you will just suck a glob of saliva to the end of the fiberoptic (that suction port is tiny!) and blind yourself.

- By blowing oxygen through the suction port, you will also provide a little supplemental oxygenation, just in case you were a little heavy-handed with the sedation and the patient has involuntarily become a facultative anaerobe.

- When the fiberoptic pops out of the end of the endotracheal tube, you ideally get the impression of a cave with a little space to look around in. Then, lo and behold, you see the epiglottis off in the distance.

- As you advance toward the epiglottis, use itty-bitty-teeny-weeny movements of the fiberoptic control to angle the end of the fiberoptic probe. Easy does it!

- Pink is the great enemy. If you just see pink, you're stuck in mucosa. Pull back until you get that cave feel. If nothing helps and you are marooned in Pinksville, USA, then pull the endotracheal tube back. The *cave* is the thing. Seek the cave, Luke!

- No luck? Have your assistant lift the chin again. Sometimes your assistant can give a little cricoid or wiggle the neck around for you. The main thing is, like any other procedure, don't reinforce failure, do something different.

- Try sitting the patients up, that will alter the terrain a little, turn their heads one way or another. Why not? If what you're doing isn't working, this can't make things any worse!

- Topical through the fiberoptic? We like it. Squirt a little in the injection port, then blast your oxygen through it.

- If you've topicalized in a major groovy fashion, you can often slip the tube in without the patient even noticing. That is the coolest, as well as being of great utility. (For example, a patient has a fractured cervical spine, and you want to do a neurologic exam after intubation.)

- Pull out the fiberoptic, hook up the circuit, check for CO_2, take the Williams Airway out (if the patients are cool and calm, they can cooperate). If you are scared you might spazz out and pull out the endotracheal tube as you are pulling out the oral airway, then slip the fiberoptic back in and keep it there as a bridge to reintubation should you pull the tube out by mistake.

And there you have it! But alas, sometimes things don't go smoothly, so let's take a look at a few problems and how to overcome them.

DIFFICULTIES AND REMEDIES

Difficulty #1: Patient bucking

- Remedy #1

Allow adequate time for the local anesthetics to work. Glycopyrrolate takes 20 minutes for a peak effect. Fentanyl is complementary to local anesthetics because it is a potent suppressant of airway reflexes. Do not topicalize before sedation. Test the gag reflex by using an oral airway or a tongue depressor.

Difficulty #2: After induction of general anesthesia, difficulty locating the glottis

- Remedy #2

Jaw thrust, apply tongue traction, cervical extension (versus flexion for direct aryngsocopy).

Difficulty #3: Difficulty inserting the tube over the fiberscope

This could be due to:

1. Anatomical factors
   a. In oral intubation, the ETT might impinge over the arytenoids (mostly right), or the esophageal inlet.
   b. In nasal intubation the main sites of obstruction are a deviated septum, or inflamed turbinate, epiglottis, or arytenoids.
   c. Large tongue, long epiglottis, or airway deformity will all lead to ETT impingement.

2. Device or procedural factors
   Includes Murphy eye of the ETT, cricoid pressure, airway intubator, or excessive jaw thrusting as it may shift the larynx anteriorly.

- Remedy #3
1. Reduction of the gap between the fiberscope and the ETT by:
   a. Use of a large-diameter fiberscope and a narrow-diameter ETT. One study showed that it was easier to intubate using a 6.0-mm ETT over a 4-mm fiberscope than an 8.0-mm ETT over the same fiberscope. Another study showed that the incidence of difficulty was lower using the larger fiberscope (diameter, 5 mm) than the smaller fiberscope (3.7 mm).
   b. Filling the gap between the fiberscope and the ETT using a thinner tube. Get a well-lubricated, 5.0-mm uncuffed and uncut tube, thread it through a 7.0- or 8.0-mm tube cut at oral length of 23 cm. The inner tube can protrude beyond the end of the bigger outer tube. Thread these two tubes over the fiberscope. After successful insertion of the scope and both tubes, remove the fiberscope and the inner tube. Two studies have confirmed the validity of this technique.

2. Use of an intubating LMA (ILMA) flexible tube:
   The bevel of the ILMA tube is made of silicone, softer than the conventional polyvinyl chloride (PVC) tube, and hemispherical with the leading edge in the center. Several studies have shown the easiness of this tube compared with the conventional PVC tube.

3. Warming the ETT with hot water or hot air.
   You might make the ETT softer to follow the curve of the fiberscope. The literature is inconclusive in this regard.

4. Loading the ETT over the fiberscope.

Value-Added Anesthesiologist

When you are released into the wild, make yourself valuable to your group. If you can do what everybody else can do, then you do not really represent a value-added member.

Get good at awake intubations!

When that Ludwig's angina or the cervical fracture come down, if you are good at awake intubations, your group will love you!

Remind them at end of the year bonus time.

When loading the fiberscope via the tube to the trachea, the fiberscope might pass through the Murphy eye and make intubation a failure. Therefore, it is always advisable to load the ETT over the fiberscope before inserting it. This might not be possible for nasal intubation; in such a case, advance the scope under direct vision until it has passed through the distal orifice of the tube.

5. Rotation of a tube.

The unrotated ETT has a bevel to the left; therefore the tip might impinge over the right arytenoid cartilage or the right vocal cord. Rotating the ETT 90 degrees anticlockwise causing the ETT tip to be away from the arytenoids, changes the curvature of the ETT posteriorly thus decreasing the incidence of esophageal intubation. This also prevents the adherence of the ETT into the inner subglottic area.

6. Use of LMA and ILMA

Intubating throughout the LMA is easier for two reasons: First, the LMA bypasses a lot of obstacles being in position such as narrowed pharyngeal orifice or epiglottis. Second, it facilitates location of the glottis using the fiberscope because the glottis is just below the grille of the mask. Many studies have shown easier intubation using LMA or ILMA in comparison to fiberoptic intubation without using LMA for intubating or ILMA.

7. Other maneuvers

Release of cricoid pressure, use of a laryngoscope to lift the tongue and epiglottis away from the fiberscope, removal of the airway intubator, and release of jaw thrust.

8. Could esophageal intubation occur despite correct fiberoptic scope placement in the trachea?

The answer is yes. If you encounter resistance during ETT advancement, the ETT might be displacing the middle segment of the fiberscope, pulling it out of the trachea, over the interarytenoid notch and into the esophagus.

But what of the physiology during all these machinations?

PHYSIOLOGY

Pulmonary mechanics and gas exchange: There are certain maneuvers during

bronchoscopy and intubation that are most stressful. These include placement of fiberscope through the vocal cords and suctioning.

Lundgren et al. found that the maximum changes in hemodynamics happened during suction and during passage of fiberscope through the larynx. Mean arterial pressure increased by 30%, heart rate by 43%, cardiac index by 28%, and mean pulmonary arteriolar occlusion pressure by 86% compared with prebronchoscopic values. A slight fall in oxygen tension occurred during bronchial suctioning, and in the postbronchoscopic period. Rate pressure product was highest during suctioning at which time three of ten patients developed ST-T segment changes. The authors attributed those changes to reflex sympathetic discharge caused by mechanical irritation of the larynx and bronchi.

Pulmonary mechanics are significantly changed during FOB. Lidholm et al. and Matsushima et al. noted a decline in vital capacity, inspiratory and expiratory flow rates for spontaneously breathing patients. A 5.2-mm bronchoscope in the adult trachea produces about a twofold increase in airway resistance, laryngoscopy and ETT alone produce threefold, while a 5.2-mm and a fiberscope with an 8.0-mm ETT produce an 11-fold increase in airway resistance. The presence of a bronchoscope in an ETT during positive pressure ventilation causes an increase in both peak ventilator pressure and true tracheal pressure. It also produces PEEP, and decreases delivered tidal volume. Consequently, there is a risk of barotrauma and hypoventilation in theses cases.

The stress of bronchoscopy in spontaneously breathing patients can be decreased by giving supplemental oxygen, and minimizing periods of suctioning. In mechanically ventilated patients, FIO$_2$ should be set at 1.0 for the entire procedure, ventilator mode should be on a mandatory setting, PEEP should be reduced. Tidal volume and minute ventilation should be monitored closely and respiratory rate increased if necessary. The ventilator pressure limit should be increased to ensure adequate tidal volume. A swivel connector would be a good idea to conserve tidal volume allowing adequate ventilation.

There is, of course, a very special form of physiology that comes into the anesthetic arena—pregnancy. And yes, pregnant patients can and do need fiberoptic intubations too.

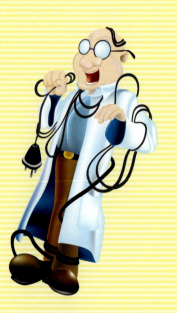

BRONCHOSCOPY AND PREGNANCY

- Elective bronchoscopy should be deferred until after pregnancy or, if not possible, until after the 28th week of gestation.

- Same principles apply for monitoring as for the nonpregnants plus fetal monitoring, if possible.

- Consider minimal doses of midazolam or equimolar $N_2O:O_2$ for conscious sedation during the procedure.

- Nasal route is ill advised in pregnancy because of capillary engorgement and risk of epistaxis.

- Maintain left-uterine tilt whenever possible. Don't get lost in the wondrous world of bronchoscopy and forget the fundamentals of pregnancy: *Don't lay them flat on their backs or the uterus will squish the vena cava.*

- Have the procedure done by the most experienced bronchoscopist.

- Consider termination of the procedure if poorly tolerated.

COMPLICATIONS

Flexible fiberoptic intubation is a relatively safe procedure. There is 0.3% incidence of major complications and a mortality rate of 0.02%. Complications include:

- Periprocedural anesthetic complications such as toxicity from local anesthetics.

- Insertion of the fiberscope through the airway will lead to a decrease in the cross-sectional area of the trachea, leading to an increase in the work of breathing, decrease in tidal volume and hypoxemia. In addition, continuous suction will lead to evacuation of respiratory gases decreasing the FRC and hypoxemia. Hypoxemia may be severer after BAL due to V/Q mismatch that occur secondary to installed liquids. Noninvasive positive pressure ventilation via a face mask can be used to treat hypoxemia.

- Arrhythmias occur mostly during the passage of the bronchoscope via the vocal cords. Cardiac arrest has occurred in some cases.

- Significant bleeding defined as more than 50 cc can occur in coagulopathic, uremic, immunosuppressed patients when biopsy or brushing is performed.

- Pneumothorax is a relatively uncommon complication.

- Fever is more common after BAL, and is believed to be due to the release of proinflammatory cytokines from alveolar macrophages.

- Patients with preexisting reactive airway disease are prone to develop bronchospasm or laryngospasm.

PHILOSOPHY OF AWAKE INTUBATIONS

- To get slick at awake intubations, you have to *embrace* awake intubations, rather than *flee* from them. If you go forever and forever and forever without doing an awake intubation, then when that awful airway comes to the OR (or ICU or ER, wherever), your brain will tell you, "Oh no! This is a bad airway, I have to do this awake! Oh my God, this is the end of life as I know it. This is an epic monstrosity! This is a fire-breathing dragon I must slay and all I've got is a butter knife!"

- If you do awake intubations on a more regular basis, you will have the right attitude, "Oh, this patient needs an awake intubation, no biggie. Doing an awake intubation freaks me out no more than any other procedure we do."

- You want to get to the point where you think along these lines: Patient needs an A-line, patient gets an A-line; patient needs a spinal, patient gets a spinal; patient needs an awake intubation, patient gets an awake intubation. There is nothing different here, an awake intubation is just plain something that some people need, so just *do it.*

- The best thing about awake intubation is that you haven't burned any bridges, you keep the patients breathing and controlling their airway reflexes as long as possible. If it takes you a while, so OK, it takes you a while, but you're not under the same time pressures you are under when you've already induced and the patient is *not* breathing!

- The next big impediment to doing awake intubations is *getting* all the stuff to topicalize the patient. If you don't have a difficult-airway kit (with local anesthetic, aerosolizing equipment, oral airways), you're more likely to shrug your shoulders and say the fateful words, "Oh, getting all this crap is too much of a pain, besides, *I think I can get it.*" Don't fall into that trap. That is lazy thinking and lazy airway management.

- Juries appear deaf to the argument, "I didn't do the awake intubation because I

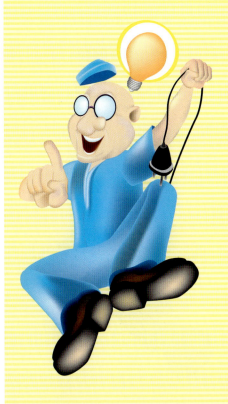

didn't want to bother getting the topicalization stuff, so instead I proceeded and killed the patient."

- Wherever you work, identify (in the light of day, with people around), where all the stuff is that you might need to do an awake intubation:

- Topicalizing drugs and equipment:

  Ovassapian, Miller, or nasal airways, whichever you like

  fiberoptics

  light sources

- If you don't have the stuff you like, buy donuts for the anesthesia techs and pharmacy, and get them on your side. Get them to order what you want, then put all the airway equipment you need in a place you can get at, reliably, day or night, holidays and weekends.

- Bad airways have a way of appearing when no one's around and you are all alone. So get the airway situation taken care of *before* you are all alone and no one's around.

- If it's easy to get the airway stuff, you're more likely to do the right thing.

- If it's easy to get the stuff, you're less likely to say, "Oh hell, I think I can get it."

THE IMPORTANCE OF ADEQUATE PREPARATION

- Dry the patient, dry the patient, dry the patient.

- If your plan is to topicalize, then consider this before you actually lay any topical on the patient's airway:

Go to your garage.

Close the door and plug up the gaps at the bottoms of all the doors.

Turn on the water.

Fill your garage up with 2 inches of water.

Now, with your garage floor under 2 inches of water, get a bucket of paint.

Paint the floor of your garage.

Ain't gonna happen.

How could you possibly get the paint to contact and bond with your garage floor? The paint will get diluted, and no matter how you thrash around and froth up your garage, you're just not going to paint that floor.

Same deal if you don't dry up the patient. Topical anesthetic only works when it lands on and soaks into the mucous

membranes you're trying to topicalize. And to do that, you've got to get your ass in gear and dry the patient up, and the sooner the better!

WHAT HAPPENS WHEN YOU DON'T ADEQUATELY PREPARE

- Secretions everywhere.

- Patient is fighting, uncomfortable, miserable, blood pressure is 10,000 and heart rate is *too numerous to count*.

- You have just arrived at the station marked "Going Nowhere Fast." The surgeon's ticked, the patient is going to hell in a handbasket, and your Option Tank is running on empty.

- Even if you start to dry the patient up now, it will take another good 20 minutes (if things go absolutely perfectly, which they won't), and by then the surgeon will be poking pins into a voodoo doll that looks just like you.

- Lesson learned. Give drying agents early.

WHAT'S THIS ABOUT GIVING DRYING AGENTS IM?

- Your target organ is the salivary glands. They secrete over time. Give an IM injection, then your drying agent sticks around for a while and you keep the salivary glands off. Long-term drying.

- If you give the glycopyrrolate IV and the levels jump up and go down again, then it's like turning off Niagara Falls for a few minutes, then letting it turn back on again. It's still wet downstream.

- Another advantage to IM: If you see a bad airway and the patient doesn't have an IV, you can get that drying agent in *now, pronto*, and let it start working. That, no kidding, is the key to good topicalization (which translates into smooth intubating).

- Anticipate!

- Get that drying agent in while the patient's in the holding area. Give it time to work! We're so used to giving drugs we forget that the toughest drug to give is *time*. Get the antisialagogue in, then go get your stuff, go recheck the room, look over the chart. You give the drying agent time to work . . . you won't regret it.

- Rush the drying agent, you *will* regret it.

- Of note, there are other agents you can give to dry out, atropine, scopolamine, or diphenhydramine. Of these, we'd shy

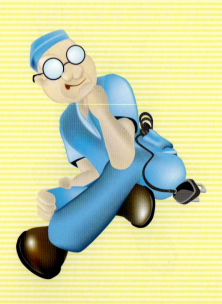

away from atropine for the tachycardia, and scopolamine for the central nervous system weirding out. Diphenhydramine is a good option because it gives you good drying and some sedation.

FOCUSING ON TOPICALIZATION

- Give the topical time to do its thing, and you'll be one happy camper.
- Rush the topical, and both you and your patient will be miserable.
- There are a ton of ways to topicalize, each with its champion and advocate. One common thread recurs—be diligent about making sure the patient actually gets numb!
- If you give lidocaine as you would an inhaled bronchodilator, don't just let the lidocaine cloud float around the patients' heads—encourage them to breathe the lidocaine into their airways.
- If you poke a mucosal atomization device (our personal favorite!) into the patients' mouth, show the patients how to breathe the stuff in, and make sure they do it.
- If you think you are done aerosolizing and you place an oral airway and the patient goes bonkers, guess what? The patient is not adequately anesthetized and you have to give more local. So give more local, and give it more time!

SEDATION

- Lot of different options, just keep this in mind: If you are doing an awake intubation, then don't do an *asleep* intubation. Don't pour so much sedative into the equation that you have lost your biggest allies, the patients themselves.
- Good explanation and good rapport go a long way to reducing anxiety and the need for sedatives.
- Midazolam with a touch, we mean a touch of fentanyl is one traditional technique. Just keep in mind the synergistic effect of drugs and the apnea potential of every drug, but especially narcotics.
- Dexmedetomidine is a dandy, dandy drug for awake intubations. It takes about 20 minutes to work if you give the loading dose and start a drip. And that's about how long you need anyway to topicalize. Patients tend to cooperate, not mind the procedure, and keep good hemodynamics.

- Dribs and drabs of propofol? Ourselves? We don't like that, it just seems too much a drift into general anesthesia land.

AWAKE FIBEROPTIC GLITCHES

- The main problem is complacency, the feeling that "I can intubate anybody."
- If we had a dime for everyone who has said, "I didn't think it would be so hard to intubate this guy," we'd be millionaires.
- The most frequent surprise comes from obese males, the soft tissue caves in on you, you can't see anything, and they desaturate in an instant.
- Practice, practice, practice. Keep doing fiberoptics, don't get out of practice.
- The biggest screw-ups in the procedure itself are failure to dry the patient and failure to take the necessary time to do a real thorough topicalization.
- If you don't topicalize or sedate well, the hemodynamics can—and do—go through the roof. If that is happening, hey, chill out! Stop the procedure! Reevaluate, retopicalize, resedate, treat the hemodynamics (nitroglycerin, labetalol, Cardene, whatever it takes). An awake intubation is an exercise in pharmacologic finesse, not a tractor pull!

Sick of all this anecdotal "This is the way I do it" stuff? Here's what the evidence says:

EVIDENCE-BASED MEDICINE

- The Williams airway provided a better view of the glottis than the Ovassapian.
- Discomfort during bronchoscopy decreased with bronchoscopist's experience and increased with patient's anxiety.
- Addition of sedation to topical anesthesia is superior to the latter alone.
- N_2O/O_2 50:50 conscious sedation during bronchoscopy is associated with less patient discomfort.
- Use of LMA as a conduit for flexible bronchoscopy is associated with a lower failure rate than the nasal route or through an ETT already placed.
- Patients who had undergone radiotherapy for the head and neck are prone to difficult fiberoptic-guided intubation and that this difficulty was predicted by the presence of preoperative laryngeal edema, hoarseness, and stridor. None of

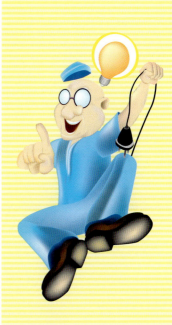

the factors predicting difficult laryngoscopy was helpful in predicting
difficulties with fiberoptic intubation.

• Caution should be exercised during
oxygen insufflation, as there is a case
report of gastric rupture secondary to
high-insufflation pressures.

• In a patient with a compromised airway,
total airway obstruction might be induced with topical airway anesthesia.

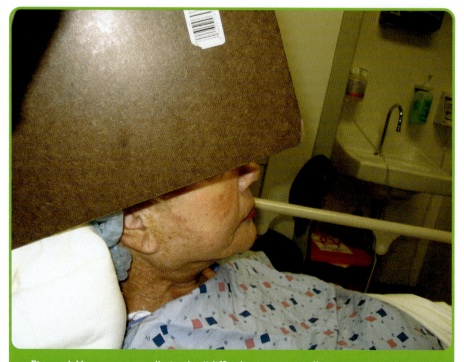

Figure 1. Your greatest ally in the "difficult airway wars" is your pre-op exam.
If the airway looks bad (she can't open her mouth much and can't
extend her neck at all, then by all means do the intubation awake.

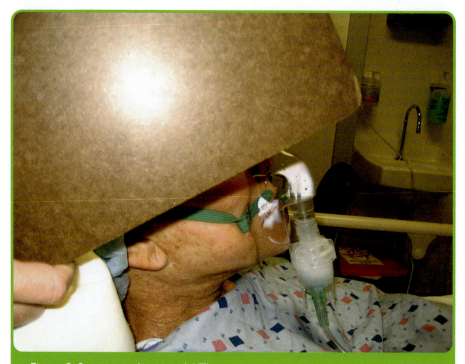

Figure 2. Start topicalizing early! The more time and care you put into making
the patient numb and comfortable, the easier will be your intubation.

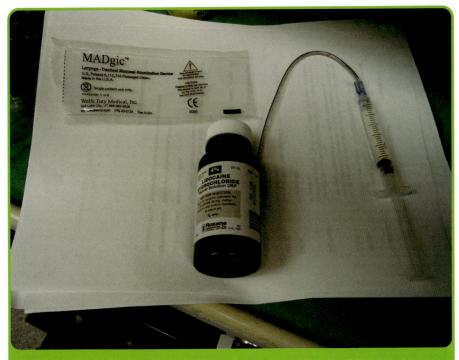

Figure 3. The Mucosal Atomization Device is just the thing! Inexpensive, disposable, and it delivers a fine mist of local (may I recommend a 2005 4% Lidocaine vintage?). Great device!

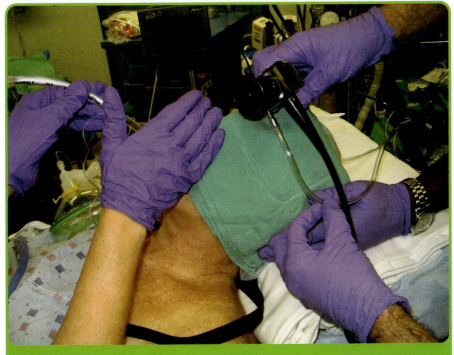

Figure 4. If you hook oxygen up to the sideport of the fiberoptic, you can blow spit and blood out of the way.

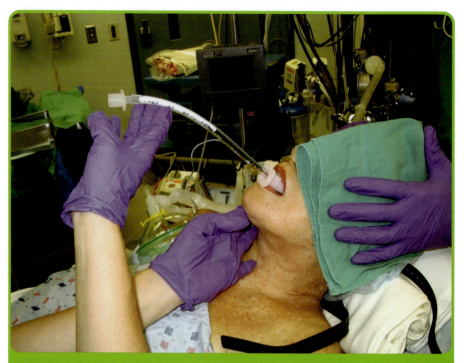

Figure 5. Load the tube into the oral airway, then you're halfway there. This also tells you how well topicalized the patient is. If they fight you at this point, pull everything out and topicalize again until they're nice and comfy cozy.

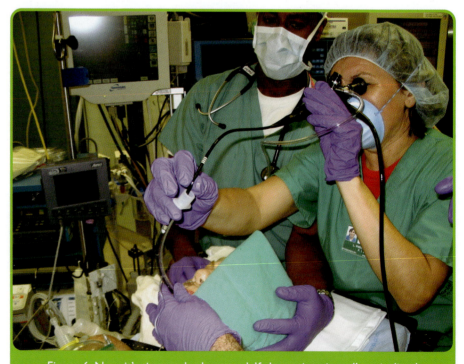

Figure 6. Now it's time to look around. If the patient is well-topicalized and sedated, then you can take your time.

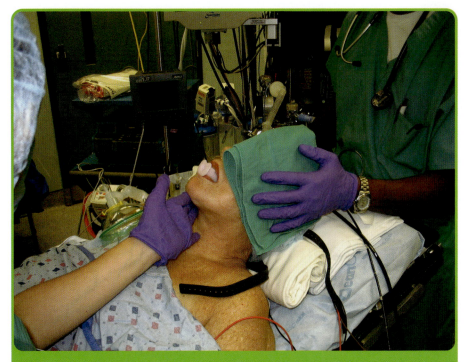

Figure 7. Great trick, lift the chin up. That will "separate" the trachea and esophagus a little and give you a better view. It also keeps everything aligned.

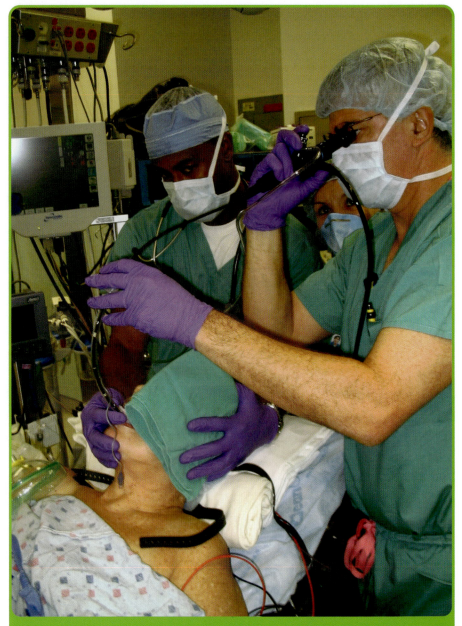

Figure 8. Look, look, look. You want to get the impression of being in a "cave" and seeing the epiglottis off in the distance. Then navigate underneath, and voila!

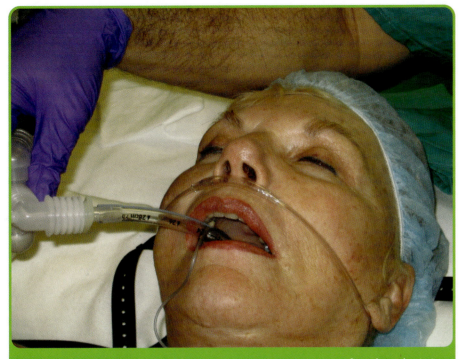

Figure 9. If all goes well, then the patient is even cooperative after the tube is in. You can do a neuro check (say you're doing a C-spine fracture case) and you can even have a patient move him/herself prone with the endotracheal tube in place. Too cool!

SUGGESTED READING

Albertini RE, Harrell JH, Kurihara N, et al. Arterial hypoxemia induced by fiberoptic bronchoscopy. *JAMA* 1974;230:1666–1667.

APIC guideline for infection prevention and control in flexible endoscopy. *AJIC Am J Infec Control* 1994;22:19–38.
- *This is a detailed review of the incidence of contamination of flexible scopes and the best ways of reprocessing them. In general, you would avoid throwing a fiberoptic into a boiling vat of Cidex, as this may adversely affect the equipment, for example.*

Asai T, Shingu K. Difficulty in advancing a tracheal tube over a fiberoptic bronchoscope: incidence, causes, and solutions. *Br J Anaesth* 2004;92:870–881.
- *This is a great article that speaks in depth on the forgotten problem of advancing the endotracheal tube over the fiberscope. In Figure 3 of the article, the authors intelligently explain how an esophageal intubation could happen even though the fiberscope was in the trachea. This has to be the most aggravating aspect of fiberoptic intubations, you're looking at the tracheal rings, but you still can't get the stupid tube in! Aaaaaarg!*

Atassi K, Mangiapan G, Fuhrman C, et al. Prefixed equimolar nitrous oxide and oxygen mixtures plus topical airway anesthesia reduces discomfort during flexible bronchoscopy in adult patients: a randomized, controlled, double-blind trial. *Chest* 2005;128:863–868.
- *This prestigious study proposed $N_2O:O_2$ 50:50 as an attractive means for minimizing discomfort, meanwhile maintaining spontaneous respiration adding to the safety of the technique. On a practical, OSHA-related note, though, you would be spilling a ton of nitrous oxide into the air during such a procedure.*

Bahhady IJ, Ernst A. Risks of and recommendations for flexible bronchoscopy in pregnancy. *Chest* 2004;126:1974–1981.
- *This article is one of the few articles on bronchoscopy during pregnancy. It ends with recommendations about the safety, use, and alternatives for bronchoscopy during pregnancy. Remember, the lost airway is the killer in obstetric anesthesia.*

British Thoracic Society Bronchoscopy Guidelines Committee, a Subcommittee of the Standards of Care Committee: British Thoracic Society guidelines on diagnostic flexible bronchoscopy. Thorax 2001;56(Suppl 1):11–21.
- *These guidelines highlighted the few absolute contraindications of flexible bronchoscopy.*

Caplan RA, Posner KL, Ward RJ, et al. Adverse respiratory events in anesthesia: a closed claims analysis. *Anesthesiology* 1990;72:828.
- *In this article the authors mentioned that an adverse respiratory event in the form of inadequate ventilation, esophageal intubation, and difficult tracheal intubation forms the largest single class of injury.*

Gonzalez R, Ramirez D, Hernandez M, et al. Should patients undergoing a bronchoscopy be sedated? *Acta Anaesthesiol Scand* 2003;47: 411–415.
- *This article found that a patient who was sedated before topicalization had better tolerance to fiberoptic intubation compared to those who did not receive sedation.*

Greenland KB, Lam MC, Irwin MG. Comparison of the Williams airway intubator and Ovasapian fiberoptic intubating airway for fiberoptic orotracheal intubation. *Anaesthesia* 2004;59:173–176.
- *This nice article showed that the Williams intubating airway had a better view of the glottis than the Ovasapian intubating airway. However both intubating airways offered similar intubating conditions once the glottis was exposed.*

Ho AM, Chung DC, Edward WH, et al. Total airway obstruction during local anesthesia in a non-sedated patient with a compromised airway. *Can J Anesth* 2004;51:838–841.
- *This is a case report about total airway obstruction following topical anesthesia in an 86-year-old patient with laryngeal cancer.*

Ho CM, Yin I.-W, Tsou K,-F et al. Gastric rupture after awake fiberoptic intubation in a patient with laryngeal carcinoma. *Br J Anaesth* 2005;94(6): 856–858.
- *Another case report that describes how oxygen insufflation under high pressure could lead to gastric rupture. Careful if you're blowing oxygen in there!*

Katz A, Michelson E, Stawicki J, et al. Cardiac arrhythmias: frequency during fiberoptic bronchoscopy and correlation with hypoxemia. *Arch Intern Med* 1981;141:603–606.

Krause A, Hohberg B, Heine F, et al. Cytokines derived from alveolar macrophages induce fever after bronchoscopy and bronchoalveolar lavage. *Am J Resp Crit Care Med* 1997;155: 1793–1797.

Lindholm CE, Ollman B, Snyder JV, et al. Cardiorespiratory effects of flexible fiberoptic bronchoscopy in critically ill patients. *Chest* 1978;74:362–368.
- *This article is one of Lindholm's series of articles studying the effects of bronchoscopy on the cardiopulmonary system.*

Lundgren R, Haggmark S, Reiz S. Hemodynamic effects of flexible fiberoptic bronchoscopy performed under topical anesthesia. *Chest* 1982;82(3):295–298.
- *This article relates bronchoscopy-induced stress to sympathetic overdischarge.*

Mitsumune T, Senou E, Adachi M. Prediction of patient discomfort during fiberoptic bronchoscopy. *Respirology* 2005;10:92–96.
- *This study predicted patients' discomfort from fiberoptic intubation based on the experience of the bronchscopist and the preprocedure anxiety level.*

Naguib ML, Streetman DS, Clifton S, et al. Use of laryngeal mask airway in flexible bronchoscopy in infants and children. *Pediatr Pulmonol* 2005;39:56–63.
- *This is a retrospective study that describes the ease of introducing the fiberscope through LMA compared to nasal introduction and introduction through endotracheal tube in the age groups, 3 months and 21 years.*

O'Brien JD, Ettinger NA, Shevlin D, et al. Safety and yield of transbronchial biopsy in mechanically ventilated patients. *Crit Care Med* 1997;25:440–446.

Reichert WW, Hall WJ, Hyde RW. A simple disposable device for performing fiberoptic bronchoscopy on patients requiring continuous artificial ventilation. *Am Rev Respir Dis* 1974;109:394–396.
- *This article points to the importance and smartness of the swivel connector in maintaining oxygenation of patients on mechanical ventilation during bronchoscopy.*

Sahn S, Scoggin C. Fiberoptic bronchoscopy in bronchial asthma: a word of caution. *Chest* 1976;69:39–42.

Schmitt HJ, Mang H, Schmitt J. Fiberoptic intubation in patients after radiotherapy for carcinoma of the head and neck: difficulty and predictability. *Eur J Anaesthesiol* 2004;21:914–927.
- *This is an interesting case report because it tells us that the factors that predict difficult laryngoscopy cannot predict difficult fiberoptic intubation. That is, of course, counterintuitive.*

Suratt P, Smiddy J, Gruber B. Deaths and complications associated with fiberoptic bronchoscopy. *Chest* 1976;69:747–751.

Articles 7-11 speak about the various complications of bronchoscopy in critically ill patients.

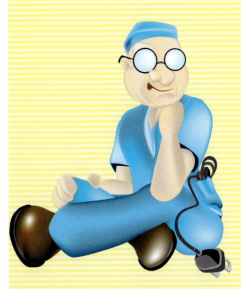

Wiretapping: The Retrograde Wire Intubation

Jong Y. Lee and
Rebecca Gilbert

INTRODUCTION

Wiretapping and you? We hope not. Few of you should place wiretaps (how many FBI anesthesiologists are there?). And few of you should have taps placed on your phones. Of course, with everything wireless now, we imagine it's easy to have your wireless wiretapped, if such a phrase makes any sense.

And, truth to tell, few of you will do the wiretap approach to securing the airway either. Let's face it, it's just not that common. But it has its place, so here's how to do it.

THE SHORT OF IT

- Get a wire and put it through the patient's neck/trachea.
- Retrieve it out from the mouth/nose.
- Place a catheter through the previous wire, and use it as a guide for placing your endotracheal tube.
- If you think this is exciting, then please read on.

SO WHO CAME UP WITH THIS ANYWAY?

- Discovered in the 1960s by Butler and Cirillo as an alternative technique to obtain an airway.
- Since then, the basic technique remains the same, but the hardware has been upgraded.

WHEN IS IT INDICATED?

- When you can't perform an endotracheal intubation by conventional oral or nasal methods because of difficulty visualizing the oropharynx secondary to blood, mass, or an unstable spine, among other reasons.
- Beware: You need time . . . usually three minutes. Less time than it takes to get halfway down that frappuccino crème caramel latte mocha.
- It is not a good idea to perform this procedure in emergency situations, that is, when your patient's saturating less than 90% and declining, or the blood pressure's going to the floor.
- If you can't intubate, you should be able to at least ventilate before considering this procedure.
- If unable to ventilate, think about cricothyrotomy or tracheostomy before the retrograde.
- Always remember the ASA Difficult Airway Guidelines.

PREPARATION: FOR YOU AND YOUR PATIENT

- What You Need
- Local anesthesia (if patient is awake).
- Minimum 18-g angiocatheter.
- 3-10 cc syringe; tuberculin syringe is *not* an option, and any size above 20 cc theoretically *can* be used, but it would be cumbersome . . .
- Long (we recommend at least 70 cm) guidewire to make the trip from the patient's neck into the patient's mouth.
- Any clamp to hold the wire in the skin (ask an OR nurse to lend you one if you need it).
- Magill forceps, or you could use your own fingers if you want to, but don't risk damaging them if you are a professional cellist or pickpocket.
- Guiding catheter (some professionals have used an ETT exchange catheter).
- Endotracheal tubes of different sizes (better first to test which will fit in the guiding catheter—it would be distracting to have to look for another ETT while the surgeon is apprehensively waiting to do the surgery).
- Retrograde intubation kits are available with all supplies included. If you are using the Cook retrograde kit, the minimum ETT size is 5 mm.
- When you don't have or want to use a guiding catheter over the wire, we recommend passing the wire through the Murphy eye so that the tip of the ETT does not get trapped in the epiglottis or the arytenoids. This hang-up at the crucial instant is the great downfall of this procedure.

> If the existing code does not permit district attorneys to have a hand in such dirty business [wiretapping], it does not permit the judge to allow such iniquities to succeed.
>
> *Oliver Wendell Holmes*
> Olmstead vs United States, 1928

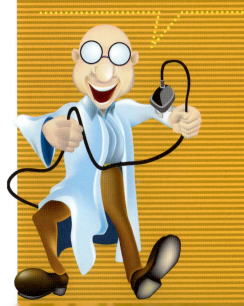

WHAT THE PATIENT NEEDS

- Normal coagulation profile because you will be going through skin, muscle, ligament, and membrane if you are lucky.
- Normal tracheal pathology, that is, no stenosis, deformity, or infections.
- These situations are not absolute contraindications, but should be evaluated in view of the clinical situation. As you saw in the earlier airway chapters, *all else* depends on the airway, so you sometimes have to buffalo through contraindications to secure the all-important *A* of *ABC*.
- Good access to the cricothyroid membrane (to attempt this procedure on a patient with a BMI of 40 and no visible neck would be very daunting). Also, patients with severe scoliosis—chin stuck on their chests—are not good candidates.

We believe that active determination of risk and benefits of the procedure should be continually evaluated during the procedure.

POSITIONING IS KEY!

- Have the patient lie supine with head extended to expose the cricothyroid membrane.
- If rolls are necessary for better neck exposure, ask for a shoulder roll.
- Finally, locate the cricothyroid membrane—remember, it's the membrane that spreads between the cricoid and thyroid cartilage.

IF YOU HAVE DECIDED FOR AN AWAKE RETROGRADE

- Topicalize the patient's oral or nasal pharynx and the airway for an invasive procedure. Choose the default airway topicalization that you are used to or use what we recommend here:
  - Antisialagogue (glycopyrrolate 0.2-0.4 mg IV will do the trick). Note, in Chapter 12, the authors make a pretty good argument for giving the antisialagogue IM. Fact is, either IM or IV will do it.
  - Cetacaine spray for the patients' pharyngeal and nasal mucosa, but don't use so freely because it quickly

causes methemoglobinemia. Read the label, it always helps.
  - 4% Lidocaine dripped down pharynx to topicalize airway above the vocal cords, transtracheal lidocaine to anesthetize the airway below the cords.

Note: If patients cough that's good; it means they're helping to spread the anesthetic in the airway for you.

  - If time permits, you should do a superior laryngeal nerve block.
  - Don't forget to make a skin weal with 2% lidocaine in the skin above the midline of the membrane before you puncture it.
  - Your patients may be sedated and airway nebulized, but will still feel pain on their skin.

Note: The retrograde technique has been done in a wide range of anesthesia from completely awake or little sedation to induced and paralyzed patients.

WHY THE CRICOTHYROID MEMBRANE YOU MIGHT ASK?

- First, it's easy to puncture.
- Most importantly, the large posterior surface of the cricoid cartilage helps prevent puncture of the esophagus if your angiocatheter is inserted too far.
- *Puncture* the midline of the cricothyroid membrane with your 18 (or larger) bore angiocatheter until you feel a loss of resistance.
- Loss of resistance indicates the end of your needle has entered the trachea.
- To confirm positioning of your needle, fill your 3-5 cc syringe with 1-2 cc of normal saline, attach the syringe to the catheter hub, and pull back on the plunger to see if bubbles appear in the fluid.
- Bubbles = Air = You're in the trachea, yea!
- No bubbles = You're not in the trachea. Redirect or start over.

Once you confirm you're in the trachea

- Angle your needle toward the head of the patient, about 45 degrees.
- Remove the needle from the angiocatheter.

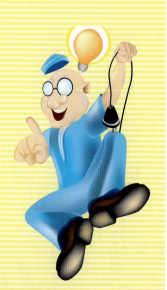

Grab your guidewire

- Thread the J end of your guidewire (loop side—the wire actually looks like a *J*) through the angiocatheter again continuing to angle toward the head of the patient.

- Look for the wire to emerge from the patient's nose or mouth.

- You may want to use the Magill forceps or your fingers, if you dare, when assisting with the emergence of the wire from the nasal or oral cavity.

- *Beware.* Do not lose the wire in the neck or, as the saying goes, you'll be stuck in a well-described creek with a boat but, alas, with no means of propulsive power.

- Remove the angiocatheter from the wire.

- Only after the guidewire has emerged from the proper orifice, secure it in the neck by clamping the wire near the skin with a Kelly or any other clamp. If the wire comes out the ear, for example, that would not be a good thing. If it drills its way out through the top of the head, this, also, is a suboptimal exit point.

Decision time . . .

- At this point, you may place the guidewire inside the lumen of your endotracheal tube (ETT) and thread the ETT down the trachea.
  - Lubricating the tube will ensure it slides easily down the patient's airway.
  - Again, ensure you don't lose your guidewire while sliding your ETT into the pharynx.

- Stop when you feel resistance. At some point, you will not be able to advance the ETT further since it is anchored by the wire in the neck, so you'll need to remove the wire.

. . . or you can choose to use the latest addition to the retrograde technique

- Use a guiding catheter over your wire before the ETT. A guiding catheter may be obtained from a premade kit, or you may use an ETT exchange catheter to facilitate the passage of the ETT through the trachea.
  - Thread the guiding catheter over the wire just as you would the ETT. The big advantage of this is you can now ventilate the patient with the ETT exchanger, and you have a stiffer surface to thread your ETT with.
  - Once your tube exchanger is in place, thread your ETT, and don't forget to lubricate your ETT.

- *Unclamp* your guidewire and remove it from the ETT out the nose or mouth.

Now confirm proper placement of the ETT

- Check for positive end-tidal CO_2.
- Bilateral breath sounds.
- Negative epigastric sounds.
- Chest X-ray.
- Secure your tube.

Celebrate! You've now completed your retrograde intubation.

NOT SO FAST! THERE ARE ALWAYS COMPLICATIONS TO BE AWARE OF

Bad

- Bleeding from trauma to the oral-nasal mucosa or underlying structures of the airway.

- Catheter threading caudal instead of cephalad could cause further damage to the lower airway structures.

- Infection of the neck tissue, but pulling out the guidewire from the mouth/nose instead of out the neck has reduced the incidence of this.

- Sore throat.

Really bad

- Puncture with the guidewire leading to pneumothorax, pneumomediastinum, subcutaneous emphysema.

- Esophageal puncture and wiring.

- The dreaded esophageal intubation.

- Failure of obtaining proper airway.

Let us reiterate, you must always assess proper placement of your ETT by multiple methods. Positive $ETCO_2$ alone is not enough—it does not prevent early detection of endobronchial intubation or a kinked or coiled tube in the airway. Check chest X-ray as soon as possible.

THINGS TO REMEMBER

- This is *not* an *emergency* technique!

- Retrograde intubation is a method for intubating patients that have failed traditional methods of intubation.

- You must have time on your side (at least three to five minutes).

- You are *not* ventilating the patient while you are threading the wire through the airway.

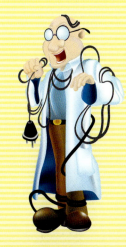

- Do not let your first retrograde intubation be on a desaturating and unstable patient.
- The old saying, "See one, do one, then teach one," exists for a reason.
- The goal is to try one on a mannequin or simulator before a real patient.

Note: This is not a very common procedure that is part of every curriculum in all universities, but studies have shown that could be very easily learned from mannequins or cadavers; the success rate has ranged from as low as 50% to more than 70%. To date, not enough literature exists to give any definitive answer.

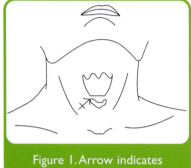

Figure 1. Arrow indicates crycothyroid membrane

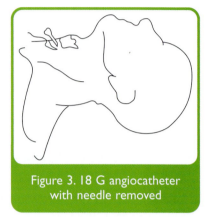

Figure 3. 18 G angiocatheter with needle removed

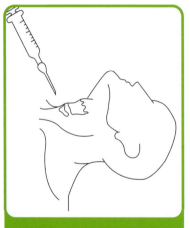

Figure 2. 18 gauge angiocatheter with syringe attached piercing crycothyroid membrane

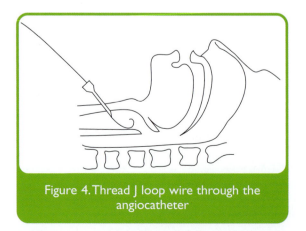

Figure 4. Thread J loop wire through the angiocatheter

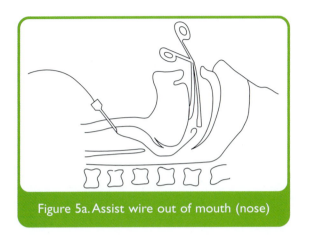

Figure 5a. Assist wire out of mouth (nose)

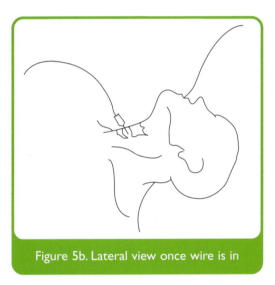

Figure 5b. Lateral view once wire is in

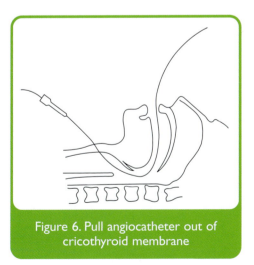

Figure 6. Pull angiocatheter out of cricothyroid membrane

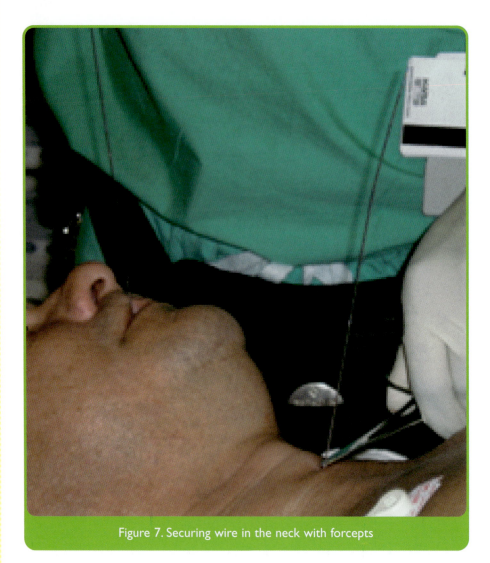

Figure 7. Securing wire in the neck with forcepts

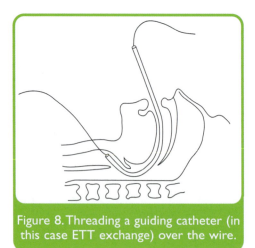

Figure 8. Threading a guiding catheter (in this case ETT exchange) over the wire.

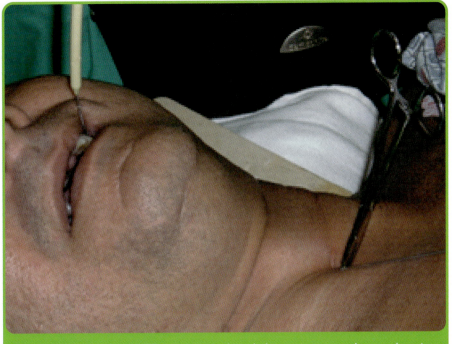

Figure 9. Live photos of ETT exachanger threaded in patients mouth over the wire.

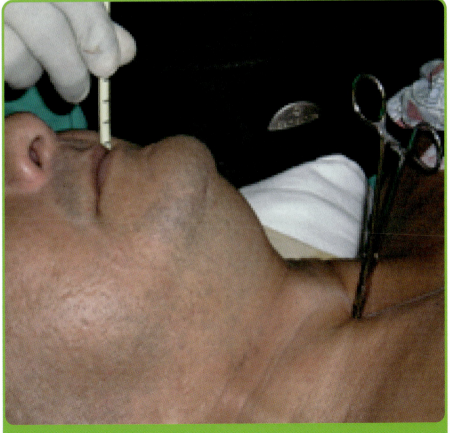

Figure 10. Live photos of ETT exachanger threaded in patients mouth over the wire.

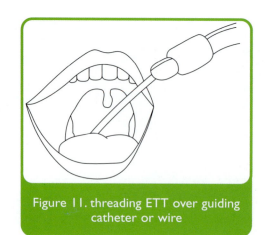

Figure 11. threading ETT over guiding catheter or wire

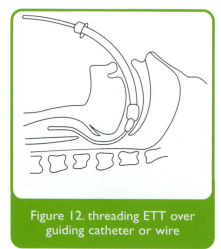

Figure 12. threading ETT over guiding catheter or wire

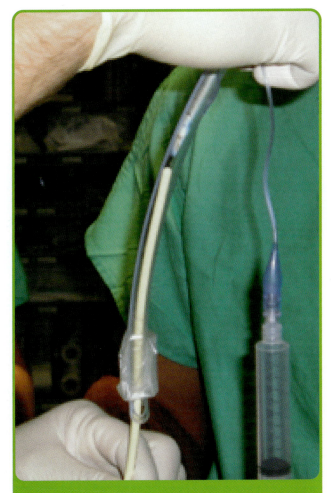

Figure 13. Threading ett over the tube exchanger.

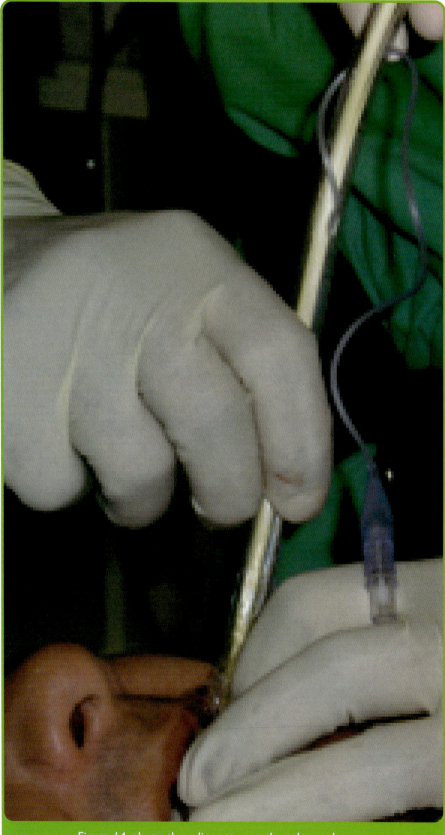

Figure 14. photo threading ett over the tube exchanger.

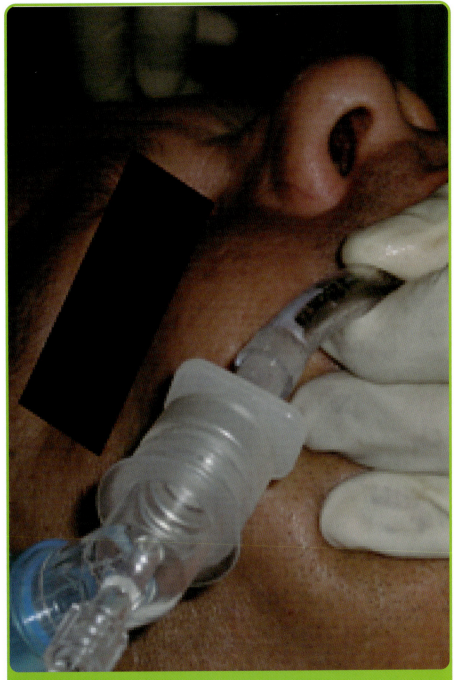

Figure 15. after wire/exchanger is removed Connect your patient to ambu bag or anesthesia circuit and confirm tube placement

SUGGESTED READING

Barash P, Slinger P, Sahoo M. *Clinical Anesthesia*, 4th ed. 2001, p 623–626.
- *This text gives a great overview of the procedure.*

Barriot P, Riou B. Retrograde technique for tracheal intubation in trauma patients. *Crit Care Med* 1988;16(7):712–713.
- *Report on 19 trauma patients intubated by retrograde technique, and the high success rate in securing the airway.*

Cook Incorporated. Cook retrograde intubation sets, suggested instructions for use. (2000) www.cookgroup.com.
- *This website has great illustrations of the technique for those of you who learn visually.*

Gill, M, Madden M, Green S. Retrograde endotracheal intubation: an investigation of indications, complications, and patient outcomes. *Am J Emerg Med* 2005;23:123–126.
- *This article goes over the multiple complications that can occur in a retrograde, and failures of the retrograde technique. Also stresses time as a big factor needed before performing this procedure. No mention is made of time required to drink a frappuccino crème caramel mocha latte.*

McNamara R. Retrograde intubation of the trachea. *Ann Emerg s*1987;16(6): 680–682.
- *Explains using the retrograde for more difficult airways, that is, cervical spine injury and anatomical distortions.*

Miller R, et al. Miller's Anesthesia, 6th ed. 2005, p 1638–1642.
- *Great section on topicalization of the airway.*

Parmet J, Metz S, Leuitt JD. Retrograde endotracheal intubation: an underutilized tool for management of the difficult airway. *Contemp Surg* Nov 1996;49(5).

- *Great article explaining the history and step-by-step technique of the retrograde intubation. The article has great illustrations.*

Shantha T. Retrograde intubation using the subcricoid region. *Brit J Anesth* June 1991;109–112.
- *This article gives another option for retrograde using subcricoid region as point of entry in the airway versus the cricothyroid membrane. Keep in mind, as you "go lower," the trachea "sinks deeper."*

Stralen D, Rogers M, Perkin RM, Fea S. Retrograde intubation training using a mannequin. *Am J Emerg Med* Jan 1995;13(1):50–52. Proof simulators work, and quick learning curve for the retrograde technique.

Chapter 30, the final chapter of this book, is "Simulators." The "prime motivator" in simulator work is, "Better to learn (and stumble) on a pretend patient than on a live patient."

Weksler N, Klein M, Sidelnick C, Chorni I. Retrograde tracheal intubation: beyond fiberoptic endotracheal intubation. *ACTA Anesthesiol Scand* 2004;48:412–416.
- *Retrospective review of retrograde intubations when the fiberoptic is not available or has failed. The day will come when the fiberoptic is broken/unavailable/stolen/in the shop, so it's worth knowing a few other tricks.*

Wijesinghe, H, Gough, J. Complications of retrograde intubation in a trauma patient. *Acad Emerg Med* 2000; (11):1267–1271.
- *Great case report of an 80-year-old, female s/p motor vehicle accident intubated with retrograde technique, but had an unrecognized inadequate intubation (tube was in the trachea, but coiled on itself). Stresses the importance of multiple checks to ensure your tube is in place.*

Fix Bayonets: The Surgical Alternative

Richard Silverman and Fani Nhuch

> Wickedness is always easier than virtue; for it takes the short cut to everything.
>
> *Samuel Johnson*
> Boswell, Journal of a Tour
> to the Hebrides
> September 17, 1773

INTRODUCTION

And the surgical alternative is the short cut (literally) to the trachea.

This route is wicked, indeed, and one we do not readily undertake. But keep in mind, we are the minders of the airway, and, as such, we have to know *all* the ways to get air into a patient. And sometimes that route involves steel.

Yipes!

This can seem awfully daunting, especially because it is so foreign to us to cut our way into the trachea. But it is doable. You just have to get the right mind-set, think through what you need to do, and when that day arrives, just do it!

INDICATIONS

- Emergent need for oxygenation.
- Emergent need for ventilation (Note: Ventilation comes second, as you can establish *oxygenation* more readily than *ventilation* in a hurry.)

CONTRAINDICATIONS

- In an emergency, with no other option available but death, there is no contraindication.
- Relative contraindication would be coagulopathy or an obstructing mass in the way, but even in these cases, if the alternative is death from hypoxemia, you'd still cut.

EQUIPMENT FOR A TRUE TRACHEOSTOMY

- For a true tracheostomy, you'd need a tracheostomy surgical tray.
- You'd rarely be called upon to do a full tracheostomy in a lost-airway emergency.

AN OUNCE OF PREVENTION

- Prevention of an airway disaster is better than treatment of an airway disaster.
- Use caution in assessing potentially difficult airways, get good at doing awake intubations, get good at using the intubating LMA, and—guess what—maybe, just maybe, you'll never have to do the surgical airway. Wouldn't that be great.

- Use the intubating LMA on a few easy airways, so you know the sequence of events, and the mechanics of the intubating LMA. Don't kid yourself into thinking you can magically do the intubating LMA right the very first time when you are in the middle of an airway catastrophe.

THE PHILOSOPHY OF THE SURGICAL AIRWAY

- Once you've decided you *must* go surgical (can't intubate, can't ventilate, can't wake the patient up and start all over, running out of time and options), then *go for it*. A surgical airway under emergency conditions may get ugly, may get bloody, but goddamn, Sam, what is the option?
- The option when you've run out of airway options is a dead patient, a brain-dead vegetative patient, *that's* the option.
- So don't get freaked or lose perspective in the middle of (what can be) a bloody mess—if you've got to cut the neck to save the patient, then cut that neck and get a move on!
- Hesitation will kill your patient.
- When things start to get sloppy, don't second-guess yourself . . . keep going. You've made your decision, now carry it out.
- When the airway is lost and you've got to go surgical, remember, hypoxemia will kill or maim the patient in just a few minutes.
- Hypercarbia will be a problem, yes, but later, many minutes later. And in an airway emergency, "a few minutes later" might as well be a hundred years later.

Okay, Now that I have Sold My Soul, Soiled My Drawers, and Promised to be a Nicer Person if All Goes Okay, How Effective is the Emergency Cricothyrotomy?

Depending on the technique and experience of the individual, the results vary greatly. But, by and large, emergency cricothyrotomy in the rescue of a failed airway always has a greater success than the alternative, death by hypoxia. A follow-up study conducted to assess the long-term outcome of 65 patients who had an emergency cricothyrotomy found that there were 27 survivors. Of the 27 patients, 13 had no subsequent airway problems, and the remaining 14 had only minor airway problems.

But this Could Never Happen to Me, I'm Too Careful

Maybe you are Caution Incarnate, but you never know when you may get called into a room where someone *else* made a bad judgment call.

Any anesthesiologist to room 2 STAT!"

You bound into the room, and there stands your partner, egg all over his face, telling you, "I can't intubate this guy and I gave 10 mg of Pavulon, and now I can't ventilate either!"

At this point, you can:

• Tell your partner, "Deal with it, it's your problem," and then leave the room.

• Do the right thing and help out. If you can't move air, even with an LMA in (better an LMA than going surgical right away!), then go surgical. Yes, you didn't cause this problem, but hell, the patient's life rides on getting oxygen now, so don't point fingers, start pointing Angiocaths at the cricothyroid membrane.

• Concentrate first on getting some oxygen in, then worry about the carbon dioxide later.

THE MENTAL LEAP THAT WILL PROVE YOUR SALVATION

• Surgical airway? "Oh God! How did it come to this? How can I do this!"

• Chill, there's a way of looking at this that will slow your pulse and steady your hand.

• All you are doing is placing an IV in a big vein—the trachea is that big, easy-to-hit vein.

• That's it! That's all you have to envision to turn this "Oh! My God! I've never done this before!" procedure into a "Hey, no big deal, I've been down this road before" procedure.

• If you've ever done a transtracheal block for an awake intubation, you've already done the hardest part of this procedure. (Incidentally, calling it a "transtracheal block" is a misnomer, it's actually a "transcricothyroid membrane block.")

• The cricothyroid membrane is shallow, it is fixed in place, and it is easy to hit. Instead of aspirating blood like you do in a vein, you aspirate air in this air-filled vein you are cannulating.

SURGICAL AIRWAY HISTORY AND PHYSICAL

• In the middle of a big disaster, you won't have time to find this stuff out.

• If by chance ahead of time you've been able to foresee this disaster, you would want to know a few things that might make cutting the neck problematic.

• Radiation.

• Neck surgery.

• Goiter or other mass obstructing access to the trachea.

• Hematoma (after a carotid endarterectomy or thyroidectomy, for example).

• Earlier tracheostomy (a tracheostomy in early childhood could be a real problem as scarring and stricture formation could make the trachea hard to hit.

• Mediastinal mass (a lost airway may not *be* a lost *upper* airway; a large mass down below could obstruct adequate ventilation and a tracheostomy won't help anything).

METHODS AND EQUIPMENT FOR A QUICK AND DIRTY EMERGENT CRICOTHYROTOMY

• IV catheter . . . very quick, but jet insufflation can get messy.

• Cannula over trocar . . . very dirty.

• Seldinger technique (commercially available kits) . . . moderately quick and not very dirty.

• Rapid four-step technique . . . questionable on quick, and definitely dirty.

• Rapid four-step technique using a Bair Claw . . . ditto of above.

• Surgical cricothyrotomy . . . not quick and definitely dirty.

IV CATHETER TECHNIQUE FOR JET-VENTILATION OXYGENATION

• Grab a 16-g or 14-g catheter.

• Connect the catheter to a 3-cc syringe.

• Palpate the cricothyroid membrane.

• Wipe alcohol on the spot if that makes you feel better.

• Insert the catheter into the midline of the cricothyroid membrane aiming in a slightly caudad direction.

• Aspirate as you go, when you get air, you have entered your air-filled vein, that is, the trachea.

• Slide the catheter in.

• Remove the needle.

• At this point, if you have a jet ventilator, you can connect it directly to the catheter and give short bursts of oxygen, always watching to make sure you don't get subcutaneous emphysema.

• Another thing you can do is to hook the 3-cc syringe to the catheter, put an endotracheal tube connector to the syringe, and then use an Ambu bag to force oxygen in there. You obviously can't ventilate through an IV catheter, but you can oxygenate through an IV catheter.

AD HOC KIT THAT, BELIEVE IT OR NOT, WILL SAVE YOUR BUTT AND IS EASY TO FIND

• Swan introducer kit

Options once you have a catheter in the trachea

A catheter in the trachea gives you lots of options:

- You can now slide a wire down into the trachea, and expand the hole.
- For example, you can grab a Swan introducer kit, slide the wire down the catheter, and place an introducer through the cricothyroid membrane, just as you would place an introducer in a vein!
- With the introducer in place, you can do more robust jet ventilation, and you can even ventilate to a small degree.
- Another option is to place a wire through the catheter and use the wire in the Seldinger-technique fashion, cutting along the wire, and sliding a small endotracheal tube (say, a 6.0) down the wire. Now you *can* ventilate.
- You can also thread a wire *up* and into the mouth, put that wire through the Murphy eye of an endotracheal tube, and slide the tube in the tracheal through the mouth. Too cool . . . but is really now a retrograde wire intubation.

CANNULA OVER LARGE-BORE NEEDLE TROCAR (COMMERCIALLY AVAILABLE) KITS

The Quicktrach by Rusch consists of a preassembled emergency cricothyrotomy unit with a 10-cc syringe attached to a padded needle and connecting tube. The system uses a plastic cannula with a fixable flange over a removable stainless steel large-bore trocar needle. These come in two sizes, 2.0 mm and 4.0 mm. While the Quicktrach was compared favorably to some other methods, concern has been raised over potential damage to the other neck structures if the operator strays from the midline. Therefore some practitioners (authors included) prefer the smaller-gauge cannula-over-needle or needle-and-guidewire techniques as inherently safer in the emergency situation.

1. Nu-Trake (by Bivona) Adult Cricothyrotomy Kit (above) and Pedia-Trake Pediatric Emergency Cricothyrotomy Kit (not pictured) uses the single large-bore puncture technique with sequential dilation. While there is significant debate about using this technique, it is the authors' preference to use a Seldinger method.

SELDINGER TECHNIQUE
Anatomy and landmarks

Frequently the patient is not calmly sitting on the table simply awaiting a cricothyrotomy. In the rare case there is some suspicion that an invasive airway would be needed, it is best to mark out the structures. In an emergency, however, simply identifying the cricothyroid membrane will suffice. Again, this is not necessarily an easy task in the face of a desaturating patient and, more particularly, in the obese. The cricothyroid membrane's dimensions are vertically 8-19 mm (mean 13.6), and width between the cricothyroid muscles from 9-19 mm (mean, 12.3 mm)—sufficient area in which to identify the space. Additionally, it has been reported that 62% of patients have an artery delineated transversely across the cricothyroid membrane.

- Once you have identified the cricothyroid membrane you are ready to access the airway. Prepare a syringe partially filled with saline and attach a needle of 18-gauge (hollow bore).
- Percutaneously pierce your needle through the skin and the cricothyroid membrane. It is recommended to stabilize the structures with your fingers on both sides of the needle. Without stabilization, it is relatively easy to get off midline and be unsuccessful.
- It is vital that you freely aspirate bubbles of air to insure that indeed you are in the airway. At this point, direct your needle slightly caudad (to the feet!). If you do not have a free flow of bubbles, stop, remove your needle, identify the landmarks, and start anew.
- Disconnect the syringe and pass a soft-tip J-wire. The wire should easily pass through the needle (bevel up), and advance 3-4 cm beyond the tip of the needle.
- Remove the needle leaving the guidewire in situ.
- Make a small vertical stab incision at the origin of the wire, and mount the cricothyrotomy tube (over its introducer) over the wire.
- With the wire secured, advance the cricothyrotomy and its dilator in a caudad direction over the guidewire. If necessary, you may taut back the skin or, alternatively, make a larger skin incision to accommodate the apparatus, or do both.

Don't Make Perfect the Enemy of Good

In the bloody mess of a surgical airway, it's worth recalling the mantra, "Don't make *perfect* the enemy of *good*." A surgeon called in to help cutting may spend a lot of time doing the down-low, routine trach—a perfect trach. Don't let the surgeon waste time doing this. Insufflate and establish oxygenation up high in the easy-to-get-at cricothyroid membrane. If you're still having trouble, establish a better airway still up high at the easy-to-get-at cricothyroid membrane.

Up there, you'll get a good, not a perfect airway. Good is good enough for now.

"Good is good enough for now." Make that the mantra of your surgical airway.

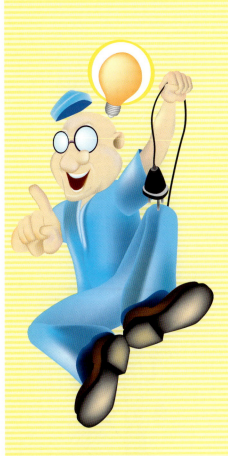

- Withdraw the guidewire and the introducer/dilator leaving the cricothyrotomy tube in place.
- Secure (suture in) the wings of the cricothyrotomy tube. At this point, you may attach the jet ventilation connection or an Ambu bag to ventilate the patient.

COMMERCIAL KITS

- These all rely on the same principle: You find the air-filled vein, then you advance a wire, then you use the Seldinger technique to put a big IV in a big air-filled vein.

There are a number of commercial kits available for the cricothyrotomy. Some are of the one-step, catheter-over-needle variety versus the Seldinger technique. While it would seem intuitive that the fewer steps would yield the fastest results, a comparison of the two methods shows conflicting outcome. The most common problem with the one-step kit was the inability to find and access the cricothyroid membrane. In the calm of an awake or stable patient this may seem unfathomable, but in the frenzied situation of losing an airway, frequently it is not as straightforward as one would hope. The Seldinger technique permits greater flexibility in this regard before introducing larger-bore apparatus.

RAPID FOUR-STEP TECHNIQUE

In 1997, BT Brofeldt described his rapid four-step technique. Simply put, the four steps are:

1. Palpation (of cricothyroid membrane)
2. Stab incision of same
3. Inferior traction of the first tracheal ring
4. Tube insertion

As described, the procedure can be completed in less than 30 seconds without the use of suction or additional light source. The only equipment needed is a #20 scalpel, a tracheal hook with a large radius, and a cuffed endotracheal tube.

RAPID FOUR-STEP TECHNIQUE WITH BAIR CLAW

This technique was an investigational adaptation of the four-step technique in which the stab and inferior traction were combined by using a scalpel with an attached (newly designed) spreading/grasping device.

There has been no manufacturing of this product. In comparison with the standard surgical cricothyrotomy on cadavers it was thought the rapid four-step with the Bair Claw was faster and appeared to be equally safe although little literature seems to indicate this method is practiced. It is mentioned here for completeness.

REAL, LIVE SURGICAL CRICOTHYROTOMY

- If you get to this point, by now you've cried "Bloody Murder" and gotten a surgeon to help you.
- If such is not the case, first go with the cricothyrotomy procedures described earlier. If you flounder through a first-time surgical cricothyrotomy without giving any oxygen, you've had it.
- God forbid you have to do this, but remember, cut high and get the easy-to-get-to cricothyroid membrane, don't go low where *real* tracheostomies are done. Real tracheostomies are too deep, and it will take too long to get in there.
- Some clever ENT can later clean up any mess you make. You are doing this to save a life, so don't fret the details right now.
- Extend the neck . . . what about the C-spine? (Don't worry too much, cricothyrotomy results in a small, but insignificant amount of movement across an unstable C-spine injury.)
- Prep and localize if you have time.
- Bluntly retract everything out of your way.
- Cut transverse across the cricothyroid membrane and insert a tracheal hook cephalad of the incision with traction applied to the thyroid cartilage.
- Place an endotracheal tube.
- Hook up to oxygen.
- Collapse and have a nervous breakdown.

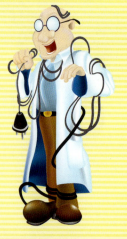

REAL, LIVE TRACHEOSTOMY

- Leave that to the surgeons.
- If they go that route, make sure you are oxygenating from above somehow while they are cutting and getting down there.

GLITCHES

- The main glitch is having to do this in the first place. Don't be lazy about keeping your fiberoptic skills up. Don't be lazy when a patient's airway looks bad from the start.
- The next glitch is the fatal hesitation halfway into the cutting: "But wait, maybe we should . . ." To hell with that. When you decide to do it, do it.
- High-pressure insufflation can cause barotraumas.
- Slashing in a hurry can cause damage to all kinds of things—vascular and neurologic—but keep in mind you are only doing this to save a life, not because you feel like it.

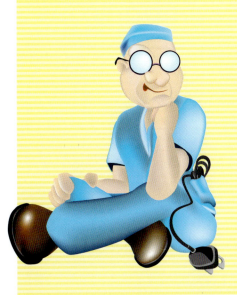

Figure 1. Patient with a serious Leforte type X fracture.

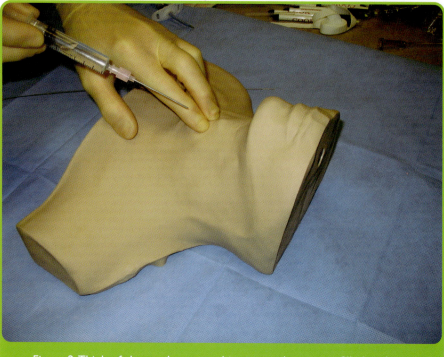

Figure 2. Think of the trachea as nothing more than a vein filled with air.

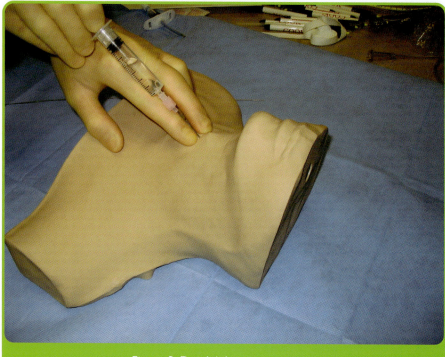

Figure 3. Doink 'til you aspirate air.

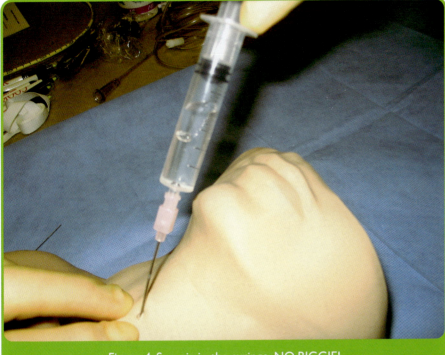

Figure 4. See, air in the syringe. NO BIGGIE!

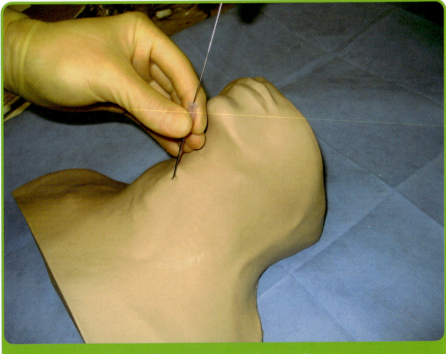

Figure 5. Now, Seldinger city. In goes the wire.

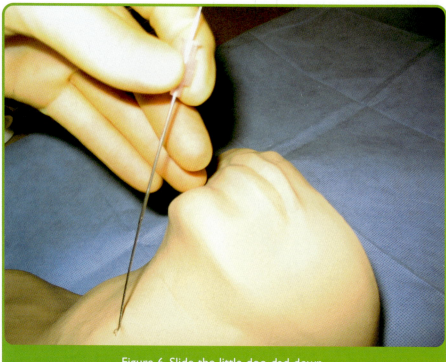

Figure 6. Slide the little doo-dad down.

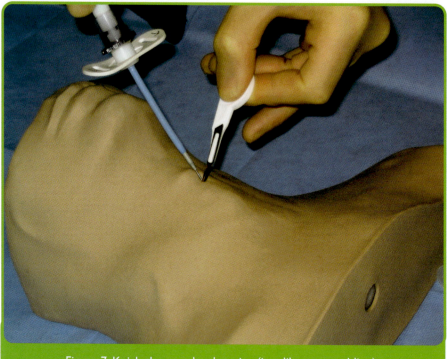

Figure 7. Knick the area by the wire (just like a central line).

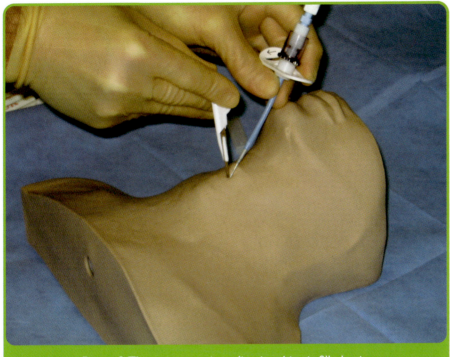

Figure 8. This is just putting a line in a big air-filled vein.

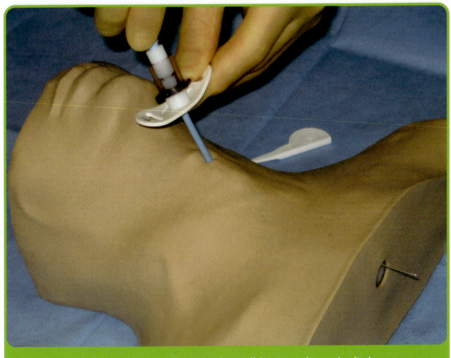

Figure 9. Shove like you mean it, this will be crunchy and a little gross.

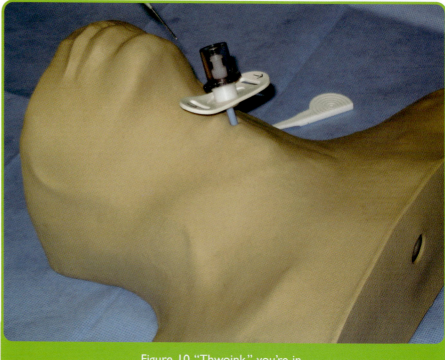

Figure 10. "Thwoink," you're in.

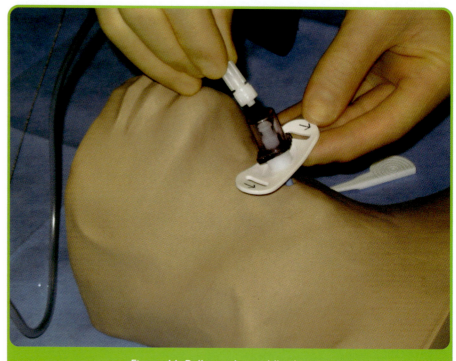

Figure 11. Pull out the middle thingie.

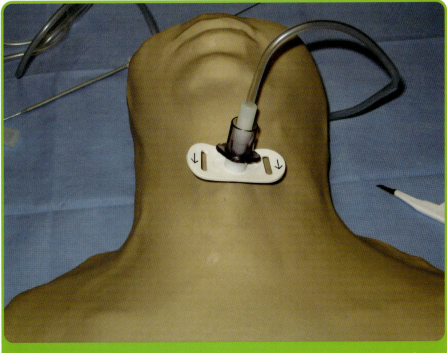

Figure 12. Hook up, and voila, your patient is no longer a facultative anaerobe.

SUGGESTED READING

Bair AE, Sakles JC. A comparison of a novel cricothyroidotomy device with a standard surgical cricothyrotomy technique; a brief report. *Acad Emerg Med* Nov 1999;6(11).
- *The authors feel there was significant improvement of this technique over a standard surgical cricothyrotomy in terms of subjective ease and time to secure an invasive airway, the need for fewer instruments, and possible safety benefits. However, the authors do caution that there was not formal assessment of hemorrhage or damage in this study.*

Bennett JD, Guha SC, Sankar AB. Cricothyroidotomy: anatomical basis. *J Roy Col Surg Edin* Feb 1996;41(1):57–60
- *In this article, cadaveric measurements were taken of the cricothyroid membrane to determine the actual surgical access in a range of clinically relevant scenarios.*

Berridge PD, Pollock KM, et al. Emergency airway equipment and training. *Anaesthesia* 2005;60:287–297.

Brofeldt BT, Panacek EA, Richards JR. An easy cricothyrotomy approach: the rapid four-step technique. *Acad Emerg Med* Nov 1996;3(11):1060–1063.
- *This article introduces us to the four-step rapid technique for emergency cricothyrotomy. This is essentially a blind surgical procedure. One of the key flaws in this trial is the use of cadaveric simulation.*

Davis DP, Bramwell KJ, Hamilton RS, et al. Safety and efficacy of the rapid four-step technique for cricothyrotomy using a Bair Claw. *J Emerg Med* 2000;19(2): 125–129.
- *This study attempted to further investigate benefits and risk of the rapid four-step procedure with the Bair Claw. The authors concluded the RFST with Bair Claw was faster than open cricothyrotomy, and appeared to be equally as safe. However, there are significant concerns in that conclusion. The trials were again under idealized conditions, cadavers. No clinical outcome data was possible and those cadavers with poorly identifiable landmarks in the test group were excluded. Furthermore, the airways were not dissected open to evaluate the posterior wall for injury.*

Fikkers BG, van Vught S, van der Hoeven JG, et al. Emergency cricothyrotomy; a randomized crossover trial comparing the wire-guided and catheter-over-needle techniques. *Anaesthesia* Oct 2004;59(10):1008.
- *This paper was an earlier comparison of the reference 1 using prepared pig larynxes. Here the investigators found the catheter over the needle technique faster than the wire-guided and subjectively easier to perform. The accuracy was not significantly different, and one complication was found in the over-the-wire technique. It should be noted that significant difference between this reference and the previous can be attributed*

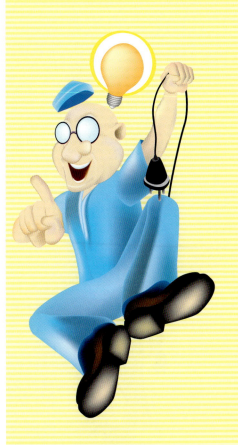

to the experiment models. The article by Schaumann used human cadaver versus prepared pig larynx. Intuitively, it would seem the human cadaver models would be more representative of a real-world situation.

Gerling MC, Davis DP, Hamilton RD, Morris GF, et al. Effect of surgical cricothyrotomy on the unstable cervical spine in a cadaver model of intubation. *J Emerg Med* 2001;20(1):1–5.

- *In cadaveric models it was found that surgical cricothyrotomy may have only 1-2 mm AP displacement and less than 1 mm of axial compression and, therefore, less than the threshold for clinical significance.*

Schaumann N, Lovenz V, Schellongowski P, et al. Evaluation of Seldinger technique emergency cricothyroidotomy versus standard surgical cricothyroidotomy in 200 cadavers *Anesthesiology* Jan 005;102(1):7–11.

- *This paper compared the two techniques with 20 emergency physicians in relation to the time to identify the location of the cricothyroid membrane, tracheal puncture, and time to first ventilation on cadavers. Both groups were monitored for injuries. The groups performing the Seldinger technique performed significantly faster and with no associated thyroid vascular injuries versus a significant number in the conventional group.*

Evaluation of Seldinger Technique Emergency Cricothyroidotomy versus Standard Surgical Cricothyroidotomy in 200 Cadavers. Schaumann, N, Lovenz V, Schellongowski P, et al. Anesthesiology 102(1):7–11, January 2005

- *This paper compared the two techniques with twenty emergency physicians in relation to the time to identify the location of the cricothyroid membrane, tracheal puncture and time to first ventilation on cadavers. Both groups were monitored for injuries. The groups performing the Seldinger technique performed significantly faster and with no associated thyroid vascular injuries versus a significant number in the conventional group.*

Emergency cricothyrotomy; a randomized crossover trial comparing the wire-guided and catheter-over-needle techniques. Fikkers BG, van Vught S, van der Hoeven JG et al. Anaesthesia 59(10) p1008- October 2004

- *This paper was an earlier comparison of the reference 1 using prepared pig larynxes. Here the investigators found the catheter over the needle technique faster than the wire guided and subjectively easier to perform. The accuracy was not significantly different and one complication was found in the over the wire technique. It should be noted*

that significant difference between this reference and the previous can be attributed to the experiment models. The article by Schaumann used human cadaver versus prepared pig larynx. Intuitively it would seem the human cadaver models would be more representative of a real world situation.

Cricothyroidotomy: anatomical basis. Bennett JD, Guha SC, Sankar AB, J Royal College of Surgeons Edinburgh. 41(1): 57–60, 1996 Feb.

- *In this article, cadaveric measurements were taken of the cricothyroid membrane to determine the actual surgical access in a range of clinically relevant scenarios.*

An easy cricothyrotomy approach: the rapid four-step technique. Brofeldt BT, Panacek EA, Richards JR, Academic Emergency Medicine, 3(11):1060-3, 1996 Nov.

- *This article introduces us to the four-step rapid technique for emergency cricothyroidotomy. This is essentially a blind surgical procedure. One of the key flaws in this trial is the use of cadaveric simulation.*

A Comparison of a Novel Cricothyroidotomy Device with a Standard Surgical Cricothyrotomy Technique; A brief report. Bair AE, Sakles JC. Academic Emergency Medicine, Vol 6(11), November 1999

- *The authors feel there was significant improvement of this technique over a standard surgical cricothyrotomy in terms of subjective ease and time to secure an invasive airway, the need for fewer instruments and possible safety benefits. However, the authors do caution that there was not formal assessment of hemorrhage or damage in this study.*

Safety and Efficacy of the Rapid Four-Step Technique for Cricothyrotomy using a Bair Claw. Davis DP, Bramwell KJ, Hamilton RS et al., J of Emergency Medicine Vol. 19 No. 2, pp125-129, 2000

- *This study attempted to further investigate benefits and risk of the rapid four-step procedure with the Bair Claw. The authors concluded the RFST with Bair Claw was faster than open cricothyrotomy and appeared to be equally as safe. However, there are significant concerns in that conclusion. The trials were again under idealized conditions, cadavers. No clinical outcome data was possible and those cadavers with poorly identifiable landmarks in the test group were excluded. Furthermore, the airways were not dissected open to evaluate the posterior wall for injury.*

Emergency airway equipment and training. Berridge PD, Pollock KM et al. Anaesthesia 2005, 60 pp.287–297

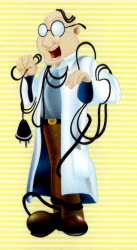

Effect of surgical cricothyrotomy on the unstable cervical spine in a cadaver model of intubation. Gerling MC, Davis DP, Hamilton RD, Morris GF et al. J of Emergency Medicine Vol 20, No. 1, pp1-5, 2001

- *In cadaveric models it was found that surgical cricothyrotomy may have only 1-2 mm AP displacement and less than 1 mm of axial compression and therefore less than the threshold for clinical significance.*

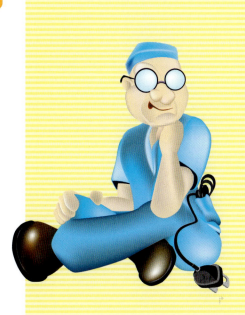

PART 4

ET TU, BRUTE?
A STAB IN
THE BACK

Oh Good, CSF! The Spinal

Christina Matadial and Jeffrey Schubert

INTRODUCTION

You will stick a few backs in your day, and when the patient complains, it will be like a penknife in your heart.

Let's find a few ways to make the spinal easier for the patient and, for that matter, easier for you.

It's like a stick across your back;
And when your back begins to smart,
It's like a penknife in your heart.

A Man of Words and Not of Deeds
Nursery rhyme,
date of origin unknown

INDICATIONS

- Anesthesia from about the midabdomen down (you can do higher abdominal operations with a spinal, but you're pushing it).
- Diagnostic withdrawal of cerebrospinal fluid (something internists do more than we do, but sometimes you'll be called to help them get it).
- Placement of a catheter for continuous spinal anesthesia (mostly done in the obstetric world, but if you get a wet tap doing an epidural, you can put the epidural catheter into the CSF and run a continuous spinal).
- Placement of a CSF catheter (again, through an epidural needle) for therapeutic drainage of CSF fluid during an aortic arch operation (for spinal cord protection).

CONTRAINDICATIONS

- Coagulopathy (risk of hematoma).
- Hypovolemia (the sympathectomy that is produced, coupled with hypovolemia, may cause catastrophic hypotension).
- Elevated intracranial pressure (could cause herniation).
- Infection at the site of injection.
- Systemic infection (relative contraindication, that is, you are concerned about seeding the CSF).
- Stenotic valvular lesion (aortic or mitral) where a sudden loss in SVR could result in a fatal drop in blood pressure.
- Mass in the spinal column (metastatic prostate CA, for example).
- Preexisting neurologic problems (relative contraindication; say you had someone with a lot of sciatica, back operations, and ongoing pain—you would hesitate to stick this person's back).

EQUIPMENT

- Spinal kit.
- Gloves, cap, mask, observing universal precautions.
- Good lighting.
- Standard ASA monitors, resuscitation, and intubation equipment.
- Someone to hold the patient in good position . . . more important than the person holding the spinal needle!

PHILOSOPHY OF SPINALS

- Spinal anesthesia provides great, reliable anesthesia for operations in the southern hemisphere of the body.
- Any spinal can fail, wear off, or can be spotty, so always be ready to go with a general anesthetic.
- A spinal is not a guarantee that you won't face the airway!
- Pushing a spinal high into the upper abdomen will compromise the patient's breathing.
- Keep in mind what the surgeon will be doing; a low operation with a lot of peritoneal stretching or tugging (insufflation, for example) won't do well under spinal anesthesia.
- No matter how you look at it, a spinal with a bigger needle (22 g) is easier to get than a spinal with a smaller needle (25 or 26 g). So, although you always want to do a spinal with the smallest caliber needle, go bigger if you are having a terrible time (obese patient, arthritis) or if you are in a hurry (C-section with a nonreassuring fetal heart tone). A resultant spinal headache can be problematic, but it's not fatal. Not getting a spinal in a C-section patient in time can be fatal.

Someday, Someday

Some day, someone smarter than you and I will develop a spinal needle with a teeny-weeny echo device at the end of it. You'll lay that needle on the skin and it will send you back a sonar picture that says one of two things:

1. Bone
2. Space

Then you'll sail that spinal needle right through the bones and *thronk* the spinal fluid first time, every time.

Oh, Brave New World that'll have such stuff in it!

But for now we're stuck doing the Singer Sewing Machine Shuffle:

- Bone, dead ahead, Captain.

- *Boink!*

- "Damn, bone."

- Redirect.

- *Boink!*

- "Damn!"

- Redirect.

- *Boink!*

Do a Spinal, It's Safer. Signed: Your Friendly Neighborhood Cardiologist

Spinals, in spite of what cardiologists and internists seem to think, are not a "safe alternative to that most dangerous of things, a general anesthetic," so don't be a weenie when it comes to optimizing your patient before a spinal.

Oh, this guy's sick as a dog, but heck, he's *just* getting a spinal, so let's roll . . . it's not like he's getting a *real* anesthetic.

Wrongo.

SPINAL HISTORY AND PHYSICAL

- Ask about earlier spinal procedures (Harrington rods, laminectomies, epidural steroids for chronic back pain).

- Review the history and labs for any contraindication, for example, coagulopathy, antiplatelet medication (clopidogrel within seven days, ticlopidine within 10 days, aspirin is ok), aortic stenosis, metastatic CA to the spine.

- The American Society for Regional Anesthesia has a website (www.asra.com) with updates on the latest anticoagulant therapy, and how long we should wait. As new and improved antiplatelet drugs are developed (we'll be seeing more variants of clopidogrel and ticlopidine in the future, no doubt), keep up-to-date through the society's latest recommendations.

- Examine the planned site of injection, looking for skin irritation or infection (beware the patient with a decubitus ulcer down low, that infection can snake up under the skin and go all over the place).

- Examine the back looking for scars, scoliosis, or arthritis that could make placement of the needle difficult.

Always have informed consent prior to starting this or any procedure.

TECHNIQUE: SITTING

- Have the room set up to induce general anesthesia—just in case—making sure you have working airway equipment.

- Make sure you have a good IV and that you have volume loaded the patient in anticipation of the coming sympathectomy and drop in blood pressure.

- Sit patients up with due care, and make sure someone stays with them to see they don't fall over (from sedation, a vagal response, or if hypotension ensues rapidly after the spinal is in). Fancy sites will have a prefabricated, stay-in-place holder device to ensure proper positioning of the patient. A sympathetic circulator or medical student will do just as well.

- A nice cooked-shrimp shape to the back is the desirous position.

- If patients have a shrimp allergy, tell them to curl up like a mad cat.

- If cats trigger asthma, tell them to curl over like a downhill skier.

- If they've never skied, are allergic to cats and shrimp, then . . . well . . . then *show* them . . . or something! How many damned curled-up analogies can you come up with?

- The holders are the key. If they get the patient to pop open those spaces, you are golden. The most often cause of failure to get a space is the holder not getting the patient in optimum position.

- Prep and drape the area and glove up.

- Get your spinal kit ready.

- Pick an appropriate needle. The pencil-point needles are less likely to give spinal headaches. If you use a Quincke-type needle, turn the bevel sideways so it *parts* the fibers rather than *pokes* the fibers.

- Find the L 3-4 or L 4-5 interspace, using the anterior superior iliac spine as your landmarks, if palpable. (You can go L 2-3, though that starts to get a little close to the spinal cord, and you can go to the L 5-S 1 interspace, the so-called Taylor approach, but most people don't.)

- If you go midline, then feel the space, put a moderate amount of local in the spot, and proceed. The key to a quiet patient is good local anesthetic administration.

- If you go paramedian, then put your local 1-2 cm lateral to the midline of the chosen interspace.

- If you choose a 25-g needle or smaller, an introducer needle may be easier to stabilize your tiny gauge one as you proceed through the tougher tissues, like skin.

- Slide the needle effortlessly into the subarachnoid space as if you had X-ray vision.

- If you hit bone, curse your fate.

- Redirect if you hit bone, aiming to *not* hit bone again and *to* hit CSF this time.

- If you hit bone again, mutter to yourself about the myriad advantages of general anesthesia, and who the hell's idea was it anyway to do this stupid spinal.

- You could write volumes about *how* to redirect.

- If you hit bone *right away*, then you've hit the superior spinous process, if you hit bone *after a while*, you've hit the inferior spinous process. All of this talk is hooey because it all just boils down to the same thing: Do something else. Try up, try down, try a little this way, try a little that way, and if none of this stuff works, then go to a different interspace because this just ain't happening, Jack.

- You can start midline and end up getting it paramedian. Fine, as long as you got it.
- You can start paramedian and end up getting it midline. Fine, as long as you get it.
- Ultimately, it's a bit of blindman's bluff, with you trying to visualize what you're hitting. Picture a spinal column (look at a plastic model), and just keep redirecting in a way that makes sense.
- Once you finally get the CSF, make sure the flow is good.
- Once the flow is good, hook up your syringe of local anesthetic.
- Master a technique, any technique, for stabilizing the hob of the needle to prevent excess movement as you attach the syringe and inject.
- Aspirate, and make sure you see a swirl (you're still in) and not a bubble (you're not in).
- Inject.
- Once you're done, pull out the needle, wipe off the area, and get the patients lying down.
- Check blood pressure right away, and talk to the patients.
- If they are talking, that is good. If they're not talking, that may not be good. Make sure they are conscious, and that they have stable vitals.
- Checking your level, temperature (using an alcohol pad), and pinpricking are the usual ways. Some more creative souls have used a nerve stimulator. Ouch!

TECHNIQUE: ON THE SIDE

- Do all the same preparatory work as for the midline approach.
- Find that interspace.
- With patients on their sides, you'll often find their backs are more relaxed and you can dig in your thumb a little deeper and get a good feel for that interspace.
- If you hit bone, keep in mind the back may be sagging and you could be hitting the side of the vertebra. Palpate again for the interspace.
- A word of note: Females tend to have a less perfectly horizontal lie (because of their curvier hips) than male patients. Be sure to trace out the direction of the spine all the way to your chosen interspace prior to starting.

VARIANTS

- You can do a hypobaric spinal by placing local anesthetic in preservative-free water. This, theoretically, will limit the sympathectomy to one side. (Adust the up leg in a fem-pop, for example, and you'll get less blood-pressure perturbation.)
- You can also do a hypobaric spinal in the jackknife position for anal surgery.
- If you are feeling absolutely wild, you can do prone, hypobaric spinal anesthesia for a laminectomy! If the local wears off, give the surgeon another spinal needle and he can put more in for you since he can see the subarachnoid space right in front of him or her. Too crazy!

GLITCHES

- The whole damn deal with spinals is bouncing off the bone and not being able to get into the CSF.
- Too bad someone doesn't invent a Site-Rite for the backbone that would help us see our way in there.
- If you've had a tough time getting in, and you hook up your syringe and aspirate, looking for the swirl, and instead get the "bubble of disappointment," then disconnect and try again. Don't inject your local thinking, "Well, I was in before, surely this will work now!" It won't.
- If you do your spinal and it is just not working at all, redo the spinal. Don't waste everyone's time hoping and praying that "it will set up soon." It won't.
- If you *pwoing* a nerve and the patient jumps, stop. Don't keep jamming and risking nerve damage.
- The peridural space contains blood vessels. So does the skin, and subcutaneous tissues. Sometimes, our needles will traverse one or the other of these. Some times we will also hit the CSF. If you see what appears to be blood, let a few drops go, and see if it clears. If it clears, yahoo! If it doesn't clear, or spurts like a bleeder, it probably *is* a bleeder. Remove the needle, and hold pressure until it stops. Try again in another place.

TO SIT OR NOT TO SIT

Sitting, or on the side?

Eventually, you want to get good at doing both, so don't fixate on one way, and become

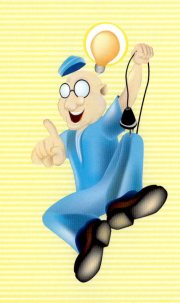

Another Word on a Little Extra Local

When you usually do a spinal, you have an itty-bitty bottle of local. That's just enough to localize if you nail this on the *first* try and don't have to move around. But, the world being the way it is, that doesn't always happen.

Then what do you do? You've already used all the local, you're gloved up, your assistant is holding the patient, and it's such a pain in the ass to get more local—you end up blowing off *more* local, and just sticking your poor patient in a different place, hoping no one notices.

I got news for you. Your patient notices.

And I, your guilty conscience looking over your shoulder, also notice.

Here's how to solve that little dilemma:

Open the kit, then *before* you glove up, draw up 10 cc of 1% lidocaine in a different syringe and squirt it into the spinal kit. That way, you have a whole lot of local already sitting in the kit. If you miss, you can just reach right down and get more local. You don't have to unglove, the nurse holding the patient doesn't have to go shopping around for you and, best of all, your patient doesn't have to hurt!

This little bit of humanity will help you out, believe me.

How Do Those Attendings Do It?

Residents often marvel that an attending gets it right away. On closer examination, what actually happens is this:

• The resident slowly, painfully slowly, slithers the needle in slower than a stalactite forms on the roof of some underground cavern.

• After an eon, the resident bonks against bone, pulls back, and then starts the glacially slow process again.

Once again, whole empires rise and fall, continents drift apart, and vast numbers of species evolve fully before the resident's spinal needle finally comes to rest against the patient's backbone again.

• The resident's head cranks around and says, "I can't get it."

• The attending throws on gloves, grabs the needle, and goes in and out like a blur, missing 17 times in two seconds then *bop!* Out rolls CSF.

The attending is no better at it; the attending just knows that you go till you hit bone then, if you hit bone, you redirect. You don't give long-winded explanations about *why* you're not getting it . . . you just soldier on until you *do* get it.

A Little Homemade Spinal Guide

On a skeleton, put the end of your left middle finger on the left iliac crest and rest your thumb right into the L 3-4 interspace (a good interspace to aim for). The crescent described from your middle finger along your palm and out to the thumb is the "hipbone-to-space" length.

This hipbone-to-space length is about the same in most adults, amazingly! With obese patients, you'll have to squish in a lot of tissue, but the distance is still about the same. Tall, short, big, small—this built-in ruler will at least get you in the ballpark when it comes to finding where to stick the needle.

On the other side, you can put your right middle finger on the right iliac crest and your thumb will plunk into the space.

position-challenged. But when you start out, sitting will prove easier.

Look at a skeleton to get a good feel for where you're going. Notice that the spinous processes are ovals when viewed from straight on. Get a marker and go ahead and draw them on the patient. This will give you a picture of the gap. Once you have those drawn, hold a little scale model of the spinal column right next to the patient so you can develop a kind of X-ray vision for your needle.

If patients are sitting up and you go midline and you hit bone, you know you just need to go up or down. (If they are on their sides and you hit bone, you may be a little baffled as to what aspect of the spinal column you hit and where you should go next.)

Much is made about going midline or paramedian. A useful distinction between these runs thusly:

"I don't give a damn where you stick, just keep going until you get CSF!"

This may seem a little cold, but that is the fact of the matter. You may start out midline, then, by the time you fish around and bounce off enough osteocytes, you may hit CSF and notice that your needle is *officially* paramedian by now.

Whatever. As long as you get the CSF.

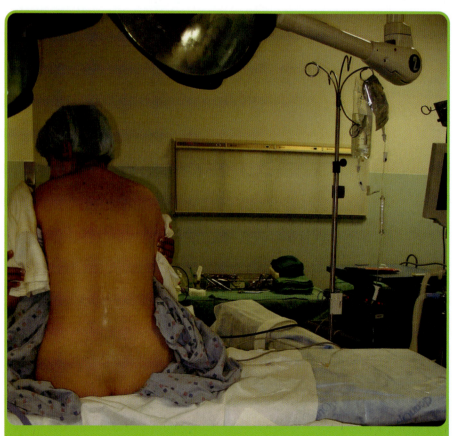
Figure 1. Sit patient up, get kit nearby, Assure good feng-shui in the room.

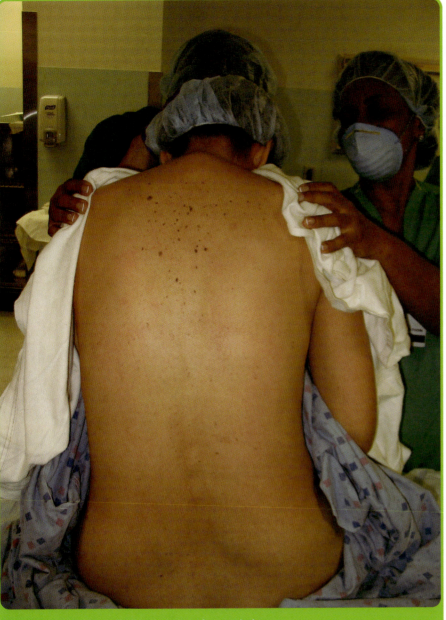

Figure 2. Bend patient forward, this opens up speces.

Gloveless Initial Marking

In a perfect world, all your patients are as skinny as supermodels and have spinous processes visible from weather satellites, but few of us get such luck. Since a lot of this is by feel, go ahead and do your feeling before you put on your gloves.

Latex can diminish the sensation, uh, some would say.

Palpate the processes, draw your landmarks. To mark the spot, take a needle, use the hub, and dent in exactly where you are going to place your spinal needle. After you prep, drape, and glove up, you can get a little lost. That dent in the skin will guide you back to the Promised Land

Headache Headaches

A small needle with a pencil point is least likely to give a headache. Next best is a regular bevel, but turned sideways so you *part* the fibers rather than leaving a hole. Small needles can be a headache in themselves, because it can be a little harder to negotiate them into the CSF. (Even if you pull back and redirect, small needles have a demonic propensity to still swerve off path and miss the CSF.)

If you're floundering, you may have to go to a bigger needle, a 22 g, dismissively called a "knitting needle" by spinal purists who look down their noses at weaklings who have to go to the big guy. Although it shouldn't really happen, you will often find that if you go in the *exact same place* and go the *exact same direction*, you will thwonk it with the 22 g where you missed it with the 25 or 26 g.

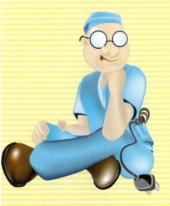

Jabba the Hutt

The trouble with food is, it tastes good.

You will encounter patients who find food downright irresistible. Here are your landmarks for these patients. You can palpate if you *want*, but you're on a fool's errand, because you won't be able to palpate anything through all that adipose. Do this instead:

• Sit them up.

• Where the good Lord split them will tell you where the midline is.

• The initial monster roll of humanity will point to the lower lumber region.

• Go up from the crack, and over from the roll. Voila and good luck.

Sidewinder

If you put the patient on the side, you will notice that the spinal column will sag a little, and that can throw off your aim. If you hit bone, you get a little more flummoxed, because ... are you hitting spinous process? Facet? And just where do you redirect? Look at a little model of the spine and you can see how you could get thrown for a loop.

If lost, step back. You can even go all the way back to Square One, take everything down, and redraw the spinous processes, that might help redirect you.

One advantage to the sidewinder approach is this: Patients can relax their backs more. When sitting, the intraspinous ligaments can get so taut that the entire back feels like one giant, fused block. (Even on skinny people!) On their sides, patients can relax more, the intraspinous ligaments don't get so tight, and you can really dig your thumb into the space.

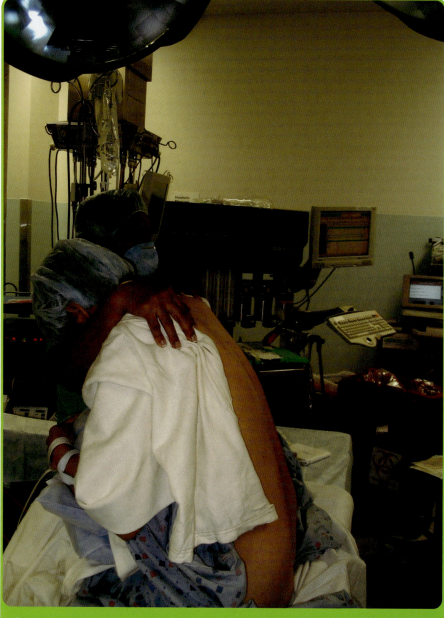

Figure 3. Assistant holds patient just so. The person holding the patient is more important than the person holding the needle.

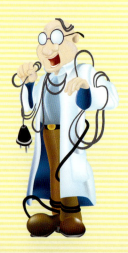

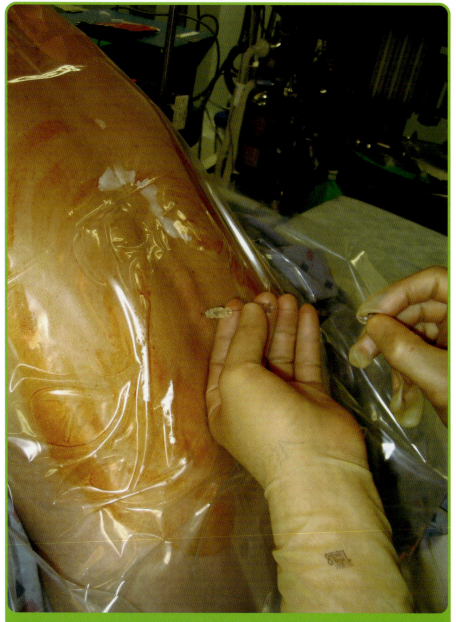

Figure 4. In you go. Avoid bone (unless you plan on a career in ortho), aortas (unless you plan on a career in vascular), and kidneys (unless you plan a career in nephrology).

Talking the Talk

Once the goods are in, check vital signs and keep talking to the patient. While the BP cuff is cycling and you're reconnecting everything, the patient's *continued ability* to carry on a discussion (on the topic of your choosing) is the world's greatest monitor. If they can talk, that means they can *breathe*, they can *cerebrate*, they must have some *perfusion*, and they are *alive*. Take none of these for granted, as a spinal anesthetic is a sympatho-guillotine.

Ooops! Didn't take into account the patient had actually bled a lot into some mysterious space and was actually hypovolemic?

Your first clue might be the patient stops talking, because his blood pressure is no more.

Ooops! Didn't pick up the history of aortic stenosis?

Your first clue might be the patient stops talking, because his life is no more.

Ooops! Didn't notice the spinal was going too high?

Your first clue might be the patient stops talking, because his breathing is no more.

Keep talking to a patient after a spinal!

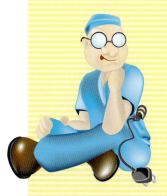

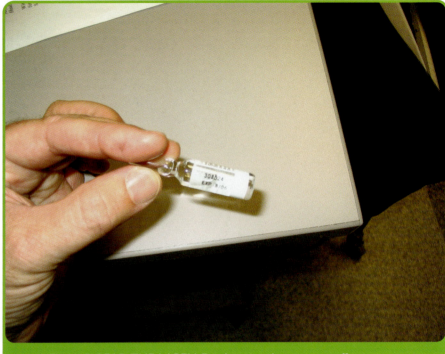

Figure 5. READ THE LABEL! Don't inject the wrong stuff or wrong concentration.

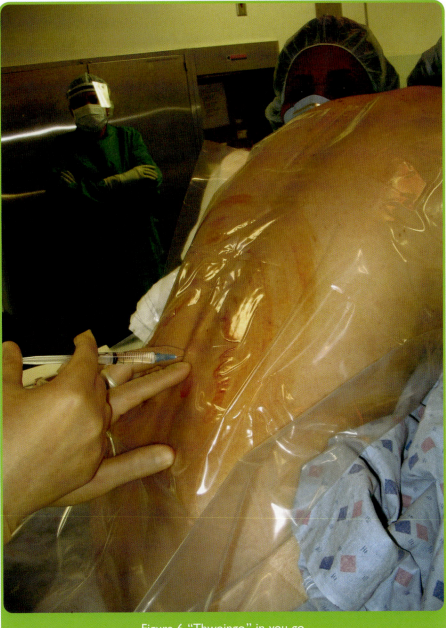

Figure 6. "Thwoingo," in you go.

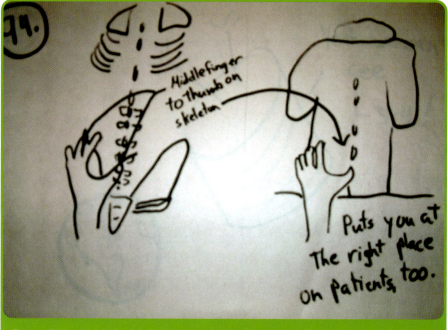

Figure 7. Using your hand as a "meaure" of where to go. And it really, really works.

SUGGESTED READING

Carpenter RL, Caplan RA, Brown DL, et al. Incidence and risk factors for side effects of spinal anesthesia. *Anesthesiology* 1992;76:906.
• *Incidence of hypotension and bradycardia is related to the block height by extent of sympathectomy.*

Chambers WA, Edstrom HH, Scott DB. Effect of baricity on spinal anesthesia with bupivicaine. *Br J Anesth* 1981;53:27.
• *Kind of self-explanatory.*

Coe AJ, Revanas B. Is crystalloid preloading useful in spinal anesthesia in the elderly? *Anesthesia* 1990;45:241.
• *About preloading patients prior to spinals, and its effectiveness.*

Colonna-Romano P, Shapiro BE. Unintentional dural puncture and prophylactic epidural blood patch in obstetrics. *Anesth Anal* 1989;69:522.
• *An effective treatment in our armamentarium.*

Drummond G, Scott D. Deflection of spinal needles by the bevel. *Anesthesia* 1980;35:854.
• *Describes the use of the introducer and different needle types.*

Graves CL, Underwood PS, Klein RL, Kim YI. Intravenous fluid administration as therapy for hypotension secondary to spinal anesthesia. *Anesth Analg* 1968;47:548.
• *What to do if something bad occurs!*

Halpern S, Preston R. Postdural puncture headache and spinal needle design. *Anesthesiology* 1994;81:1376.
• *Which to use, and which not.*

Kennedy WF Jr, Bonica JJ, Akamatsu TJ, et al. Cardiovascular and respiratory effects of subarachnoid block in the presence of acute blood loss. *Anesthesiology* 1968;29:29.
• *What not to do when pt is volume depleted.*

Leighton BL, Norris MC, Sosis M, et al. Limitations of epinephrine as a marker of intravascular injection in laboring women. *Anesthesiology* 1987;66:688.
• *Describes possible transfer of intrathecal medications through small meningeal hole during CSE technique.*

Phero JC, Bridenbaugh PO, Edstrom HH, et al. Hypotension in spinal anesthesia: a comparison of isobaric bupiviaine without epinephrine. *Anesth Analg* 1987;66:549.

Reiman A, Anson B. Vertebral level of termination of the spinal cord with report of a case of sacral cord. *Anat Rec* 1944;88:127.
• *Anatomical end of spinal cord as well as landmarks.*

Schneider M, Ettlin T, Kaufmann M, et al. Transient neurologic toxicity after hyperbaric subarachnoid anesthesia with 5% lidocaine. *Anesth Anal* 1993;76(5):1154.
• *Something you don't want to see.*

Sinclair CJ, Scott DB, Edstrom H. Effect of the Trendelenburg position on spinal anesthesia with hyperbaric bupivicaine. *Br J Anesth* 1982;54:497.
• *Also rather self-explanatory.*

Tarkkila P, Isola J. A regression model for identifying patients at high risk of hy-

potension, bradycardia and nausea during spinal anesthesia. *Acta Anesthesiol Scand* 1992;36:554.
• *Side effects of spinals.*

Thornburn J, Louden J, Vallance R Spinal and general anesthesia in total hip replacement: frequency of deep vein thrombosis. *Br J Anesth* 1980;52:1117.
• *Shows how spinal can blunt the stress response to surgery.*

Oh Damn, CSF! The Epidural

Christina Matadial and Stephanie Katz

A grievous burden was thy birth to me.

William Shakespeare
King Richard III, Act IV, scene iv, 168
Late 1500s, early 1600s

INTRODUCTION

Epidurals Are Great

You can use epidurals for lots of cases, from foot cases to orthopedic cases to big vascular cases. You can put epidurals in for combined general-epidural cases, using the epidural for postoperative pain relief as well as intraoperative management. You can put epidurals in the thoracic region to manage those painful and often taxing thoracotomies. So the epidural can do what most spinals can do, plus the catheter stays in for redosing, to be used after the case . . . all kinds of wonderful things.

But who are we kidding? The most frequent use of epidurals is on the labor deck. "Yea, I have heard the voice of woman in travail," says the Good Book, and, if you are an anesthesiologist, "Yeah, ye too will hear the voice of woman in travail."

And they will be asking for pain relief from "the grievous burden of birth."

And that means you.

And that means an epidural.

INDICATIONS

- Delivery of local anesthetic to provide anesthesia
- Delivery of local anesthetic to provide analgesia
- Delivery of narcotic to provide analgesia
- In a few special cases, delivery of other medications for analgesia (clonidine, for example)
- Placement of epidural steroids for pain relief
- Placement of epidural devices for chronic pain relief (these last two more in the realm of a pain textbook)

CONTRAINDICATIONS

- Coagulopathy.
- Infection at the site.
- Systemic infection (relative; for example, the pregnant patient with chorioamnionitis runs a risk of infection, but a functioning epidural makes her a safer C-section in case of a sudden need to cut, so you may place the epidural even in the face of an infection).
- Mass in back, such as metastatic CA. Keep in the mind the cancers that often spread to the back, such as prostate CA.
- Earlier neurologic problems or procedures (relative; a pregnant patient with a lot of sciatica may benefit from the safety of a well-placed and functioning epidural, even though you are loathe to instrument the back of someone who has chronic back pain).
- Increased intracranial pressure. You could get a wet tap, then the patient could herniate.
- Hypovolemia (where the sympathectomy could finish them off).
- Stenotic valve lesion (where the sympathectomy could finish them off, but even this is relative, since you could argue that you could dose *very* slowly, watch the volume status, and still pull this off in a safe fashion. It's hard to make absolute statements in the world of medicine!)

EQUIPMENT

- Epidural kit, dealer's choice.
- Beware the "new kit that they just ordered." The needle may be sharper than you're used to and oops, here comes the wet tap.
- Someone to watch the patients and hold them in good position (crucial, crucial, crucial).
- On OB, a fetal heart monitor that's sending a good, reliable signal (don't place an epidural if you're not picking up a good signal, the baby could get in trouble and you'd never know it).

BEWARE THE ALREADY-IN EPIDURAL

- Just make sure it's still in by doing a test dose. People wiggle around and those epidurals find a way to fall out, or worse, are not too far out, they're actually IV the CSF.

Don't Think About It

Most of the epidurals you do will be on the labor deck. Now, some of you lucky saps will perform epidurals on yuppie mummies who take good care of themselves, gain 15 pounds during their pregnancy, hold perfectly still, and brim over with motivation and understanding.

The rest of you will do epidurals in the setting that is *not* conducive to a regional anesthetic:

- Can't give sedative as that will go to babykins.

- Ofttimes a body habitus reflecting a somewhat robust antepartum weight gain.

- Youth, ah, carefree youth, with the attendant nonmaturity and nonhold-still-itude of youth.

- Ongoing painful contractions leading to yet more nonhold-still-itudeness coupled with tympano-shattering cries of joy at the miracle of childbirth.

- And the pièce de résistance? Your fallback of a general anesthetic in case of regional failure is fraught with hazard: a guaranteed full stomach, guaranteed swollen and friable airway, guaranteed rapid desaturation, and 16 times increased chance of death.

So, the less you think about this, the better.

- Make equally sure the damn thing hasn't wiggled into a vessel. (Test dose again!)

- Of particular danger is this scene: You get a wet tap, thread a catheter into the CSF, use the epidural as a continuous spinal, then you get relieved and somehow the message doesn't get relayed. Then someone forgets, gives an epidural dose through a continuous spinal . . . and *bad news!*

PHILOSOPHY

- Outside of the OB setting, you can sedate patients when you place epidurals.

- When you sedate patients, don't overdo it. You need their cooperation and you need to hear if you spear a nerve root.

- We hesitate to place these in the patient under general anesthesia (the exception being a kiddie caudal), because a patient under general anesthesia cannot report to you that you have nailed a nerve root!

- In OB, don't sedate, because any sedative you give mummerkins will go to babykins.

- The exception on OB? If you have a completely out-of-control patient due to innate or acquired cerebral pathology, you may be better off sedating and getting an epidural in rather than just saying, "To hell with it." Such a to-hell-with-it attitude can paint you in the corner of having to do a stat C-section under general anesthesia later on, with the grave risk of losing the airway in the pregnant patient.

- If you do have to give sedative to a pregnant patient, let the pediatricians know about it since they may have to support the baby's ventilation.

- On OB, when you place the epidural, you have to keep your third eye (cf., the guy behind the diner counter in the best Twilight Zone episode ever) on the fetal heart rate at all times, or deputize the holding person to watch it.

- Getting an epidural on a wiggling, pain-wracked OB patient will tax you. Pray to the patience gods.

- When a woman has a contraction, she almost invariably wants to extend her back, rather than scrunch forward. This does not help.

- Do your best to keep the patient from extending, and when that doesn't work, then do your epidural work between contractions when she will lean forward—you may be able to strike a deal

---

with her—she'll tell you when a contraction is starting, and you'll stop and let her wiggle and breathe through it.

- On OB, if you see trouble coming (very large patient, potential bad airway, preeclampsia), get your epidural in *early*, even if that means you just place the catheter, but don't dose it. Remember, you are working hard to prevent a disaster:

  - fetal trouble
  - back to OR
  - stat C-section
  - no time for a regional or can't get it in under pressure
  - induce general anesthesia
  - lose the airway
  - *catastrophe*

- No kidding, no kidding this happens, so don your proactive shoes and get ready early on. An epidural that works and that you have confidence in will go a long way toward heading off this very real threat.

- Thoracic epidurals for thoracotomies provide great pain relief, and a thoracotomy is a most painful procedure. So this is one regional technique we encourage patients to accept.

- If you are placing an epidural for a vascular case, think carefully about dosing of heparin, and think carefully about when you will pull the catheter out. If, for example, an AAA turns into a bloodbath and the patient develops a coagulopathy, then make sure the coagulation system is back to normal before you remove the catheter.

- If you ever get a *hint* of epidural trouble—hematoma or abscess— *drop everything!* Get neurosurgery and get a study (MRI or CT) *right away! Don't* let someone else take care of this! *Don't* send orders and hope they'll get done! *Don't* continue your normal workday! Absolutely make this the Number One priority in your life—*this minute, this second.* A short stretch of time separates complete recovery from complete paralysis and *you* have got to make it happen!

EPIDURAL HISTORY AND PHYSICAL

- Ask about and look for the contraindications to an epidural.

- Easy bleeding and bruising? On Plavix? On Coumadin?

- If they are on aspirin, that's OK, as long as they aren't on all sorts of other stuff.
- Systolic murmur no one heard about before? Get an echo and make sure they don't have aortic or mitral stenosis.
- Look at the back for masses, infections, and old scars from surgery.

TECHNIQUE

- All the wizardry you employ to find the space between the bones for a spinal, apply here.
- Palpate that back, getting a feel for where the spinous processes are.
- Look again at a model of the vertebrae, so your mind's eye will be able to navigate the twists and turns and avoid bone.
- Feel the space with your bare hand and make a dent in the skin with the hub of a needle, which often gives you a better first shot.
- You can go midline or paramedian, keeping in mind that the paramedian approach is a little more likely to get you into a blood vessel.
- For a lumbar approach, go L 3-4 or L 4-5, as you do for a spinal. For a thoracic approach, you can place the epidural almost anywhere, the idea is: Make sure you will cover the area of the incision.
- For the thoracic approach, the higher you go in the thorax, the steeper the angle. The lower you go in the thorax, the shallower the angle. Thus, a low thoracic epidural is not much different than a high lumbar.
- You can place epidurals sitting or on the side, just as with a spinal.
- Place your local midline for a midline approach.
- Place your local 1-2 cm lateral for a paramedian approach.
- Place the epidural needle.
- Attach a syringe filled with air or saline. This syringe should be a special epidural syringe that has an easy-slide plunger that will give you a good feel for the loss of resistance. We think glass syringes give the best feel.
- You can use air or saline, however bear in mind that saline and CSF look the same, and if there's any question that you have a wet tap, a syringe that was previously filled with air, now filled with fluid, will leave little doubt as to what has transpired.

- Advance the needle slowly, applying pressure to the plunger, until you feel a give. This is damned hard to describe in words, and it's something you just have to do to get that Aha! feeling.
- Some describe it as if the needle went through a leather wallet, then came through the other side and went *whoosh*.
- Don't advance any more. You are damned close to CSF and a wet tap.
- Remove the syringe and look for the tidal wave of damnation (warm CSF telling you that you got a wet tap).
- Advance the epidural catheter into the epidural space. Place it no more than 3-4 cm or so.
- Placing the catheter too shallow runs the risk of the catheter pulling out.
- Placing the catheter too deep runs the risk of sticking it in a nerve root.
- The catheter should go easily.
- Once the catheter's in, pull the needle back. Never pull the catheter back through the needle, because you may sheer the catheter off.
- Discard the needle, and secure the catheter.
- Make sure you use a transparent dressing because you will want to inspect the site.
- Aspirate the catheter, looking for blood (a red substance) or CSF (a clear substance). If you get either of these, remove the catheter and start over.
- Alternately, if you get CSF, you can use this as a continuous spinal catheter, but make damned sure everybody knows! Label *everywhere*: the catheter, the infusion pump, even the infusion tubing! An epidural dose of local anesthetic delivered into the CSF is a vast overdose, and will result in a high spinal, respiratory arrest, and circulatory collapse.
- The above-mentioned three items are not good things.
- Your test-dose solution will consist of a quick-onset local anesthetic, and usually 1:100,000 epinephrine.
- Give the test dose of local anesthetic, looking for signs of intra-CSF injection (you get a complete block similar to a spinal) or an intravascular injection (ringing in the ears, funny feeling, tingling around the mouth, or tachycardia).
- If the test dose is OK, then you are in business.
- Keep in mind, though, that *every* dose you give is a test dose, and that a

Prepare ye the Way of the Airway

As you will do a lot of these in labor rooms, rather than operating rooms, you will have to be like a turtle, carrying your house around on your back. Or, in this case, you will have to carry your house around on that red cart.

Make sure the cart has airway stuff, including pentothal and SUX, and know where the suction apparatus is in the room. When you get into badness (a seizure, high spinal, cardiovascular collapse—all possibilities you need to consider), you will need to move like lightning. That is no time to be finding stuff, checking the light on the laryngoscope, or spiking the stylet into an ETT.

It's not a bad idea to make sure you have an Eschmann intubating stylet and an LMA on that cart too. Remember, every obstetric patient is a potential difficult airway, so have some special equipment around to help you with the airway in case you can't get it with the usual stuff. To reiterate, if patients suddenly seize and you need to secure their airways, there's no time to say, "Oh, I can't see anything, can you go find me a (fill in the blank)."

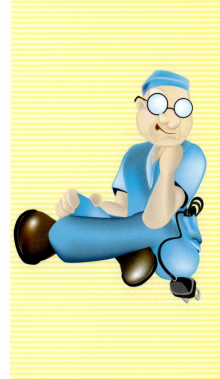

Sit or Side, the Eternal Question

As with spinals, you want to make sure that you can do both. Especially in obstetrics, you'll see a lot of patients where sitting is just not an option. You'll sit the patient up, the fetal heart rate trace will look nonreassuring (I love that phrase, Bill Clinton could have made it up), and you'll have to lay the patient on her side. This should not come as a big surprise. Pregnant patients can get supine hypotensive syndrome from laying flat on their backs. Internal vena cava squishalage is the culprit. So if you sit someone up and scrunchulate them forward like a shrimp, that same internal vena cava squishalage can occur, causing hypotension or placental insufficiency.

There are some other advantages to the side position in pregnant patients. God forbid something should go wrong and the patient should lose consciousness, that's a lot easier to manage with the patient already down than with the patient toppling forward on the nurse and ripping out all lines and monitors as she crashes to the linoleum while the horrified father, looking on, picks up his cell phone and speed dials 1-800-SUE A DOC saying, "I got another 50 million dollar case for you!"

Another, less dramatic advantage, is this: If patients are uncomfortable during contractions, they tend to wiggle and straighten up less when they are on their sides.

Sitting has the usual advantage—you're less likely to get lost. If the patients are heroically enormous, and they sometimes are, you go with the usual "up from the crack, over from the fold" to hit the spot. Hit bone? Go up or down, those are the only options you need to consider. On their sides, with many hundreds of pounds sagging and the mattress sagging and the midline sagging and your spirits sagging, your epidural needle can get lost in space. You hit bone, but you're not sure whether to go rostrad, caudad, leftad, rightad, crawdad, or just plain out-of-your-mind mad.

catheter that *was* in the right place may *now* be in the wrong place. Have a healthy respect for epidurals, and always look at them as maybe, just maybe, not still in the epidural space.

GLITCHES

- After you place an epidural in pregnant patients, they should feel relief within a few contractions. If, by the time you finish your paperwork, they are groaning just as loudly with each contraction, troubleshoot the epidural.

- It's faster to redo an epidural than to hem and haw about how it "might be in, let's just give it some time."

- Ideally, you give just enough analgesia to make the patient comfortable, but not so much that she can't push. Every recipe and concentration in the world has been used. The best titration is done at bedside with frequent revisits, going up or down on your dosage depending on the patient's response.

- Don't place a labor epidural and disappear. Check up on it, keep abreast of developments, and be there for delivery. Your patients will appreciate it and, why by coy about it? They'll be a little more

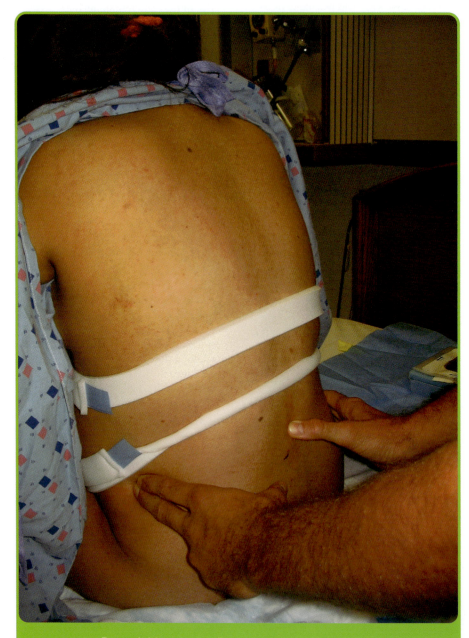

Figure 1. No surprise. Positioning is just like a spinal.

likely to pay the bill if you were part of the process rather than just there for the needle part.

- Thoracic epidurals can be a little touchy. If you put a lot of local in during a case, and the surgeon does a lot of mediastinal manipulation, you can lose your blood pressure. Is it the surgeon? The local anesthetic from the epidural? To make your life easier, wait to put the local anesthetic in when all the mediastinal manipulation is over and the surgeon is closing. There will be less going on, less confusion about what is causing the blood pressure drop, and you should have time for the local to set in and have the patient wake up comfortable.

- With narcotic infusions, be sure and write orders for monitoring and treating respiratory depression (disastrous) and pruritus (bothersome, but rarely fatal).

- If you get a wet tap, either slide in a catheter and use it as a continuous spinal, or remove it and go elsewhere. There is now evidence to suggest that a wet tap with a 17-g Touhy, which is used as a spinal catheter will have a lower chance of causing a postdural puncture headache than a hole in the dura which wasn't used as a continuous spinal. Either way, tell the patient and be ready to treat a spinal headache later.

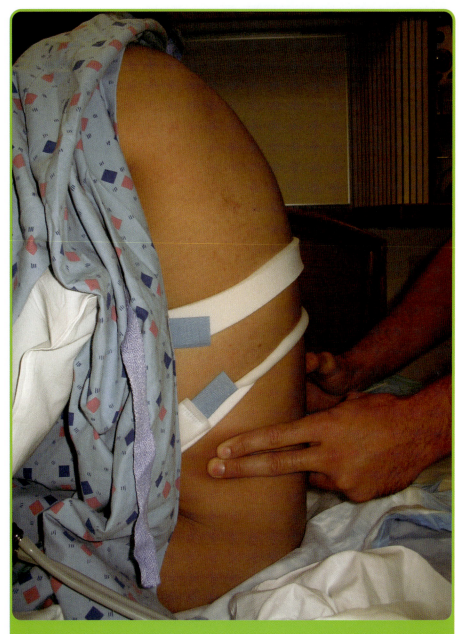

Figure 2. Left hand pegs the hip bone.

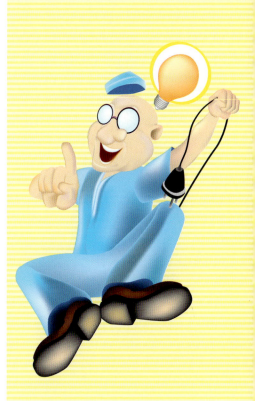

Go Loco with Local

Myself, I open up a bottle of local and pour it into one of the little trays in the epidural kit. Just as, during a spinal, I want extra local in case I miss, so also with an epidural. If I miss, I want to reach down and draw up some more local right away, rather than waiting for the hassle of having someone else open up my local. Plus, if the patient is plus-sized, you are likely to have to fish around a little. The more local you have, the easier it is to localize anew in a new spot.

Block a big space, too. Go straight in, localize along the path you envision, then localize a little above and below that path. After all, if you hit bone, you will redirect. Better to have that new area localized already.

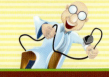

The Actual Stick

If there's anywhere that a book falls short, it's describing the feel of the loss of resistance. You have Touhy to do it to know it. You *can* practice before you do it for real, though. Take a needle and give an epidural to an orange. (Navel, Valencia, doesn't matter). As you advance through the peel, you will feel a give when you get through the peel and into the juicy fruit part of the orange.

That is sort of what the "loss of resistance" is.

It's been described as "going through leather." However you describe it, the idea of an epidural stick is always the same: Advance the needle slowly, pressing in the plunger of the syringe, until you feel a pop and the plunger slides in effortlessly. Some people advance with constant pressure on the plunger, others push the needle in a little, recheck, then push in a little more, recheck. Either way is fine.

An alternative technique is the "hanging-drop" technique. You put a drop of fluid in the hub, then advance until the drop sucks in. The epidural space, being a potential space, has a little negativity associated with it. So when you enter it, that drop of fluid goes *zip*, right in there. (It's cool to see it.)

Once you're in the space, disconnect the needle from the syringe, and engage in the "look of truth." This is when you hold your breath and hope to hell that warm CSF fluid doesn't gush out of the needle, meaning you went too far and got a wet tap. If just a little fluid drips out, and it's cool to touch, then that is just the saline you used in your syringe. But if it's body temperature, and it keeps on coming, then damn, you done did it.

Assuming the look of truth yields a happy result, thread your epidural catheter in about 3 to 4 centimeters. Thread it in much more, and you may slide out a nerve root and get a crummy block. Slide it in less, and the line-migration zombies may attack, and the catheter may come out. The catheter should slide in easy but easy. If you *bonk bonk bonk* and try to force it, then you are trying to unlock a door with a wet noodle, that is, you are engaging in futility.

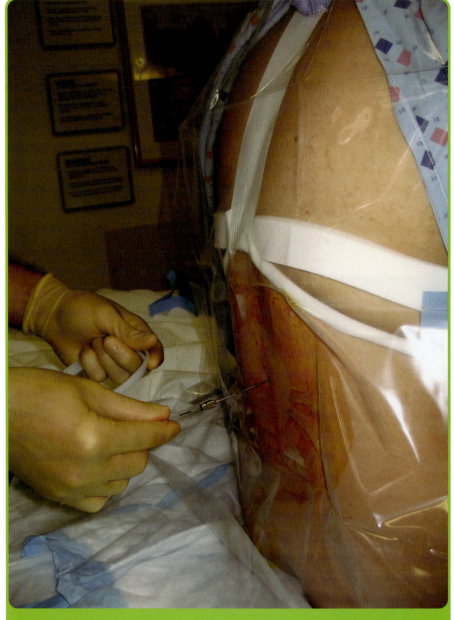

Figure 3. Sterile prep, drape, then go for it.

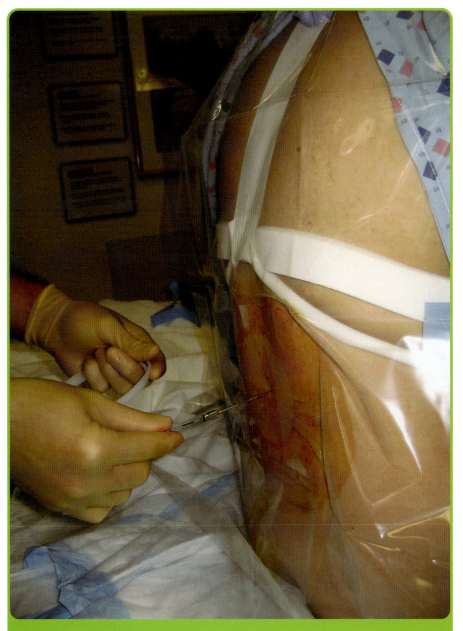

Figure 4. Slide in the catheter. Shouldn't have to force it or pound it in with a ballpeen hammer.

Remember that the epidural space is a potential space—it's not an actual space that the patient is born with, waiting for you to come along and pop your catheter into; a lot of folks actually inject a small amount of saline, 3-4 cc, to expand the potential space into an actual space, which also theoretically makes it easier to slide your catheter in.

Once you slide it in, measure and make sure you're in the correct depth, slide the needle out (making sure you don't pull the catheter out), remeasure and make sure you're still in the correct depth, then secure the catheter. Make sure when you secure it that you can see the entry site and the marks on the catheter. If you cover it with duct tape and manhole covers, you'll never be able to see it if you have to adjust the catheter.

Dosing the Epidural

Aspirate before every injection, and follow the dictum: "Every dose is a test dose." If you did something bad in your last life, and that catheter goes intravascular, and you don't pick it up by aspirating (it happens), then make sure that you never give a fatal dose *boom*, all at once. Give a few cc's, watch the patients, talk to them, see if they're weirding out on you, wait a little, then give a few more cc's. You will never regret dosing slowly, but you sure as hell will regret dosing *quickly*.

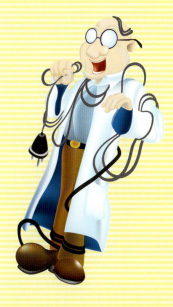

Thoracic Epidurals

Go back to your skeleton, well, preferably some other poor sap's skeleton, and look at the thoracic vertebrae. The lower thoracic vertebrae have lumbar-like spinous processes, pointing straight out. Getting between these spinous processes is no harder than doing a lumbar epidural.

Now look at the higher thoracic vertebrae. Those damned spinous processes nearly overlap like armor plating! To sneak between those, you either have to go paramedian and squeak in from the side (a tough shot, plus if you *zink* off to the side you can drop a lung), or else you have to do a supertough steep angle to creep between those overlapping spinous processes.

Plus, if you think about it, if you place the epidural low, say T 10, slide it up a few centimeters, allow for spread of local, you can pretty much take care of most thoracic cases. Hey, Perry Mason couldn't make a better case.

If you place a thoracic epidural, and you're the world's greatest and slickest, by all means put it in real high. Amen and all praise and honor to you!

If you don't do a lot of thoracic epidurals, if you're more of an occasional thoracic epidural type, then make your life a little easier and place them low.

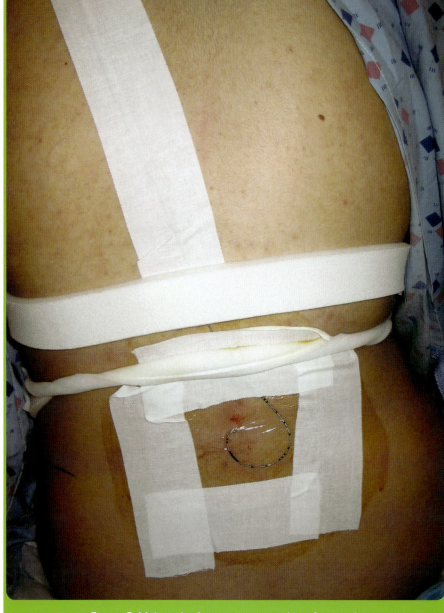

Figure 5. Make it look neat, sweet, and professional.

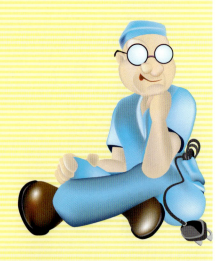

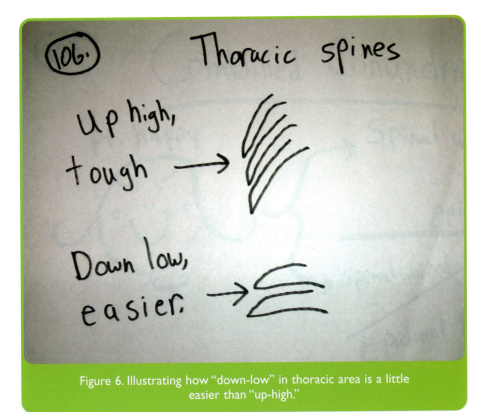

Figure 6. Illustrating how "down-low" in thoracic area is a little easier than "up-high."

Cervical Epidurals

Doing one of these for surgical anesthesia is as rare as rocking-horse manure. Most cervical epidurals in the real world are for pain-relief procedures.

How do you do one of these?

The usual, prep and drape sterile technique, (gloves, vasectomy), local, then advance the epidural needle as for the other locales. I insult your intelligence by saying, make sure you're superfacile with lumbar epidurals before you go to the neck. Better yet, leave this frightening procedure to the pain experts. Many pain people don't even do these without being guided by fluoroscopy.

SUGGESTED READING

Deschamps A. Autonomic nervous system response to epidural analgesia in laboring patients by wavelet transform of heart rate and blood pressure variability. *Anesthesiology* Jul 1;2004;101(1):21–27.
- *Indices of parasympathetic and sympathetic activity after neuraxial blockade in laboring patients can be obtained by analysis of both heart rate and blood pressure variability.*

Eltzschig HK, Lieberman ES, Camann WR. Medical progress: regional anesthesia and analgesia for labor and delivery. *N Engl J Med* Jan 23;2003;348:319–332.
- *Epidural analgesia has been shown to be a safe, widely used, effective means of pain relief during labor and cesarean delivery.*

Higuchi H. Factors affecting the spread and duration of epidural anesthesia with ropivacaine. *Anesthesiology* Aug 1;2004;101(2):4514–60.
- *Epidural anesthesia can have an unpredictable extent and duration. Differences in the surface area of the dura, epidural fat volume, and epidural venous plexus velocity may explain the variability in the extent and duration of epidural anesthesia.*

Holte K. Epidural anesthesia, hypotension, and changes in intravascular volume. *Anesthesiology* Feb 1; 2004; 00(2):281–286.
- *One of the most common side effects of epidural anesthesia is hypotension with relative hypovolemia, requiring fluid boluses or administration of vasopressors.*

Miller RM. Miller's Anesthesia, 6th ed. NY: Elsevier/Churchill Livingston; 2005.
- *What can you say, I mean, Miller. It's all there. (Once at an ASA meeting many moons ago, a nondescript anesthesiologist crossed out his own name on his name tag and wrote "Ron Miller" on it. Perhaps it was some vain attempt at horning in on Professor Miller's fame and glory. Alas, this sad sack then ran into the famous Dr. Miller in an elevator! Aag! Busted! With complete non-chalance and utter class, Dr. Miller looked at this name tag, raised his eyebrows, and said, "Interesting name.")*

Portnoy D. Mechanisms and management of an incomplete epidural block for cesarean section. *Anesthesiol Clin North Am* Mar 1;2003;21(1):39–57.
- *When inadequate epidural block becomes apparent during surgery there are limited alternatives. Depending on the degree of inadequate anesthesia, options include patient reassurance, supplementation with a variety of inhalational and intravenous agents, and local anesthetic infiltration. General anesthesia is typically left as a backup option, but must be considered if the patient continues to have discomfort.*

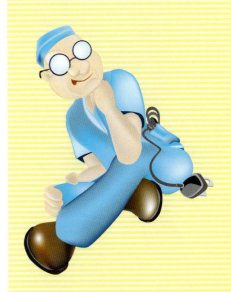

Parting Words?

- Have a never-ending respect for every epidural that you, or someone else, places.

- When you arrive at a bedside, never trust any catheter you find attached to a patient—not even yours.

- Test dose everything, every time.

- Remember setup and backup won't keep the badness away, but they will stave it off for longer.

- Altered sensorimotor exam in a patient with an epidural catheter history (with no medication on board) is an emergency.

- If bleeding and coagulopathy were an issue during surgery or postop, get coags on the patient before you touch the catheter.

- Epidurals, like all regional anesthetic techniques, have a failure rate. Even the slickest hands occasionally have to redo a catheter or two.

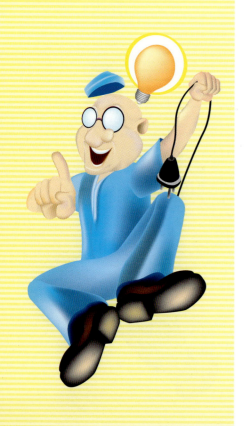

Sielenkämper AW. Thoracic epidural anesthesia: more than just anesthesia/analgesia. *Anesthesiology* Sep 1;2003;99(3):523–525.

- *Thoracic epidural blockade may be useful in providing protection against splanchnic hypoperfusion under the conditions of ischemia and reperfusion, which may occur during trauma, hemorrhage, or circulatory shock.*

Visalyaputra S, Rodanant O, Somboonviboon W, Tantivitayatan K, Thienthong S, Saengchote W. *Anesth Analg* Sep;2005;101(3):862-868.

- *In severely preeclamptic patients undergoing regional anesthesia it was found that there was a statistically significant difference in mean arterial pressure, with more patients in the spinal group exhibiting hypotension, in comparison to those that had received epidural anesthesia.*

Mix and Match: The Combined Spinal-Epidural

Allison Lee and Andres Missair

For surely this is the best of all possible worlds.

Voltaire
Candide, 1759

INTRODUCTION

Science writer, James Gleick, in his 2000 book, *Faster: The Acceleration of Just About Everything*, touches a nerve. What is the big rush with everything? Do we need to be always and everywhere in instantaneous communication with everything? Has our attention span so shortened that we can only watch two-second dance shots, one after the other, on MTV? Must political discourse devolve to the 15-second sound bite?

Must the entire universe be *now*, this *second*, this *nanosecond*?

Enter the combined spinal-epidural, used most commonly on OB. No more waiting a few minutes for the epidural to kick in, now we zap pain in an instant with the super-quick onset spinal, and then we have the epidural to keep the good thing going throughout labor.

James Gleick would be proud that *The Acceleration of Just About Everything* now includes *The Acceleration of Labor Analgesia*.

Read on.

And be quick about it!

INDICATIONS

- Labor analgesia.
- Cesarean section.
- Other gynecologic surgery.
- Urologic surgery.
- General surgery.
- Orthopedic and trauma surgery of the lower extremities.
- CSE technique is especially useful for high-risk cases, such as the morbidly obese patient where spinal anesthesia is indicated, but there is concern about a too-high spinal block. In such cases, a lower than usual dose of intrathecal local anesthetic can be given and then the epidural catheter used to slowly raise the level of the block.
- In cases where you're worried a spinal won't last long enough, the epidural acts as backup.
- Where spinal anesthesia is indicated and the epidural is desired for postoperative pain relief. The epidural may be left in place in order to run an infusion of local anesthetic or a local anesthetic/opioid mixture postoperatively.

Long-acting epidural morphine (morphine sulfate extended-release liposome injection) following CSE is another good option. Bear in mind, though, that if this is used, only the local anesthetic test dose can be given, at least 15 minutes before the morphine is injected, and that local anesthetics should not be injected afterward. The interaction between local anesthetics and the drug may lead to increased serum concentrations of morphine. The advantage is that the epidural catheter can be removed immediately postoperatively while knowing the patient's pain is taken care of for the next couple of days.

CONTRAINDICATIONS

- Coagulopathy.
- Infection at the site.
- Systemic infection. This is a relative contraindication. For example, a common occurrence is the pregnant patient with chorioamnionitis. Labor epidurals are frequently placed in this scenario.

The concern with placing an epidural or spinal in the presence of bacteremia is a potentially increased risk of epidural abscess or meningitis. A functioning labor epidural, however, has numerous benefits, not least among which is making the patient a safer C-section in case of a sudden need to cut. One retrospective study looked at over 500 women in whom labor epidurals were placed and, even in those who had bacteremia, no cases of epidural abscess were reported.

Another study looked at the occurrence of meningitis following dural puncture in bacteremic rats. One finding was that a dose of antibiotics prior to dural puncture eliminated the risk of infection. It is advisable to ensure the patient has received a dose of antibiotics prior to performing neuraxial anesthesia in the presence of suspected bacteremia. It has also been advised that the patient should be informed of the potentially increased risk of infection when obtaining consent for the procedure.

- Mass in back, such as metastatic CA.
- Earlier neurologic problems or procedures: relative.

Neuraxial anesthesia is not a good idea in someone with evolving neurologic deficits, but may be fine, for example, in patients with scoliosis and Harrington rods. Doing a CSE or epidural following back surgery may be much more challenging or even impossible if the epidural space has been compromised, and this should be explained to the patient. A one-shot spinal may be easier.

- Hypovolemia (where the sympathectomy could finish them off).
- Stenotic valve lesion (where the sympathectomy could finish them off, but even this is relative, since you could argue that you could dose *very* slowly, watch the volume status, and still pull this off in a safe fashion. It's hard to make absolute statements in the world of medicine!
- If that looks a lot like the earlier contraindications, this should come as no surprise.

COMBINED SPINAL-EPIDURAL HISTORY AND PHYSICAL

(Same as for earlier epidurals, and included here so you don't have to flip back to the previous chapter.)

- Ask about and look for the contraindications to an epidural.
- Easy bleeding and bruising? Patient on Plavix? Coumadin? Low molecular weight heparin?
- In obstetrics, the most common problem would be a low platelet count in a preeclamptic patient, prolonged PT/PTT in a patient with HELPP syndrome, or both.
- If they are on aspirin, that is OK as long as they aren't on all sorts of other stuff.
- Systolic murmur no one heard about before? An echocardiogram will pick up valvular lesions like aortic or mitral stenosis.
- The most common murmur you'll hear on OB is a flow murmur.
- However, if obstetric patients have truly severe valvular disease, they are usually already showing up extremely sick from the volume overload of pregnancy by the second trimester.

- Look at the back for masses, infections, and old scars from surgery.

EQUIPMENT

- As for any regional anesthetic, basic resuscitation equipment must always be on hand.
- These include devices for management of the airway, a source of oxygen, suction, vasopressors, and other emergency drugs necessary to deal with intravenous injection of local anesthetics or a high spinal.
- The patient must have a well-functioning IV in place.
- Standard monitors are a requirement: pulse oximetry, intermittent blood pressure, and electrocardiography.
- Prior to initiating labor analgesia, there should be at least noninvasive blood pressure measurement.
- Fetal heart rate monitor in OB. Always, always, have your antennae up for signs of fetal trouble!
- Be sure to obtain informed consent from your patient, of course.
- Have assistants watch the patients and hold them in good position. In the obstetric patient, they will also be able to help monitor the fetal heart rate.
- An experienced OB nurse who knows how to spot trouble, knows how to hold the patient in position, and has a good rapport with the patient is a godsend. (Be sure and bring such a nurse goodies periodically and always pay for the pizza on call nights).
- Epidural kit: dealer's choice. A variety of options exist.
- Several specialized CSE kits are commercially available.
- However, a basic epidural kit containing, say, a 17-g or 18-g Touhy or Hustead epidural needle may be used along with a separately acquired extra-long 24-g to 27-g spinal needle.
- Most importantly, the epidural needle in the kit should be able to admit the spinal needle.
- And the spinal needle must be able to protrude at least 13-15 mm from the tip of the epidural needle.
- The distance from the tip of the epidural needle to the subarachnoid space can range from 0.3–1.05 cm.

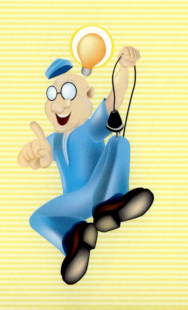

- To decrease the risk of postdural puncture headache, the needle should be a small-gauge pencil point spinal needle.
- Special CSE needles are available, however claims of superior performance are unconfirmed.
- The Eldor needle allows the passage of a spinal needle along the outer wall of the epidural needle.
- The Torrieri-Aldrete pair (TA pair) needle consists of an 18-g epidural and a 22-g spinal needle welded together with a common tip. The epidural needlepoints, cephalad, and the spinal needle, caudad, allow passage of a smaller-gauge spinal needle.
- The E-SP needle is similar, but has an over-under configuration as opposed to side-by-side in the above two.
- The Espocan epidural needle is designed with a back eye near the bevel to allow passage of the spinal needle. The spinal needle is kept along the central axis of the epidural needle by a centering plastic sleeve.
- The theory behind these modifications is that the spinal needle and catheter will have different trajectories and that this will therefore decrease the already insignificant risk of the catheter entering the dura through the spinal needle puncture site.
- The Becton-Dickinson needle has an adjustable interlocking device between the hub of the epidural and spinal needle. This device stabilizes the spinal needle within the epidural needle during intrathecal injection.
- Finally, the intrathecal and epidural drugs to be administered must be prepared ahead of time under strict aseptic precautions.

Resuscitation

- Ambu bag
  - Oxygen source
  - Laryngoscope with blades (straight/curved) in different sizes
- Endotracheal tubes (sizes 6-7.5)
  - Intubating stylets
  - Oral/nasal airways
  - Laryngeal mask airways
  - Suction catheters
  - Emergency drugs: ephedrine, phenylephrine, epinephrine, atropine, naloxone, thiopental, succinylcholine, labetalol, hydralazine, nitroglycerin, calcium
  - IV fluids, catheters, and tubing

- Defibrillator readily available
- Bed capable of Trendelenburg position

PHILOSOPHY OF THE COMBINED SPINAL EPIDURAL

- All the philosophy of a regular epidural applies (see the previous chapter).
- CSE provides the best of both worlds.
- For surgery, it combines the advantages of spinal anesthesia with a rapid and reliable onset of dense sensory and motor blockade with the flexibility provided by an epidural catheter of adjusting the level of the block and extending the duration of anesthesia.
- For labor analgesia, it provides rapid onset of pain relief (within five minutes) with a smooth transition to epidural analgesia.
- For labor, adding the spinal to the mix really does speed up pain relief. It seems the very minute you put that local anesthetic or local anesthetic/opioid mix in, patients start to feel better.
- The CSE technique also allows the possibility of ambulation by the patient during labor.
- The use of low-dose local anesthetics alone or in combination with opioids can produce selective sensory blockade with minimal motor blockade and preservation of proprioception.
- Some women enjoy the option of being able to ambulate during labor and it has been suggested that analgesic requirements may be decreased.
- It is uncertain whether or not the duration of labor is shortened.
- The so-called walking epidural must be carried out with care.
- The patient must be accompanied at all times.
- Patients must be assessed to determine the degree of motor blockade following CSE. Muscle groups innervated by L 1 to S 5 should have normal or nearnormal motor power and proprioception should be intact.
- There should be no postural hypotension.
- There should be no fetal heart rate decelerations
- Facilities for continuous fetal monitoring should be present: remote/cordless (telemetry).

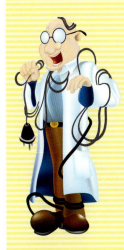

- Maternal blood pressure should be recorded at frequent intervals, say, every 15 minutes.
- It has been suggested that the use of CSE in early labor results in more rapid cervical dilatation in nulliparous women compared with conventional epidurals. There was no difference found in mode of delivery or obstetric outcome.

TECHNIQUE

- Historically multiple approaches exist.
- The most common technique is known as the "needle-through-needle" technique.
- Have the patient either sitting or lying on the side. Patient positioning is not only determined by preference, but may also be dictated by the clinical scenario.
- For example, the OB patient with fetal heart rate decelerations every time she sits up should be done on her side.
- Get the epidural needle into the epidural space as described in the previous chapter.
- Once the epidural space has been detected by loss of resistance, place your spinal needle through the epidural needle.
- There should be a give as the needle traverses the dura.
- Here lies one advantage of this technique: In the event of uncertainty about the position of your epidural needle, you have objective evidence via CSF spouting from your spinal needle and are hence able to verify your location.
- Once you get CSF, attach your syringe securely to the spinal needle while keeping it in place.
- This can be challenging because the spinal needle has the tendency to move within the larger epidural needle.
- Make sure to steady the back of your hand against the patient's back and, with your thumb and forefinger, hold the hubs of both needles in place.
- Aspirate, looking for a *swirl* and not a *bubble*.
- Inject your local anesthetic or local anesthetic/opioid mixture through the spinal needle.
- Withdraw the spinal needle.
- Thread the epidural catheter. You may inject 3-5 mL of saline in the epidural space first to facilitate passage of the catheter.

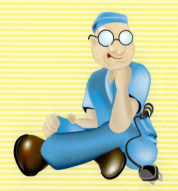

- Look at the markings on the epidural needle and determine the depth at which you found loss of resistance.
- Withdraw the needle carefully, holding the catheter during withdrawal.
- Measure the catheter and make sure you leave a length of about 3-5 cm into the epidural space.
- Bear in mind that too long a length increases the risk of a one-sided or single dermatome block, while too short a length increases the risk of dislodgement of the catheter.
- Secure the catheter with a transparent dressing.
- When applying the tape, ensure that the dressing allows you to peek-a-boo at the site.
- Return the patient to the desired position for the procedure. In the laboring patient, ensure that the patient is in left lateral uterine tilt to avoid hypotension.
- In the OR you have no choice but to be there. But, remember in the labor patient, you should hang around to monitor the patient, her vital signs, and the fetal heart rate for at least 20 minutes when all the bad stuff that can happen will happen (i.e., fetal bradycardia, hypotension, respiratory depression).
- Aspirate and give a test dose, looking for toxicity or signs of subarachnoid injection.
- Remember that negative aspiration for CSF or blood does not always guarantee your catheter is not in the subarachnoid space or in a blood vessel.
- It is claimed that multiorifice catheters will more accurately detect intravascular placement with aspiration than single end-hole catheters.
- The most commonly used test dose is 3-4 mL of lidocaine 1.5% with 1:200,000 epinephrine.
- Use of the test dose with epinephrine in the laboring patient is an area of some controversy due to the high incidence of false-positive and false-negative results and possible deleterious effects on uterine blood flow.
- To improve the sensitivity of the test dose, it is best given in-between contractions.
- Some practitioners forego the test dose altogether in CSEs for labor, feeling that with the dilute local anesthetics solutions we use today, intrathecal placement in the well-monitored patient will be detected as slow onset of a motor block. Alternatively, intravenous placement

would be noticed as regression of analgesia with minimal risk of toxicity.

- Another area of controversy is the inability to accurately test the catheter when a combined spinal epidural has been performed.

- For this reason, it may be advisable in cases where knowing a properly working catheter is in place is critical (such as a severely preeclamptic patient with rapidly falling platelets), to place a conventional epidural.

- Regardless of all this test-dose controversy, it is safest to treat every injection of the catheter as a test dose, aspirating first and giving no more than 5 mL at a time.

- For labor, many practitioners begin the local anesthetic infusion immediately after CSE, allowing an adequate level to build as the effect of the intrathecal medication begins to wane.

- For surgery, you have to bear in mind the duration of action of your chosen drug and start bolusing the epidural as the intrathecal local anesthetic wears off.

GLITCHE

- The same glitches as for any epidural or spinal.
- Loss of resistance, but no CSF!
- This can happen if your epidural needle is not quite in the midline.
- If you reassess your landmarks and adjust the needle appropriately to the left or right, you will probably hit the jackpot.
- Asking patients if they feel the needle off to the right or left usually helps in locating the midline in patients with ambiguous landmarks.
- There is the concern about PDPH in combined spinal epidurals, especially in parturients who experience a higher incidence of spinal headache even with the use of small-gauge needles.
- There are no controlled studies that look at the incidence of PDPH following CSE, but the reported incidence is very low (less than 1%).
- There are several theories why this may be, some of which are:
- The Touhy needle as introducer may allow meticulous puncture of the dura without necessitating multiple attempts.
- The increased pressure in the epidural space following administration of local

anesthetic solutions may limit the leakage of CSF.

- The entry of the spinal needle may be at an angle as it is deflected against the tip of the epidural needle. The holes in the dura and subarachnoid may therefore overlap and result in decreased risk of leakage.

- Another potential fly in the ointment is this: If they get good pain relief, then how do you know your epidural went in the right place? In the traditional setting, you knew your epidural was good, or was not good, based on pain relief.

- Now, with a spinal providing, say, two hours of pain relief, you might not *know* what's going on with your epidural for just that long.

- For this reason, many practitioners avoid CSE in patients when a functioning catheter needs to be identified early, for example, in cases of severe preeclampsia and decreasing platelet count, morbidly obese patients, stress patterns on the fetal heart tracing, and in other patients where concern exists for emergent cesarean section.

- Bear in mind, though, that even apparently well-functioning labor epidural catheters can turn out to provide inadequate anesthesia for surgery.

- One study reported a decreased failure rate for epidural catheters placed via CSE.

- This may be because use of the spinal needle for dural puncture provides an additional verification step in the event of unclear loss of resistance.

- Several studies have reported an association between intrathecal opioids and transient fetal bradycardia.

- The incidence is unclear, but it occurs infrequently.

- Although the reason is uncertain, one theory is that the rapid onset of analgesia results in a sudden decrease in circulating catecholamines, which decreases the beta effects on the uterus and may lead to increased intensity and frequency of uterine contractions.

- When it does occur, it is rapid in onset—within 15 minutes of injection—and is transient, lasting approximately 30 minutes.

- If this occurs, place the mother in left uterine displacement (LUD), give supplemental oxygen, start an IV fluid bolus, and hold the oxytocin.

- Diagnose and treat any maternal hypotension.

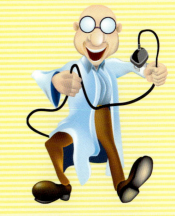

- Uterine hyperstimulation may be helped by IV ephedrine even in the absence of hypotension, subcutaneous terbutaline, or IV/sublingual nitroglycerin.
- Of note, several reports have shown no increase in the emergency cesarean section rate associated with fetal bradycardia following CSE.
- Respiratory depression (very rare).
- Hypotension (5%-10% with intrathecal fentanyl/sufentanil).
- The incidence of hypotension with CSE in labor is no higher than with a routine labor epidural.
- Pruritus (80% of patients receiving intrathecal sufentanil).
- The etiology is unclear.
- The intrathecal bupivacaine-fentanyl combination has been shown to decrease the incidence of pruritus.
- Be prepared to manage pruritus if severe (less than 5%) and reassure the patient that it is usually short-lived. Most patients do not require treatment.
- Treatment includes IV naloxone boluses or infusion, diphenhydramine (even though the etiology is not related to histamine release), nalbuphine, and small propofol boluses.
- Nausea, vomiting (2%-3%).
- Urinary retention.
- Studies have been divided, but some investigators indicated that the initiation of neuraxial analgesia early in labor was associated with an increased rate of cesarean delivery, or that there are slightly prolonged labors in the presence of labor epidurals.
- A recent study of nulliparous women at term showed that initiation of neuraxial analgesia early in labor did not increase the rate of cesarean delivery, provided better analgesia, and resulted in shorter duration of labor than systemic analgesia.
- Those women studied were with cervical dilatation less than 4.0 cm, when they had CSE performed with intrathecal fentanyl only, followed by initiation of epidural analgesia on the second request for analgesia. They were compared with a group receiving systemic hydromorphone until cervical dilatation of 4.0 cm or more, or the third request for analgesia, when epidural analgesia was begun.

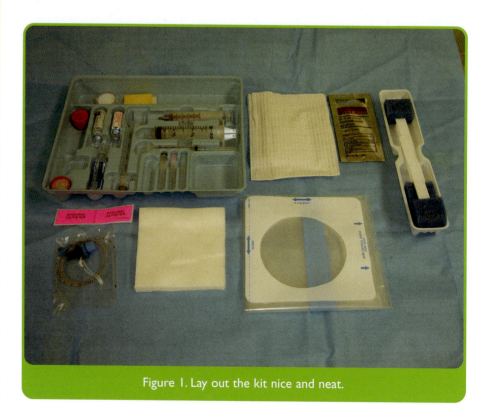

Figure 1. Lay out the kit nice and neat.

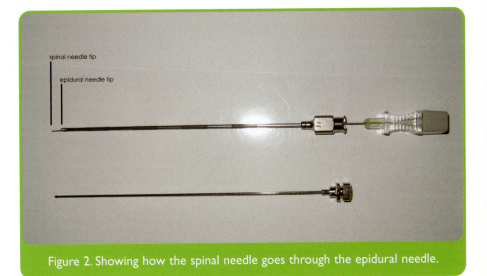

spinal needle tip

epidural needle tip

Figure 2. Showing how the spinal needle goes through the epidural needle.

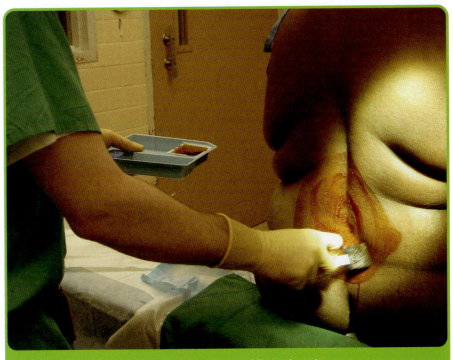

Figure 3. Prep starting at meddle and circling out.

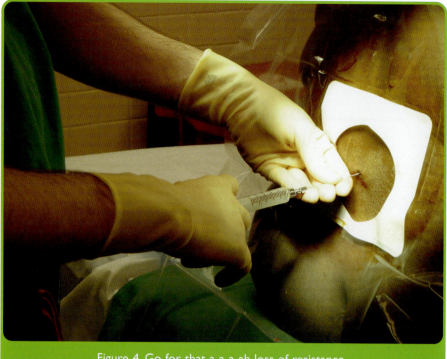

Figure 4. Go for that a-a-a-ah loss of resistance.

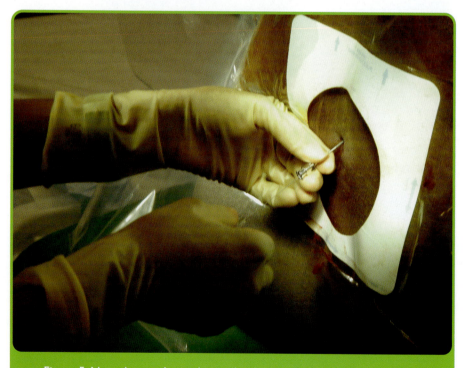

Figure 5. Now that you're in the epidural space, put the spinal needle in.

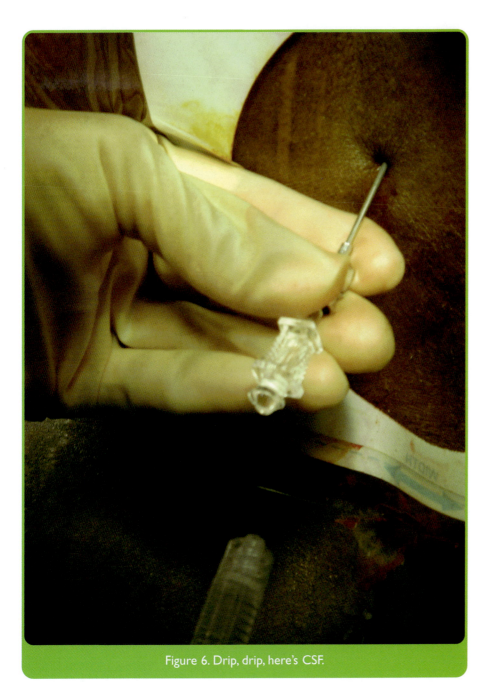

Figure 6. Drip, drip, here's CSF.

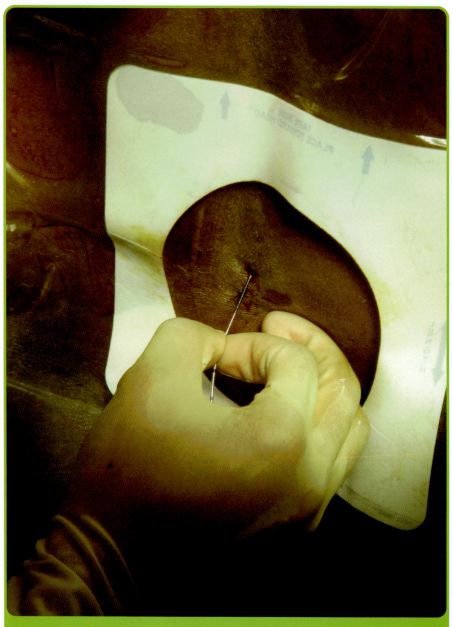

Figure 7. Once spinal stuff's injected, out with that needle, and thread the catheter.

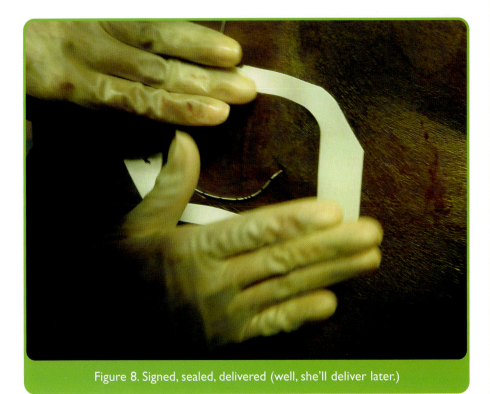

Figure 8. Signed, sealed, delivered (well, she'll deliver later.)

SUGGESTED READING

Allbright GA, Forster RM. The safety and efficacy of combined spinal and epidural analgesia/anesthesia (6,002 blocks) in a community hospital. *Reg Anesth Pain Med* 1999;24:117–125.
- *Retrospective study showing CSE safe for labor, and also finding a lower failure rate for analgesia/anesthesia than epidurals alone.*

Birnbach D, Gatt S, Datta S. *Textbook of Obstetric Anesthesia*. NY: Churchill Livingstone. 2000, p 157–182.
- *Comprehensive discussion of CSE including history, different techniques, and different needles.*

Calimiaran AL, Strauss-Hoder TP, Wang WY, McCarthy RJ, Wong CA. The effect of epidural test-dose on motor function after a combined spinal-epidural technique for labor analgesia. *Anesth Analg* Apr;2003;96(4):1167–1172.
- *Study concluding epidural test dose should be avoided after CSE for labor if ambulation is desired.*

Carp H, Bailey S. The association between meningitis and dural puncture in bacteremic rats. *Anesthesiology* 1992;May;76(5): 739–742.
- *Study showing a single dose of gentamicin prior to dural puncture in bacteremic rats eliminated the risk of meningitis.*

Chestnut DH. Spinal anesthesia in the febrile patient. *Anesthesiology*. May;1992; 76(5):667–669.

Eisenach, J. Combined Spinal-Epidural Analgesia in Obstetrics. *Anesthesiology* 1999;91:299–302.
- *Classic article discussing use of CSE for labor.*

Frenea S, Chirossel C, Rodriguez R, Baguette JP, Racinet C, Payen JF. The effects of prolonged ambulation on labor with epidural analgesia. *Anesth Analg* Jan;2004;98(1):224–229.
- *Study suggesting ambulation may be beneficial during labor.*

Goodman EJ, De Horta E, Taguiam JM. Safety of spinal and epidural anesthesia in parturients with chorioamnionitis. *Reg Anesth Pain Med* Sep-Oct;1996;l;21(5): 436–441.
- *Retrospective study of women who got spinals or epidurals whose placentas were later found to have chorioamnionitis. The researchers concluded that conduction anesthesia may be safe in parturients with chorioamnionitis without prior antibiotic therapy.*

Holstrom B, Laugaland K, Rawal N, et al. Combined spinal-epidural block versus spinal and epidural block for orthopedic surgery. *Can J Anaesth* 1993;40:601–606.
- *Study comparing spinal and CSE vs epidurals for orthopedic surgery finding spinal and CSE superior to epidurals alone.*

Hughes S, Levinson, G, Rosen M. *Schnider and Levinson's Anesthesia for Obstetrics*, 4th ed. Philadelphia:Lippincott Williams & Wilkins; 2002, p 158–167.
- *OB anesthesia text - explains use of intrathecal opioids in CSE for labor.*

Katz J: Spinal and epidural anatomy. In: Katz J, ed. *Atlas of Regional Anesthesia*. Norwalk, CT: Appleton-Century-Crofts;1985,168–169.
- *Road map to what we're working with.*

Norris MC, Grieco WM, Borkowski M, et al.: Complications of labor analgesia: epidural versus combined spinal epidural techniques. *Anesth Analg* 1994;79:529–537.
- *Study showing the CSE technique is a safe alternative to epidurals.*

Tsen LC, Thue B, Datta S, Segal S. Is combined spinal-epidural analgesia associated with more rapid cervical dilation in nulliparous patients when compared with conventional epidural analgesia? *Anesthesiology* Oct;1999;90:920–925.
- *Study showing CSE is associated with faster cervical dilatation compared with epidurals.*

Urmey WF, Stanton J.. Combined spinal epidural vs epidural anesthesia for outpatient knee arthroscopy [abstract]. *Reg Anesth Pain Med* 1997;222(suppl):6.
- *Study finding CSE's good for outpatient orthopedic surgery.*

Vallejo MC, Firestone LL, Mandell GL, Jaime F, Makishima S, Ramanathan S. Effect of epidural analgesia with ambulation on labor duration. *Anesthesiology.* Oct;2001;95(4):857–861.
- *Study of ambulatory epidural analgesia concluding that walking or sitting does not shorten labor.*

Wong C, Scavone B, Peaceman A, McCarthy R, et al. The risk of cesarean delivery with neuraxial analgesia given early versus late in labor. *New Engl J Med* 2005;352(7):655–665.
- *Study finding no increased risk of cesarean delivery, better analgesia, and shorter duration of labors with CSE. What more could you want?*

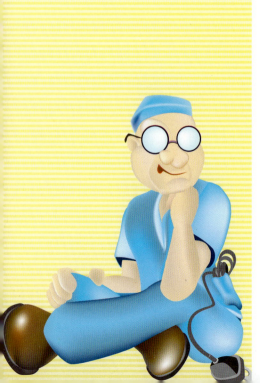

Mending Fences: The Blood Patch

Allison Lee and Amy Gruen

Patch grief with proverbs.

William Shakespeare
Much Ado About Nothing

When the head aches, all the members partake of the pain.

Miguel de Cervantes Saavedra
Don Quixote

INTRODUCTION

In sooth, you'll know why you are so sad the first time you see that clear gush of CSF coming out the hub of your Touhy needle. Things are bad enough with a patient in labor moving all over creation, blood-curdling screams following each contraction, and now this—a wet tap.

She sits up the next day and the hands go up to her head. "Aaagh! I've got the worst headache!"

I should have been a cowboy.

I should have become a guide on Mount Everest.

I should have kept at my accordion lessons and worked bar mitzvahs.

I should have done ANYTHING BUT ANESTHESIA!

But you're in it now, time to mend fences and take care of that post-dural puncture headache. Time to patch things up.

INDICATIONS

- Post-dural puncture headache (PDPH)
- PDPH is the most common adverse complication of dural puncture.
- The most important factor in the development of PDPH is needle size. In fact, the incidence of headache after dural puncture with 18G needles has been reported as up to 80%.
- PDPHs occur after spinals, too. The incidence has been reported between 2% and 12% with 26G Quincke needles and less than 2% with 29G needles.
- Pencil-point needles have been shown to reduce the incidence of PDPH.
- Several studies also support the hypothesis that placing the epidural or spinal needle with the bevel sideways also reduces the incidence.
- An epidural blood patch has been used in the treatment of spontaneous intracranial hypotension syndrome, which is due to CSF leakage, usually in the cervical or upper thoracic spine.

CONTRAINDICATIONS

- Patient refusal (no surprise—look how much trouble you caused the last time you worked on her back)
- I say "her" although, obviously, you can get a wet tap on men, too. Parturients are at particular risk of PDPH because of their gender, young age, and the widespread use of epidural anesthesia. Women who have been actively pushing during the second stage of labor also have a greater incidence of headache, probably due to greater CSF loss.

- Infection—this is the real McCoy of a contraindication. You don't want to be drawing septic blood out of a patient and putting it into her epidural space.
- You should probably avoid a blood patch in the presence of fever and a raised white cell count.
- It is appropriate to perform a blood patch in patients with HIV as long as no other active bacterial or viral illnesses are present.
- Coagulopathy
- Then all the usual contraindications to placement of an epidural, which in this case you have thought about before because you were doing an epidural when you got the wet tap!

EQUIPMENT

- Epidural kit
- Stuff to draw 20 cc of blood in a sterile fashion (tourniquet, 20-cc syringe, needle, iodine prep)
- Someone to hold the patient still while you place the epidural (at this point you're not so worried about fetal heart rates—as the kiddo is out and about somewhere—but Mummykins can still get vagal and pitch over on you)
- An assistant to draw the blood for you

PHILOSOPHY

- Like anything we do in medicine, you want the diagnosis before you effect the cure—make sure this really is a spinal headache.

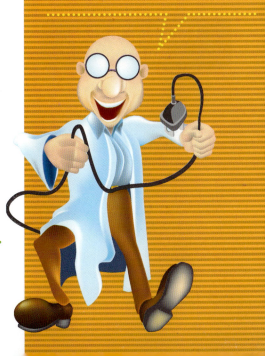

A Headache of a Different Color

A physician was playing golf one day when he felt a tremendous pain in his head that was triggered by his swing. He ordered a head CT for himself that showed two small pockets of fluid in the frontal region. The doctor was a healthy guy who had begun going to the gym and working out on the treadmill and with light weights. A week into his exercise regimen, he had noticed severe neck pain, which he treated with heat and ibuprofen. The neck pain was followed by intense headaches that came on suddenly with certain head movements and were most intense with leaning forward. They lasted minutes to hours, but this one on the golf course lasted for days.

Over the following two months and after several consults, neither the headaches nor the serial CT scans changed. Finally, a neurologist suggested intracranial hypotension based on the finding of thickened meninges on the CT, which can lead to the formation of tiny fluid pockets. A visit to a neurosurgeon confirmed the diagnosis. He was sent to an interventional neuroradiologist to locate the spontaneous leak and a blood patch was successfully performed to treat the tear that had been caused by lifting weights.

(Story originally published in *The New York Times Magazine*, September 11, 2005, Section 6)

How Not to Live Your Life

A friend (who will remain nameless) once had knee surgery. Instead of getting a general anesthetic, he demanded he get an epidural and, guess what, got a wet tap. Later, he went in for a blood patch. Miraculously, he was cured.

To celebrate this miracle cure, he went home and blazed up. Unlike President Clinton, he did inhale, precipitating a violent coughing jag, disrupting the blood patch. His headache came back and he had to go in for another blood patch.

Lesson learned: Be careful after you get a blood patch.

- Weird neurologic things happen in pregnancy—under all the pressure and straining, aneurysms leak; with all the hypercoagulable hormonal changes, vessels clot.

- You must rule out nonspecific causes, migraine, hypertension-related, caffeine withdrawal, pneumocephalus, infection, cortical vein thrombosis, intracranial subarachnoid hemorrhage, and increased intracranial pressure (e.g., mass lesions, pseudotumor cerebri).

- Perform a good neurologic exam and make sure "something else" isn't happening.

- The good news about doing a blood patch is that the pressure is no longer on you. Baby's out. Mom's not wiggling and suffering during contractions. You're not looking at a sudden crash C-section and maybe a need for general anesthesia, where maybe you'll lose the airway and maybe it's the end of the universe. No, you're just doing a blood patch in a much less demanding setting.

- Because a blood patch is such a low-pressure situation, you should not fear the need for a blood patch. It's more important to get the baby out safely and get Mom safely through the delivery than it is to "prevent a blood patch."

- In other words, if the day before when Mom needed a C-section, you couldn't get the spinal in with a 25G needle, and you really needed to get that spinal in urgently, then go to a 22G needle if you must.

- Also, an intentional wet tap and placing an intrathecal catheter is a great option in certain high-risk patients, like the morbidly obese. It is reliable and can give you exquisite control, allowing you to titrate the intrathecal medications to get the desired sensory level.

- You can always do a blood patch. You can never bring back someone from the dead.

- Should you go right to a blood patch, or should you choose "conservative measures"? That's a controversial question.

- In the majority of cases, a PDPH is a self-limiting event. The largest study reported that 72% of headaches resolved within seven days. Knowing this and conveying this to the patient may affect the choice of treatment, especially in less severe cases. (There have been reports of headaches persisting for as long as six months successfully treated with epidural blood patch.)

- Conservative measures include bed rest (shown to have no benefit), analgesics, intravenous hydration, and other medications (IV or oral caffeine, sumatriptan).

- Some people will say to hell with the conservative stuff—do the patch. It's low risk and it makes them better. Jacking Mom on heavy caffeine prevents her from sleeping plus she's running to the bathroom all the time with all the fluids and caffeine's diuretic properties.

- The epidural blood patch has had a great safety record. Theoretically, excessive volumes of injected blood could impair spinal cord blood flow. There is always the concern of epidural or paraspinous abscess because of the injection of a culture medium; however, there have been no published reports of this happening.

- Complications of the blood patch include back pain (occurring during the first 48 hours in 35% of patients and persistent in 16% of patients for an average of 27 days), bradycardia, cauda equina syndrome, pneumocephalus, and cerebral ischemia.

- The timing of the blood patch is debatable. Studies suggest greater success when the blood patch is delayed for 24 to 48 hours; however, this may be related to the severity of the headache.

- Prophylactic blood patches are another controversial area. This involves the injection of blood through the epidural catheter prior to the development of a headache. This technique is not routinely used in the majority of centers but there are reports of success.

- Not all patients will develop PDPH and some patients will be needlessly exposed to the risks associated with blood patches.

- There was one report of an immediate total spinal following a prophylactic blood patch. Presumably, local anesthetic-laden CSF was pushed cephalad due to compression by the injected blood outside the dura.

- There have been many alternative attempts to try to treat or prevent PDPH.

- Epidural saline has been used but is ineffective in patients following dural puncture with a 17G needle and relief is only temporary. Dextran has been used but has not found widespread acceptance.

- Intrathecal catheter placement following a wet tap with removal after 24 hours has been reported to reduce the incidence of PDPH.

- In one small study, the injection of 10 ml of intrathecal saline appeared to decrease the severity of PDPH.
- PDPH is very distressing to most patients. They can't nurse and care for their baby. Their expectation of a wonderful birth experience has been shattered. Showing concern, explaining the reasons for the headache, the expected time course, and treatment options goes a long way toward lowering the patient's fears and stress.
- When getting consent for spinals or epidurals, always mention the risk of PDPH. Of course, after you get a wet tap you need to discuss the possibility of PDPH and assure the patient that you will follow up and explain the therapeutic options ahead of time.

BLOOD PATCH HISTORY AND PHYSICAL

- Is the headache worse when sitting upright? Postural headache is the hallmark feature of PDPH—worse in the upright position within 15 minutes and relief when supine within 30 minutes.
- In about half of all cases, the headache is frontal but may also be occipital, both, or generalized.
- Neck pain and stiffness and upper shoulder pain may be present. This can mimic meningitis.
- When did it start? Within the first 24 hours, PDPH will manifest in 38% to 65% of patients. Most cases will be reported within the first three days but it can occur later in up to 25% of cases.
- Diplopia? PDPH may have associated signs suggesting cranial nerve involvement. Visual disturbances (incidence 14%) are related to cranial nerve paresis of CN III, IV, and VI (92–95%).
- Hearing changes or tinnitus? These are related to vestibulocochlear dysfunction. The decrease in CSF pressure is transmitted to the inner ear, disrupting the balance between the endolymphatic and perilymphatic pressures.
- Nausea, vomiting, dizziness, ataxia, and loss of appetite are sometimes present.
- Neurologic symptoms—motor or sensory loss? This would point to some intracranial or spinal cord pathology.
- Fever? Suggests infection. Differential: meningitis, chronic or acute sinusitis.

- Hypertension? History of preeclampsia? Remember, 44% of eclamptic seizures occur postpartum without other premonitory signs.
- Ask about a history of migraines and caffeine consumption.
- Do a thorough physical exam and make sure there are no hard findings. If there are, then do the appropriate studies.
- Intracranial subdural hematomas and dural venous sinus thrombosis are rare. Persistent headache may occur in the presence of a tumor or space-occupying lesion.

TECHNIQUE

- Have a well-functioning IV in place.
- Make sure you have your usual emergency drugs for resuscitation and equipment for airway management and suction readily available.
- Place the patient in a good position. This is critical in case, God forbid, you blow it and give them a second wet tap.
- Although having the patient in the sitting position is usually easier for the person performing the blood patch, the headache may be so severe that you have little choice but to do the procedure with the patient lying on their side.
- At this point, because the baby is out you can sedate the patient, if necessary. However, if the mother is breastfeeding, you may want to limit how much sedation you give her.
- Look over the arm where you will draw blood and make sure you will be able to draw blood from somewhere.
- Your assistant should prep the arm and prepare to draw the blood while you are locating the epidural space.
- Choose the interspace at the level of or one below the original site.
- Perform a sterile prep and drape and infiltrate the area with local anesthetic.
- Once the epidural space is located, have your assistant draw 20 ml of blood in a sterile fashion.
- Slowly inject 15 ml to 20 ml of the blood into the epidural space, or until the patient feels pressure in the back, buttocks, or legs.
- Pull the needle out and take a bow.
- Relief is damned near miraculous.
- The patient should remain spine for about one hour.

An Ounce of Prevention

"Don't get a wet tap!" is about as useful as saying "Don't double fault" or "Don't miss easy putts." EVERYONE KNOWS you shouldn't get wet taps—it's not like you do it on purpose. So is there anything you can do to avoid it?

Mmmmm ... maybe.

If you're in an interspace and really floundering, and you can feel the sweat rings forming in your axillae, and your arm and shoulder muscles are getting tense and starting to cramp, and your fingertips holding the needle are getting numb, and you're getting so ticked off that your calvarium is about to explode like Mount St. Helen's, then perhaps it's time to reconsider.

Pull back, go to a different interspace, take a breather.

As your Frustrat-o-Meter goes into the red zone, you are more likely to, as the rock-and-roll song says, "Break on through to the other side."

The other side of the dura, that is.

Spinals

When it comes to spinals, use the smallest needle you can, and use a pencil point. If you use a non-pencil point needle, arrange the needle so that it "separates" the fibers rather than "cuts a hole" in the dura. So if the patient is sitting, turn the bevel sideways. If the patient is on their side, keep the bevel pointed toward the ceiling.

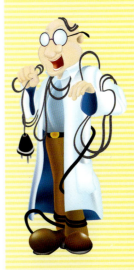

Hammering Home the Point about General Anesthesia and OB

You know from OB that a general anesthetic has 16 times the risk of a fatal outcome.

The patient is as big as Montana and both intubation and a spinal look like they'll be tough.

Time is of the essence.

You can't get the spinal with a skinny needle.

So do you:

1. Go to general anesthesia?

2. Keep floundering with the little needle?

3. Avoid the it's-easier-to-get-it-in 22G spinal needle for fear of subsequent headache and blood patch?

4. Just go for the bigger needle if you must. And don't forget the option of just going for broke and getting an intentional wet tap and placing an intrathecal catheter.

5. Say, "Damn the headache! I can always do a blood patch later in the cool, calm, no one's-life-is-at-risk, postpartum period."

Yes, this is a loaded question. Keep that in mind until you're dribbling oatmeal down your bib and they're debating whether to make you a no-code or not.

A BLOOD PATCH IS PREFERABLE TO BOXING THE PATIENT!

Go for the bigger needle and get a move on.

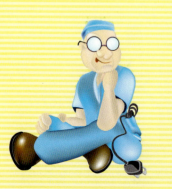

GLITCHES

• When trying to do a blood patch, if you nail the CSF again, then go up a space and try again. If you hit it again, go get counseling and start medication for yourself.

• If you locate the epidural space and can't get blood anywhere, you're in a bad way.

Look over the "vein situation" before you stick the back.

• If it looks super-tough, you might want to place an IV cannula with a short length of tubing before locating the epidural space. However, these can clot sometimes and then you're back to square one.

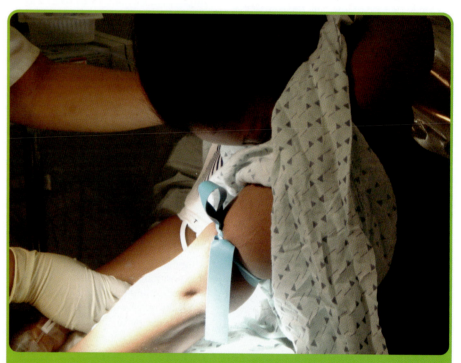

Figure 1. While this may look like modern art, this is actually getting a patient ready for a blood patch.

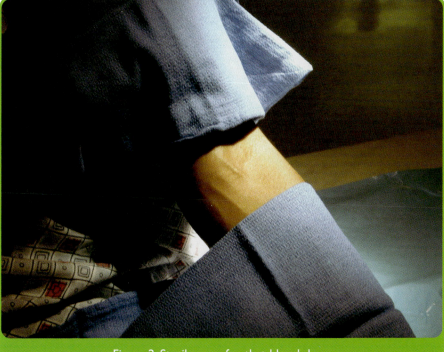

Figure 2. Sterile prep for that blood draw.

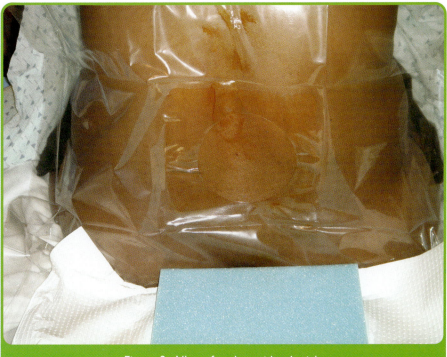

Figure 3. All set for the epidural stick.

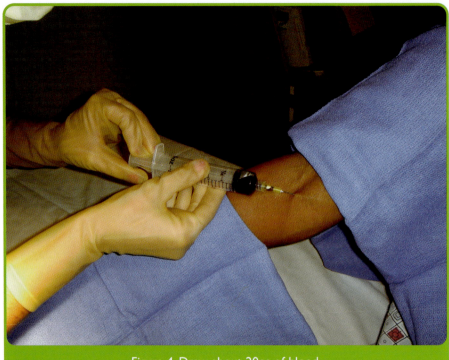

Figure 4. Draw about 20cc of blood.

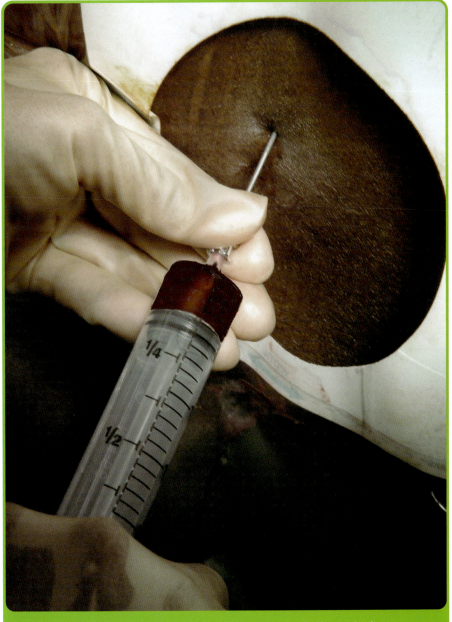

Figure 5. Get the loss of resistance, praying to God you don't get another wet tap. Then, inject the blood.

SUGGESTED READING

Abouleish PJD, Vega S, Blendinger I, et al. Long-term follow-up of epidural blood patch. Anesth Analg 1975;54:459–63.

- *Study finding relief of PDPH in 97.5% overall following blood patch (including those with second blood patch) and procedure safe after two-year follow up.*

Aldrete JA, Brown TL. Intrathecal hematoma and arachnoiditis after prophylactic blood patch through a catheter. Anesth Analg 1997;84:233–4.

Andrews PJD, Ackerman WE, Juneja M, et al. Transient bradycardia associated with extradural blood patch after inadvertent dural puncture in parturients. Br J Anaesth 1992;69:401–3.

- *Small study demonstrating significant drop in heart rate of patients undergoing blood patch.*

Angle P, Thompson D, Halpern S, Wilson DB. Second stage pushing correlates with headache after unintentional dural puncture in parturients. Can J Anesth 1999;46:861–66.

- *Bearing down to squeeze out that bundle of joy probably makes the headache worse.*

Birnbach D, Gatt S, Datta S. *Textbook of Obstetric Anesthesia*. Churchill Livingstone, 2000, 487–503.
- *Everything you wanted to know about PDPH but were afraid to ask.*

Camann WR, Murray RS, Mushlin PS, et al. Effects of oral caffeine on postdural puncture headache: A double-blind, placebo-controlled trial. Anesth Analg 1990;70:181–4.
- *Study finding caffeine provides transient relief of symptoms of PDPH.*

Carter, BL, Paspuleti, R. Use of intravenous cosyntropin in the treatment of postdural puncture headache. Anesthesiology 2000;92(1):272–4.
- *Case report. Maybe ACTH helps by stimulating adrenal glands to increase CSF production or by increased beta-endorphin output? Based on thoughts of Collier.*

Charsley MM, Abram SE. The injection of intrathecal normal saline reduces the severity of postdural puncture headache. Reg Anesth Pain Med 2001;26:301–5.
- *Reduced PDPH and need for blood patch found when investigators injected 10 ml normal saline through the epidural needle or intrathecal catheter after wet tap. Those with injection through the catheter before removal did better.*

Collier, BB. Treatment for postdural puncture headache. Br J Anaesth 1994;72:366–7.

Cornwall RD, Dolan WM. Radicular back pain after lumbar epidural blood patch. Anesthesiology 1975;43:692–3.

Diaz JH. Permanent paraparesis and cauda equina syndrome after epidural blood patch for post-dural puncture headache. Anesthesiology 2002;96:1515–7.
- *Case report. Bad stuff has been associated with blood patch.*

Evans RW, Armon C, Frohman EM, et al. Assessment and prevention of post-lumbar puncture headaches. Report of the Therapeutics and Technology Assessment Subcommittee of the Academy of Neurology. Neurology 2000;55:909–14.
- *The neurologist's take on the matter.*

Fog J, Wang LP, Sundberg A, Mucchiano C. Hearing loss after spinal anesthesia is related to needle size. Anesth Analg 1990;70:517–22.

Hughes S, Levinson G, Rosen M. *Schnider and Levinson's Anesthesia for Obstetrics*, 4th Edition, Lippincott Williams and Wilkins, 2002, 415–7.
- *Text discusses risks associated with PDPH and blood patch.*

Kawamata T, Omote K, Matsumoto M, et al. Pneumocephalus following an epidural blood patch. Acta Anaesth Scand 2003;47:907–9.
- *And it just keeps coming . . .*

Loeser EA, Hill GE, Bennett GM, et al. Time vs. success rate for epidural blood patch. Anesthesiology 1978;49(2):147–8.
- *Answers the question of when to patch.*

Mercieri M, Mercieri A, Paolini S, et al. Postpartum cerebral ischaemia after accidental dural puncture and epidural blood patch. Br J Anaesth 2003;90:98–100.
- *Case report. Can cerebral vasospasm occur with anatomical brain displacement after wet tap or be secondary to blood spreading through the dura mater?*

Nishio I, Williams B, Williams J. Diplopia: A complication of dural puncture. Anesthesiology 2004;100:158–64.

Oh J, Camann W. Severe, acute meningeal irritative reaction after epidural blood patch. Anesth Analg 1998;87:1139–40.
- *More bad stuff.*

Palmer JH, Wilson DW, Brown CM. Lumbovertebral syndrome after repeat epidural blood patch. Br J Anaesth 1997;78:334–6.

Safa-Tiesseront V, Thormann F, Malassine P, et al. Effectiveness of epidural blood patch in the management of post-dural puncture headache. Anesthesiology 2001;95:334–9.
- *Observational study concluded that epidural blood patch is effective for PDPH and the effectiveness is less with dural puncture from a large-bore needle.*

Rucklidge MW, Yentis SM, Paech MJ. Synacthen Depot for the treatment of postdural puncture headache. Anaesthesia. 2004 Feb;59(2):138–41.
- *Investigators found no difference with synacthen depot for PDPH.*

Turnbull, DK, Shepherd DB. Post-dural puncture headache: Pathogenesis, prevention and treatment. Br J Anaesth 2003;91(5):718–29.
- *Great comprehensive discussion of PDPH and management—from the history to weird and wonderful alternatives to blood patch.*

Vandam LD, Dripps RD. Long-term follow-up of patients who received 10,098 spinal anesthetics. Failure to discover major neurological sequelae. JAMA 1954;156:1486–91.
- *Classic article.*

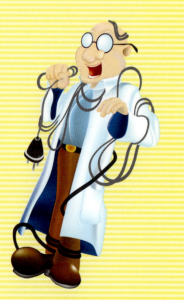

Wang LP, Schmidt JF. Central nervous side effects after lumbar puncture. Dan Med Bull 1997;44:79–81.

• *All the things that happen with doing an LP.*

Williams EJ, Beaulieu P, Fawcett WJ, Jenkins JG. Efficacy of epidural blood patch in the obstetric population. Tnt J Obstet Anesth 1999;8:105–9.

• *Discussion of how well blood patches really work.*

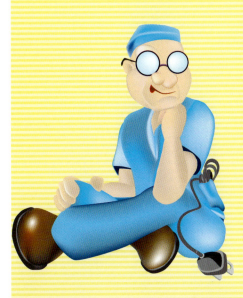

Oh, The Little Darlin's: Kiddie Caudal

James Halliday and Ramiro Gumucio

INTRODUCTION

An anesthesiologist dies and goes to Heaven. Upon entering, she reads, "Welcome to Heaven: Everyone is equal here." She becomes famished upon completion of her tour through Heaven. Once in the cafeteria, a man dressed in green scrubs rushes past her, a policeman, a firefighter, a schoolteacher, and a 70-year-old housewife.

"Hey I thought everyone is equal here!"

"Oh him?" replied the angel. "That's God; he thinks he's a surgeon."

Ramiro Gumucio, M.D.

Never let a surgeon come between you and your procedure!

I digress and step off the anesthesiologist pedestal to render a few helpful hints on the easiest procedure in pediatric regional anesthesia.

True enough, but if a kid hurts, you will hear about it! No stoic suffering in silence in this age group. You will hear their displeasure across the room.

This block has predictable postoperative pain relief. Many of us do a "single shot caudal" after induction of general anesthesia for surgery below the diaphragm.

> No one ever keeps a secret so well as a child.
>
> *Victor Hugo*
> Les Miserables, Book VIII,
> Ch. 8, 1862

SIMPLE, EFFECTIVE, LOW COMPLICATION RATE, GREAT FOR A VARIETY OF PROCEDURES

Regional enthusiasts will point to a zillion regional blocks you can do in children (psoas sheath continuous block, axillary blocks in various flavors, you name it). But unless you're in a real specialty place, you won't see so many of those.

Kiddie caudals? Those you will see. Those everyone does.

INDICATIONS

- Caudal block is a useful adjunct to general anesthesia in most procedures performed below the umbilicus. Remember, in children the sacral ligament is noncalcified and the hiatus is wide, further contributing to the ease of caudal needle placement.

- In larger volumes (0.8 ml/kg to 1.25 ml/kg) and in younger children, it has been described for use in upper abdominal and lower thoracic procedures.

- Pain relief for procedures below the diaphragm (the lower abdomen and lower extremities) is optimized.

- The caudal can provide surgical anesthesia but caudals are most often placed while children are under general anesthesia. Once the caudal is placed, you could let the child emerge from general anesthesia and perform the rest of the case with caudal alone but most often the general anesthetic is continued until the end of the procedure.

- Of course, the general anesthesia you provide can be very light.

- Operations that can benefit from caudal analgesia include herniorrhaphy, orchiopexy, GU procedures, anal/rectal cases, and orthopedic procedures on the lower extremities, hip, and pelvis.

- More adventuresome souls place caudals and slide the epidural catheter farther up, providing analgesia for procedures in the upper abdomen and even thorax. This is a specialty procedure performed mostly by that pediatric anesthesiologist in your practice who watched episodes of *McGyver* during residency.

- Timing is everything. It is better to place the block at the beginning of the case when the patient will reap the benefit of the anesthesia-sparing effects and be monitored post-block. Placing it at the end of the procedure may result in pain immediately postoperatively and bad things going unnoticed as the child is taken to the PACU.

CONTRAINDICATIONS

- Few and similar to those in adults
- You are going to stick a needle where? (Parent or guardian refusal)
- Doctor, this baby bleeds like a stuck pig. (Coagulopathy)

- Why does the sacral cornu have cheese on it? (Sepsis/meningitis or infection localized to the site of entry)
- Doctor, this baby's fontanelle is *deep*. (Uncorrected hypovolemia; hemodynamically, the sympathectomy could put the kid over the edge.)
- There goes her chance to strut down a New York runway for Calvin Klein. (Malformations of the sacrum)
- Myelomeningocele: malposition of the cord or dural sac
- Hydrocephalus
- Doctor, my child sets off the metal detectors at the airport. (S/P implant, such as Harrington's rods or similar implants)
- Risks and benefits in these patients should be carefully considered on an individual basis.

EQUIPMENT

- A caudal block can be performed with just about any kind of needle. An IV or butterfly needle are your weapons of choice.
- A short or intermediate bevel is preferable to a real sharp needle because the more blunt needle gives a better "feel" when the sacrococcygeal membrane is penetrated.
- You can use a specific epidural catheter for this procedure (Crawford), although people often use a 20G or 22G IV cannula. Stylette needles prevent the introduction of a skin plug into the epidural space that may later develop into an epidermal inclusion cyst. Intravenous catheters offer the advantage of confirmation of correct placement if the catheter easily slides off the needle.

Epican Caudal Needle Options

- 25G × 1¼ in. without wings
- 22G × 1-3/8 in. without wings
- 20G × 2 in. without wings

PHILOSOPHY

- No kidding (pardon the pun), this block is easy to do.
- Kids emerge from anesthesia so nicely with this procedure; it makes pediatric anesthesia most rewarding.
- Of course, parents are thrilled when their child wakes up pain-free. This is a real win-win kind of a block, and so well worth doing.

- A word of caution: The apparent simplicity of this block and technical ease is where the potential danger arises—that is, the unseen *intravascular* injection of local anesthetic.

TECHNIQUE

- Induce the child: inhalational or IV (if you are fortunate to have a kid with an IV)

MONITORING

- Monitors should be applied and their function confirmed before the block is performed. In particular, the electrocardiogram should be adjusted so that the P wave, QRS complex, and upright T wave are present. One should monitor initial vitals before the procedure.
- An ETT/LMA or mask airway is fine as long as you can maintain adequate ventilation and oxygenation with the patient on their side.

STERILE TECHNIQUE

- Bacterial colonization of caudal catheters in children occurs at a rate of 6% to 35%. Gram-positive organisms are most common although gram-negative colonization can occur, particularly with caudal catheters. Children under three years of age are most likely to have colonization of caudal catheters. Chlorhexidine is better than povidone iodine for reducing the risk of catheter colonization in children. Remember, this is an *epidural* and should be respected as such in terms of sterile technique.
- Palpate the sacrococcygeal membrane, which is in the triangular space bordered by the sacral cornua laterally and the sacrococcygeal joint caudally. The sacrococcygeal membrane is just a little above the coccyx (see figure).
- Want another way? The right spot is often just at the beginning of the crease in the buttocks (see figure).

CAUDAL TECHNIQUE

- The posterior superior iliac spines and the sacral hiatus form an equilateral triangle, the apex of which points inferiorly. The sacral cornua are easily

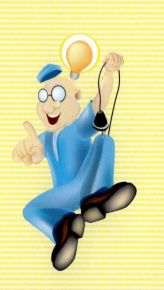

palpated on either side of the sacral hiatus, approximately 0.5 cm to 1 cm apart.

- Take an intravenous needle, an intravenous catheter, or a Crawford needle (kiddie epidural needle) of appropriate size. Palpate the sacral hiatus. Advance through the skin at about 45° until you feel a pop.

- Reduce the angle of the needle and advance into the caudal canal.

- If you're going to do an epidural, slide the catheter up now. If you're using an IV catheter, slide the catheter up the caudal canal. It should pass easily; if not, you're not in. Remove the needle and aspirate.

- After negative aspiration, inject your dose of local anesthetic. The local should inject easily. If resistance is felt or you feel crepitance, then you are subcutaneous.

GOT YOU!

Test dose: The authors strongly recommend the use of a test dose to decrease the likelihood of intravascular injection. However, it is not 100% reliable and dosing with careful attention to vital signs is recommended. A test dose should be 0.1 ml/kg of a local anesthetic solution with 5 μg/ml of epinephrine to a maximum volume of 3 ml. An increase in heart rate of 10 beats per minute above baseline within 1 minute is a reasonable predictor of intravascular injection.

FIVE GOLDEN RULES TO STAY OUT OF TROUBLE

1. Aspiration test before injection (blood, CSF)

2. Evaluation of test dose (ST/T wave changes, brady-tachycardia)

3. Inject slowly or incrementally. A huge bolus of IV local will result in much more plasma-free drug and be much more hazardous than the same quantity given time to bond with intravascular proteins and such, not that you ever want to inject intravascularly.

4. No change in resistance to injection

5. Repeat aspiration prior to incremental injection and following catheter placement.

LOCAL ANESTHETICS

- Bupivicaine 0.25% or 0.125%. A lower concentration is better for kids three years old and older where urinary retention may be an issue with a higher concentration.

- Levobupivicaine may have less cardiovascular consequences if there is an inadvertent IV injection.

DOSAGE

- Sacrolumbar (T11) 0.5 ml/kg
- Lumbothoracic (T8) 0.75 ml/kg
- Midthoracic (T6—maybe you should not be performing a caudal) 1 ml/kg

CAUDAL-TO-THORACIC TECHNIQUE

The caudal approach to thoracic epidural has been used in infants and even in children up to 10 years of age. Success in this age group is related to the less densely packed epidural fat that allows free cephalad passage of the catheter. Some authors also suggest ease of removal of the stylet from a stylette-type catheter, ease of injection, negative aspiration, and test doses predict successful placement, whereas others suggest radiographic confirmation.

CONTINUOUS CAUDAL CATHETER

Equipment

- An 18G or 19G needle (Crawford type) with a 20G or 21G catheter is used in patients of all sizes.

- Smaller catheters tend to kink either at placement or during postoperative use.

- A stylette catheter has been reported to increase the successful passage of catheters to the thoracic level.

- After placement, care must be taken to prevent fecal contamination because of the proximity of the anus to the insertion site.

- It is prudent to keep them in for no longer than three days.

Glitches

- 119 children's hospitals
- 150,000 caudals
- 1:40,000 catastrophic complications (namely, IV injection of local anesthetics)

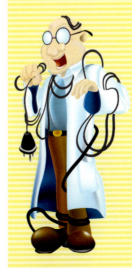

- Complications are unusual—1 out of 1000 procedures—and usually minor.
- Most complications result from the misplacement of the needle into superficial soft tissues or sacral foramina, resulting in block failure, intrathecal puncture with subsequent spinal anesthesia, or intravascular or intraosseous injections, leading to systemic toxicity.

- You inject, feel crepitance, you're subcutaneous.
- In patients under five years old, an epidural catheter should advance easily. Older than that, passing the catheter gets more problematic.
- As with any other regional procedure, the local can go in the wrong place—intravascular or intraosseous.

THINGS TO REMEMBER

- The most common glitch is from—what else—inexperience.

Major Complications	What to Look for
Excessively high block	Hypotension/respiratory difficulties/
	SpO$_2$/bradycardia
Total spinal	Above symptoms and LOC
Intravascular migration of catheter	Numbness, blurred vision, tinnitus
Infection	Visual (transparent dressing)
Bleeding with development of epidural hematoma	Back pain, increased sensory and motor block

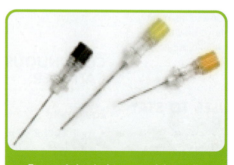

Figure 1. Little bitty caudal needle things for the little varmints.

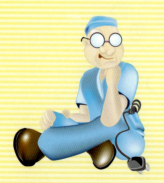

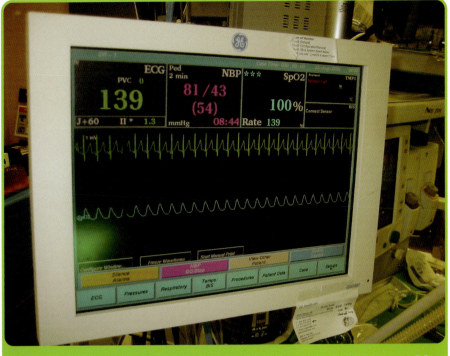

Figure 2. Breathe them down (or IV them down if you're lucky and have an IV).

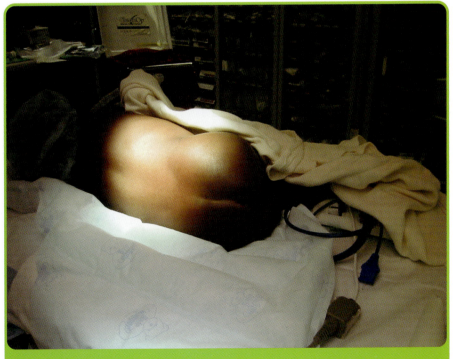

Figure 3. Flex the patient's hips up; this will expose the insertion site.

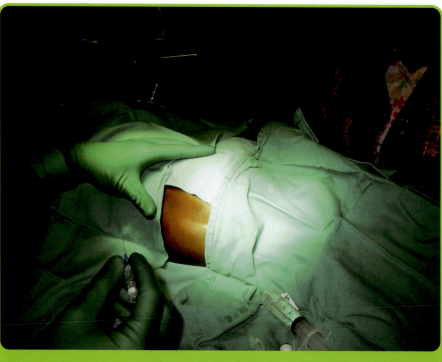

Figure 4. Are your hands clean doctor?

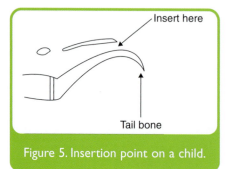

Figure 5. Insertion point on a child.

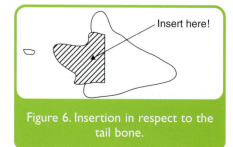

Figure 6. Insertion in respect to the tail bone.

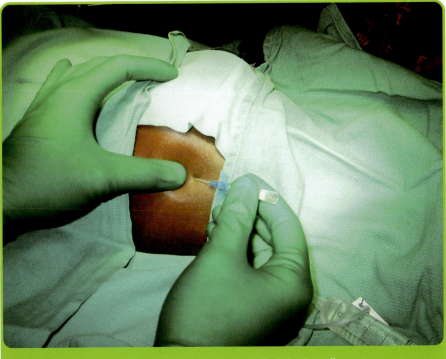

Figure 7. Go shallow 'til you feel the "pop."

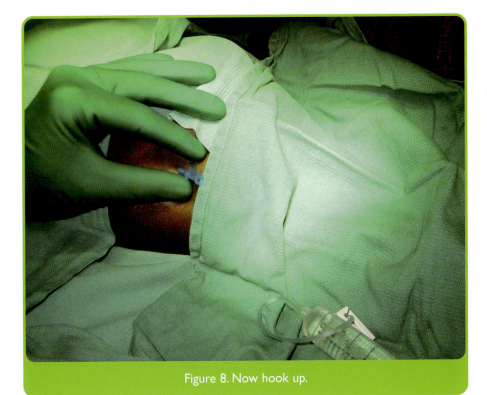

Figure 8. Now hook up.

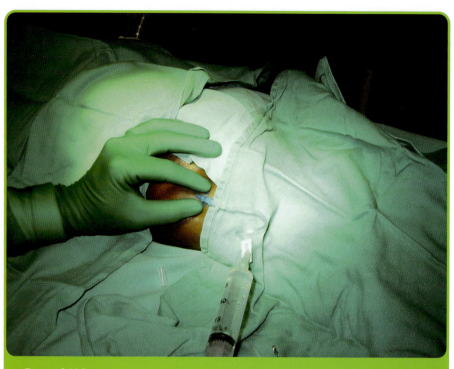

Figure 9. When you inject, make sure you don't feel crepitance. That indicates you're sub-q.

SUGGESTED READING

Gunter JB. Thoracic epidural anesthesia via the caudal approach in children. Anesthesiology 1992;76(6):935–8.
Sounds wild but they can slither that catheter way up there.

Inagawa G, Miwa T, et al. Unanticipated dural tap in caudal anesthesia: A case of intrasacral meningocele. Anesth Analg 2005;101:302.
Damnation, it seems there's a snake under every rock.

Ivanni G, De Negri P, et al. Caudal anesthesia for minor pediatric surgery: A prospective randomized comparison of ropivicaine 0.2% vs levobupivicaine 0.2%. Pedi Anesth 2005;15(6):491–4.

Miller, R. *Miller's Anesthesia*, 6th edition. 1673–4, 1732–4.
What would we do without Miller?

Seefelder C, Hill, D, et al. Awake caudal anesthesia or inguinal surgery in one conjoined twin. Anesth Analg 2003;96:412–3.
Just when you thought there couldn't be something new in anesthesia.

Suresh S, Wheeler M. Practical pediatric regional anesthesia. Anesth Clin N Am 2002;20:83–113.
Walks you right through it.

Tobias J. Caudal epidural block: A review of test dosing and recognition of systemic injection in children. Anesth Analg 2001;93: 1156–61.

Verghese S, Hannalalah R, et al. Caudal anesthesia in children: Effect of volume vs concentration of bupivicaine on blocking spermatic cord traction response during orchiodopexy. Anesth Analg 2002;95: 1219–23.

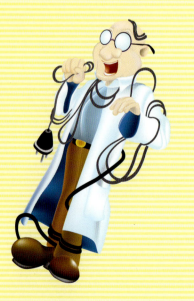

PART 5

EFFICIENCY-VILLE

Getting a Case Going at a Greater-than-Glacial Pace

Jas Katariya and Samir Kulkarni

This time, like all times, is a very good one, if we but know what to do with it.

Ralph Waldo Emerson
The American Scholar, 1837

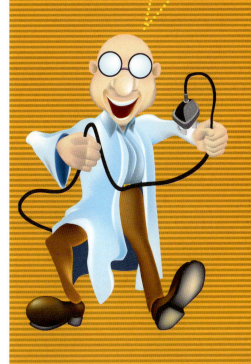

INTRODUCTION

If you can't get a case going in private practice, they will chew you up and spit you out. Do not deceive yourself—efficiency matters. A surgeon may like you, a surgeon may admire your brilliance and skill, but more than anything else a surgeon wants to get going.

Go so fast you're unsafe? Never.
Skip crucial steps? Never.
Treat the patient dismissively? Never.
Rush the OR staff and treat them in a snippy fashion? Never.
Cut out unnecessary steps and move in a logical fashion to get the case going? Always!

INDICATIONS

- Getting home eventually! The sooner you get going on the case, the sooner you get going home.

CONTRAINDICATIONS

- When would you not want to be efficient? I can't think of that time.

PHILOSOPHY OF EFFICIENCY

- By definition, efficiency is "the production of the desired results with minimum wastage of time, effort or skill." There's nothing earth-shaking or MENSA-like going on here. Just think through your movements and remove the excess.
- Efficiency begins in the preoperative suite: Teamwork, organization, and communication are key.
- A timely and thorough review of the chart and medical history is essential. This includes all preoperative testing and any required specialist evaluations. In case of possible concerns regarding patient optimization, the surgeon's office must be informed a few days in advance so that timely interventions can lead to a timely start of an elective case on the day of surgery.
- Get those insurance companies on board early. Pre-approval for the procedure should be secured prior to the day of surgery. Plus, it's unseemly to hold the patient upside-down and shake them in the hopes of getting some spare change on the day of surgery.

TEAMWORK

- The team consists of the anesthesiologist, surgeon, pre- and postoperative area staff, OR nurses, and environmental services each performing to ensure rapid patient movement in and out of the OR.
- From an economic standpoint, don't forget the environmental services personnel. It doesn't make sense to hold up a $600/hour OR plus all kinds of pricey specialists because you are short one minimum-wage person to mop the floor between cases. You should have the largest supply of these people so that they never constitute a "roadblock" to starting a case or turning over a room.

GET YOUR ACT TOGETHER

- The key to the kingdom here is *preparation*.
- Get all the stuff you need ahead of time. Running around with the patient in the room is low class.
- Scout your surroundings so *you* know where the special equipment is located.
- A well-trained anesthesia technician is always a major asset. This person can be trained to keep stock of the inventory, keep the OR well-stocked, be vigilant with the upkeep of the difficult airway cart, MH cart, fiberoptic carts, and so on. They know the rest can also be trained to recognize cases in which invasive monitoring is required so as to set them up for the next day.
- However, over-reliance on technicians will invariably bite you in the butt because one day the tech is gone, the tech is sick, or the tech just bailed out and went elsewhere for bigger bucks and you don't know where anything is located.

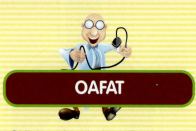

OAFAT

Obligatory Anesthesia, uh, Fool-Around(?) Time.

This is the time we, of the anesthesia persuasion, use up prior to handing the anesthetized patient over to the surgeons. As far as surgeons are concerned, OAFAT is all wasted time. Forget that we are frittering away our time doing trivial things like establishing an airway, getting adequate lines, and assuring a stable and insensate patient.

"Let's get going," say our surgical confreres. "Let's get going, whatever it takes."

Do we ignore this surgical badgering? Well, to quote many a politician, yes and no.

Yes, ignore the surgical badgering. Never let a surgeon rush you when you are doing something life-saving (intubating awake, getting a needed central line, stabilizing vital signs).

No, don't ignore the surgical badgering. There is no getting around it—the surgeon is your referral base and any surgeon wants to get going. Hey, who can blame them? The sooner we go, the sooner we go! (And that means you get to go home too, so everyone wins if you move along efficiently.)

Develop a slick start to your case. That doesn't mean you skip any safety measures or cut corners but it does mean you move smoothly and efficiently, getting the case going as soon as you safely can.

- Have extras with you. For example, if you are doing an art line, have an extra catheter with you in case you miss the first time. Not that *I* ever miss, heaven forbid, but we include this useful tidbit for the lesser mortals out there.

- Clean up as you go along; don't leave dirty sharps lying around. You might get hurt or someone else might get hurt. Be especially aware of the "dirty sharp lying under a drape" syndrome. You go to lift up the drape and *bazingo*! You lift up your hand and it looks like a porcupine's quill is stuck in it.

- Check, oh check, oh please Lordy Lordy, check that consent before you give some midazolam. Nothing like a "No wait! We have to change the consent!" and there you stand with a now-empty midazolam syringe, a patient with glazed eyes, and a real problem on your hands.

- Once patient and chart are checked and cleared by you and a working IV is ensured (remember Chapter 1: Don't trust a crummy IV from the floor—make sure you have a real, live, good-enough-for-anesthesia IV), anxiolytics and amnestics are administered as the patient is wheeled to the OR. All your movements from here on should come like clockwork

TECHNIQUE

- Do a little shadowboxing to see just how inefficient you are. Go into an empty room and "imagine yourself" performing a case and do all the walking you usually do.
- Note that you make about five "round trips" around the table.
- Figure out how to make five round trips into one round trip.
- Go around to the right side, put the EKG monitors on that side, place the pulse oximeter, and strap the arm down. Now swing around to the left, place the EKG pads there, the art line, make sure the IV is OK, place the blood pressure cuff, strap the arm down, and go to the head of the bed. Voila! One trip rather than running back and forth, back and forth.
- Once you're ready to start, note how long you will have to stand there, doing nothing, while the patient pre-oxygenates. But wait! There's a solution to that too.
- Before you go around the patient, use the black face strap and put the mask on

the patient. That way, the patient pre-oxygenates *while* you are putting on EKG pads and other monitors.

- With the patient already pre-oxygenated, once you get to the head of the bed, you can go right into your induction.
- To make injecting easy, place some stopcocks within easy reach.
- Think and think and rethink what you do, always asking, "How can I streamline this procedure?"
- Have extras with you. For example, if you are working with an art line, have an extra catheter with you in case you miss the first time. Sound familiar? We who place lines from the Olympian heights of "Never Do I Miss" Land really *are* laughing at those of you who do.
- Clean up as you go along; don't leave dirty sharps lying around. You might get hurt or someone else might get hurt. (Yes, this is repetitive but it bears repeating. One moment's inattention in exchange for months of anguish, blood tests, and who knows what.)
- So far so good; no rocket science here. It's the same thing every day, day after day—repetition of an efficient sequence ensures that nothing gets missed in times of crises. Now you can focus on the vital part: the induction.
- Always have a backup plan in case of a crisis. Take control of the situation while calling for help and give out specific, coherent instructions to the nursing staff, anesthesia personnel, and surgeon (who will often be present).
- If you move well and convey a professional attitude, then you *are* a professional. OR staff appreciate this—people like to work with professionals. They are not so fond of working with Bozo the Clown.

GLITCHES

- You screw up when you think "shortcut" rather than "streamline." Of course, you can get going faster if you don't pre-oxygenate. But that is a dangerous shortcut, not a streamline maneuver.
- Don't push OR staff. That will always come back to haunt you. You need to work with these people and treating them as underlings to be bossed around is both wrong and counterproductive.
- Work *with* the OR staff to get cases going. The spirit of cooperation will do you right in the long run.

- On those occasions when you *do* have to push the staff (cath lab emergency coming down in full arrest and there is no time to set up the room properly), then the OR staff will understand. Push them *all the time, every day*, and you won't get that understanding from them. It's the "Boy Who Cried Wolf" syndrome: Because you're *always* yelling at them to get a move on, when you really *do* need them to get a move on, they will just say, "Oh, that again."

- Don't panic in a super-bad case (such as that cath lab disaster in full arrest coming down to the OR). If everything is chaos and madness, then that is the time to *slow down*. Make sure the oxygen is on, make sure the ventilator is working, and make sure the lines are all hooked up. Perform a methodical assessment of everything or you will miss something big.

- An efficient, organized, and motivated anesthesiologist commands respect from the patients, OR staff, and surgeons

alike. If that doesn't work, then give everyone a lot of money at holiday time and try to buy some friends.

BEWARE TOO MUCH EFFICIENCY IN CERTAIN SITUATIONS

- In a busy private practice, rooms are switched around all the time.
- Surgeons will have multiple cases lined up, often at more than one site, storming in and out of ORs and hospitals
- *Always* double-check consent and side of surgery but especially when your normal lineup has been disrupted. This is where mix-ups occur, so always take a few seconds to make sure the right thing is being performed on the right person.
- You always have time to *think*, no matter how fast you're moving.

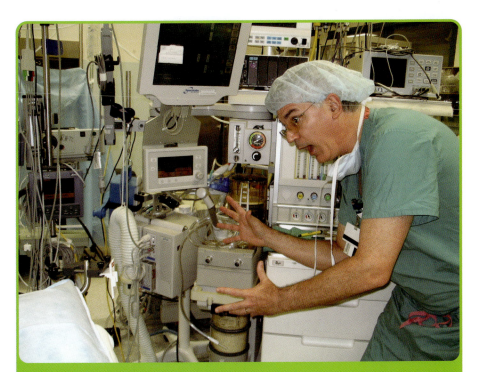

Figure 1. When setting up your room, try to use what little remnants of a frontal lobe that you still have.

A Typical Start

In comes the patient.

"Damn, where's the armboard?"

You leave the room.

"What, no armstraps?"

Again, you leave the room.

You swing around to the right, then come over to the left, then swing back to the right, tripping over wires and compression tubing.

After floundering around all over the place, *now* you start pre-oxygenating, so everyone gets to sit around for even more time—all because you didn't think through this stuff ahead of time.

A floundering, inefficient, time-consuming launch is not safer, either! In your chicken-with-head-recently-detached modality, you are more likely to overlook or "shortchange" stuff.

Forget to strap an arm down, then you induce and the arm flops off the armboard.

You are so "behind" that you do an incomplete pre-oxygenation. Ack! Remember the mantra, "Trouble doesn't ring a bell." This will be the very patient whose airway gets lost and you end up in the soup.

You're in such a tizzy that you forget to look at the chart and miss something major (MH, spinal cord injury, allergy). It sounds impossible but it happens! Especially in a busy practice where rooms are switched around and sometimes the patient even gets "put on the OR bed for you, all you have to do is put him to sleep." You can overlook *major* stuff.

Remember, no matter the time constraints, you *always* have time to *think* before you induce.

Ongoing Efficiency

Once you've induced, your "move to efficiency" should not stop.

As soon as the patient is induced, you can tell the surgeon or nurse, "OK, place the Foley," if the case requires a Foley. The idea is to keep doing as many things at once as you can. Do more than one thing at once rather than plod along, one "procedure" at a time.

Say the circulator is placing the Foley; you can handle the airway alone most of the time. If, by chance, you need a hand, tell the circulator, "Oops, hold off a second on that Foley and give me a hand here." Yes, yes, a purist would say you cannot possibly liberate the circulator a nanosecond before you are completely done, but come on. If you can safely send the circulator on to the next task, then do it.

Does the surgeon need to stand there like a statue while you place extra lines?

No.

The surgeon can prep while you place an A-line or a CVP. At some crucial point, you might ask, "Stop wiggling the patient for a second here, and let me get this wire in." Then you, and everybody, move on.

Keep moving, keep moving, and keep doing stuff.

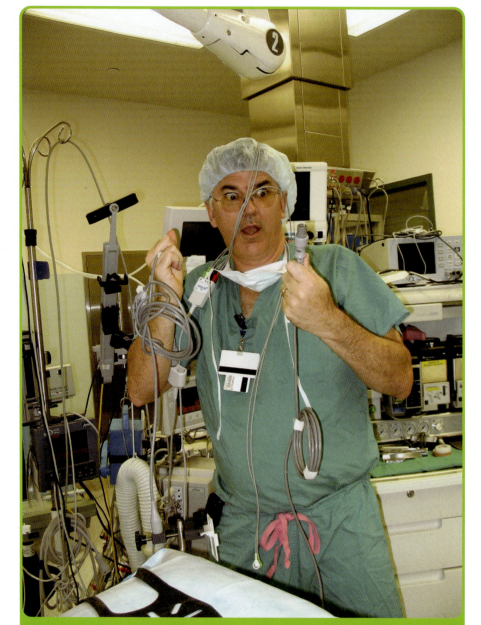

Figure 2. Don't fall into the trap of going into congestive line failure. Oh what a tangled web we weave.

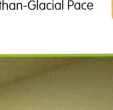

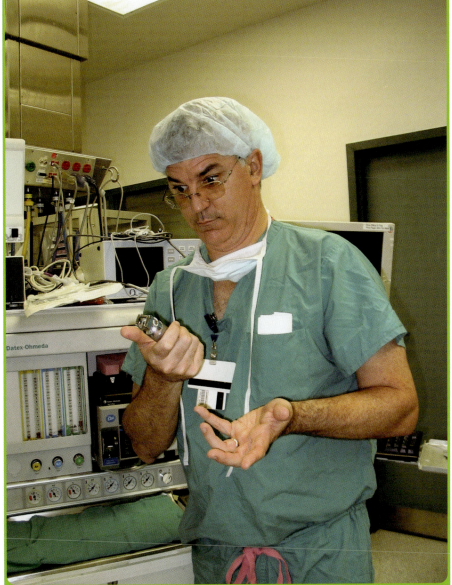

Figure 3. Get the stuff you need ahead of time. You don't want to be looking at a malfunctioning, or for that matter, non-existent blade at the moment of truth.

Getting People to Help You

Can you rope anyone into this Efficiency-ville you are building? By all means!

Work with the staff in your room. For example, see if they can at least put the EKG leads on for you. Show them how to "tee up" the wrist for an A-line (wrist board with rolled up 4 X 4s, wrist placed in extension). That way, if you are having trouble with an A-line on the left, you can say, "Tee up the right wrist for me while I clean up here," and you can diminish "down time" between line attempts.

In-service yourself on where all the "stuff" is. Wander around central supply or the central core and find for yourself the awake intubation equipment, CVP and spinal trays, extra stopcocks, and pressure tubing. In the tiny hours of the night, tech help is hard to come by, so the more "auto-anesthesia-teching" you can do, the better.

Nothing would tick off a surgeon more than you running from pillar to post, looking for some routine equipment and delaying the start of the case.

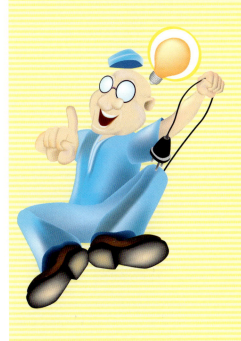

Efficiency Outside the OR

- The ORs have traditionally been a very significant source of revenue generation, not only for the OR-related specialties but for hospitals in general. In this era of declining profits and increasing costs, inefficiency leading to large scale cancellations or wasted OR time further reduces profits.

- More hospitals are now looking to *anesthesiologists* to assume the role of OR managers, often with a formal title as such as "Medical Director of Perioperative Services" or "MDPS," which is either impossible to pronounce or will be a creature in the next *Harry Potter* book.

- An anesthesiologist with an extensive knowledge of the workings of the OR may work as a liaison between the surgeons, nursing staff, and hospital administrators. Let's see, such a beast would be called, um, "Liaison Between Surgeons, Nursing Staff and Hospital Administrators" or "LB-SNSHA." J.K. Rowling, take note.

- An efficient administrator needs to ensure that OR time is allocated based on a service's and surgeon's requirement of total hours of all elective cases. If there is a fluctuating need for time allocation, as is the case in most operating rooms, the cases need to be accommodated in a manner that uses staff or rooms in the most efficient manner possible. Statistically derived staffing solutions are available to calculate staffing requirements for each service, thereby minimizing under- or over-utilization of ORs and staff.

- In this constantly evolving and changing job description, other aspects such as quality improvement also become very important. This entails monitoring the accurate collection of data regarding timely starts, reasons for delay, cancellations, turnover times, hold times, either under- or over-utilization of allocated time to a service, and so on. Each of these issues will affect revenues and therefore early recognition and efficient correction of the same affects the bottom line.

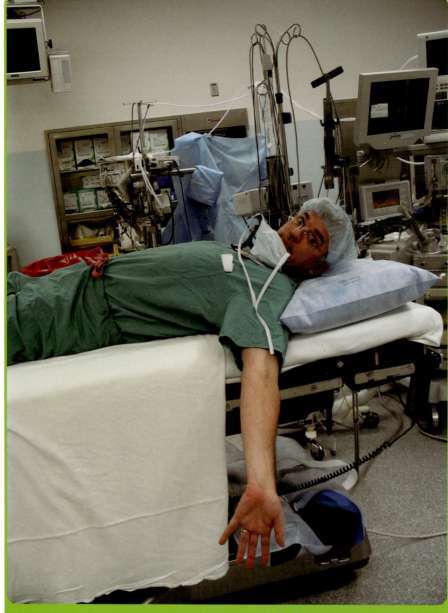

Figure 4. No armboards on the table? Oh that's great, where will the patient put his or her arms? Remember, each step you DON'T take care of ahead of time, is a step you will have to take care of when the patient is in the room. And that wastes valuable OR time.

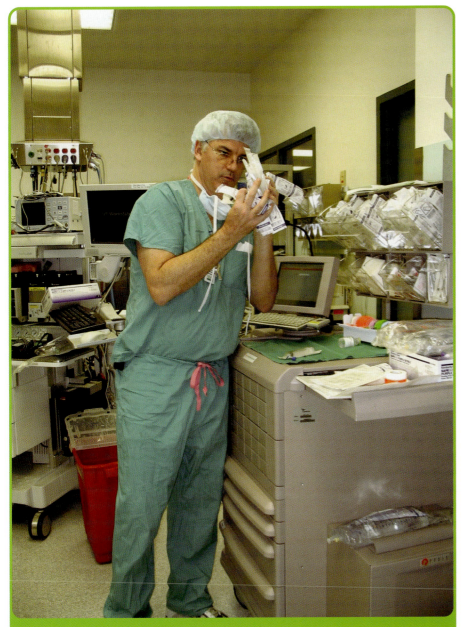

Figure 5. Drawing up all your drugs when the patient is in the room. No good! Again, you are wasting time and looking like a ninny! Do all you can ahead of time so when the patient hits the room, you are all efficiency.

- Previously, we weren't so scientific about all this stuff—we just fumed and fussed at the front desk, saying "That bastard said he'd be done in two hours and here we are, five hours later and he's still ankle deep in chitlins in there. Get me the MDPS! Better yet, get me the LBSNSHA!" Now we collect data, send angry e-mails, then stand at the front desk fussing and fuming.

- High-quality information systems must be incorporated into the working OR. These provide a broad database, enabling retrieval and linking of information between the areas of pre-operative testing, intraoperative charting, quality assurance, laboratories, radiology, and anesthesia billing. This is an emerging trend, one that promises to enable anesthesiologists to have vital patient information available instantly. Another application of the information systems would be patient safety by facilitating adherence to guidelines, warnings, and alerts and decision support, thereby reducing medical errors.

- Of course, such a system has its detractors who point out that automated systems require battalions of computer-savvy gurus to flit around the ORs like wraiths at all hours of the day and night as computer systems sputter, choke, gag, and die at the worst possible times.

- In the face of declining reimbursements and sky rocketing costs, anesthesiologists must know how the money flows and know how to make the ink become black so the hospital can get some green.

- In this day and age, a good anesthesiologist is therefore not only a good, efficient, and caring doctor but also a business manager par excellence. That's why, as you might have noticed, every other anesthesiologist now has an MBA, and even those who don't have an MBA are starting to use "MBA-speak"—prioritization, institutionalization of goal-directed manifestations, ad-hoc committees to further investigate variegated subsets of . . . you get the drift.

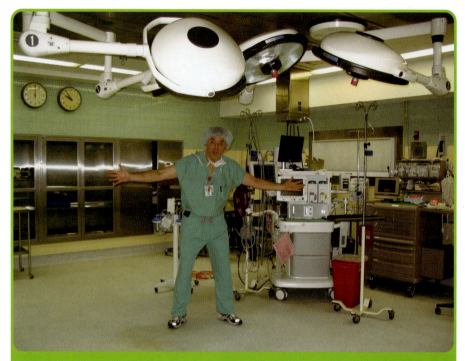

Figure 6. Oh yeah, don't forget little things, like making sure there is, say, SOMETHING FOR THE PATIENT TO LIE DOWN ON! (No kidding, this has happened. You roll into the room and there is, well, no bed in the room. A more common glitch is this, they get on the table and the electrical signals don't work. Look over the table and make sure it works!)

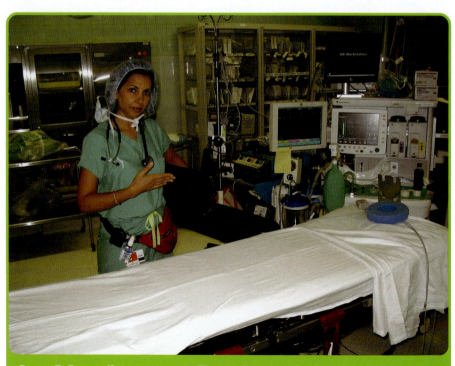

Figure 7. Enter efficieny-incarnate. The armboard is already on the side opposite 'patient arrival', and the other armboard is right there, not lost somewhere in Tibet or Greenland.

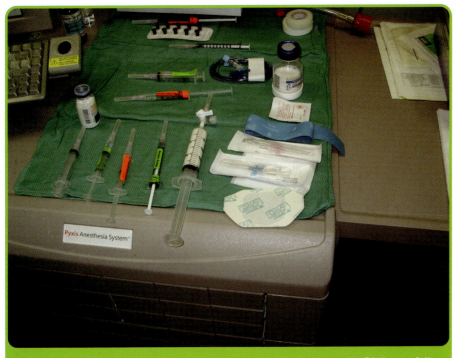

Figure 8. Drugs, ah, nice and neat. Labeled, laid out, ready to go. Oh be joyful!

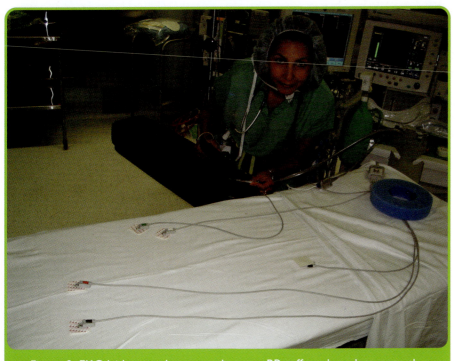

Figure 9. EKG laid out, pulse ox ready to go, BP cuff ready to leap onto the patient. This is living! Why can't everyone be as organized and brilliant as this practitioner?

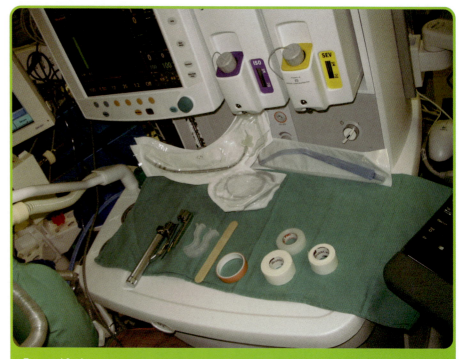

Figure 10. Airway equipment, par excellence. No clutter, just what you need and where yo need it.

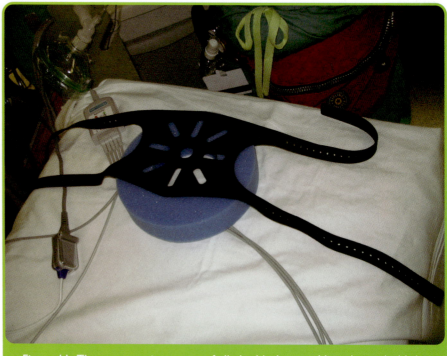

Figure 11. The greatest time saver of all, the black strap. Use this to hold the mask in place so you can pre-oxygenate the patient WHILE you do other stuff. Then, when you've got all your monitors on, presto chango, the patient is already pre-oxygenated and you are ready to induce.

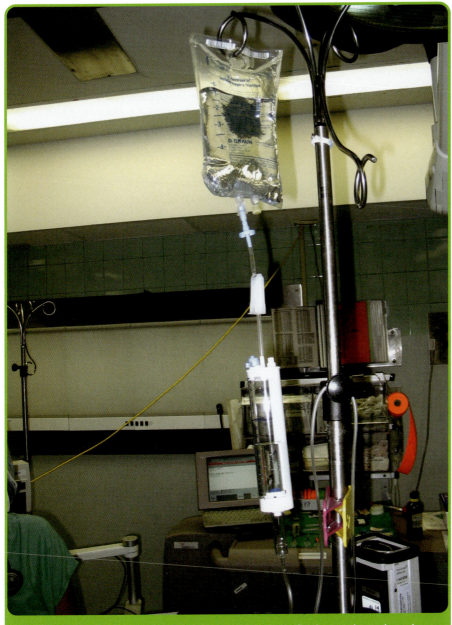

Figure 12. Don't forget the IV, have that ready to go, fluids run through, and you are READY TO ROCK!

SUGGESTED READING

Abouleish AE. Responding to 'You're inefficient—work faster!' ASA newsletter April 2003;67.

- *This article was written in April 2003. It discusses in detail important issues involved in OR efficiency and common misconceptions about anesthesiologists as seen from the standpoint of surgeons, OR managers, and hospital administrators. The points the author discusses are "we don't work fast because we get paid by time," "if the turnover time was shorter, more cases would be done," and "according to benchmarks, you don't need*

more people to cover more ORs." The author carefully dissects each of these issues and correctly shows why they are incorrect.

Dexter F. Allocating operating room time and scheduling surgical cases to maximize

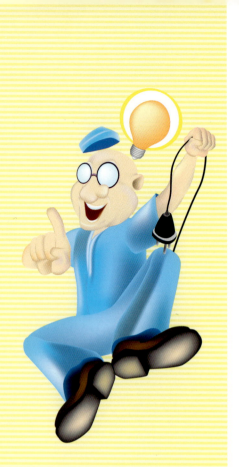

operating room efficiency. 54th annual refresher course lectures, clinical updates and Basic Science Reviews

- *A concise and scientific approach to tackling efficiency-related issues and thereby reducing costs. He details appropriate usage of all resources including the staff and writes about optimal OR time allocation.*

Malhotra VV. Nuts and bolts of O.R. management. ASA annual meeting refresher course lectures 2002

- *This lecture covers a wide array of OR-related issues including operational and financial topics, leadership, importance of adherence to schedule, data management, quality improvement, and so on. A nice easy read yet very informative.*

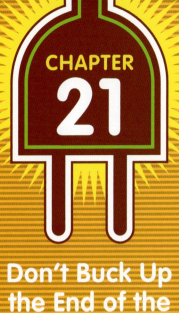

CHAPTER 21

Don't Buck Up the End of the Case: The Smooth Wake Up

John Sciarra and Codruta Soneru

Hail, ye small, sweet courtesies of life! For smooth do ye make the road of it.

Laurence Sterne
Tristram Shandy, 1760

INTRODUCTION

What is a procedure?

When we think of a procedure, we think of "sticking something somewhere"—art line, central line, or axillary deposition of local anesthetic. Somehow a "smooth wakeup" doesn't fit into the "procedure" bailiwick.

But think about it for a second:

- A procedure requires some thought.
- A procedure requires some skill.
- A procedure serves a purpose.

So hell, a smooth wake up *is* a procedure. And if you've ever gotten in trouble during a *stormy* wake up, you know just how valuable a *smooth* wake up can be. So what do you think of when I say smooth?

Smooth as a baby's bottom.

Smooth as butter.

Smooth as glass.

Smooth as [insert your name here]'s wake ups. Now wouldn't that be nice to hear?

INDICATIONS

- A big muscular brute who used to play tackle for Oklahoma. If he wakes up thrashing, he might clock you. Also, his heavily muscled chest could generate monster negative pressure pulmonary edema if he goes into laryngospasm.

- An obese patient. Similarly, a stormy wake up with 4+ thrashing could bring the patient's bulk over the edge of the OR table with disastrous consequences. Also, if you extubate during a smash-o-rama with this obese patient, you could end up with quick desaturation as you struggle to mask assist with ventilation.

- Blood in the upper airway. If a patient post-ethmoidectomy or rhinoplasty decides to "emerge like thunder," you can end up with severe bleeding in the airway. Now you may extubate amidst a spray of blood, a quick obstruction, and a catastrophic smashing-on-of-mask-on-freshly-sculpted nose. Bad news!

- Asthmatic with a difficult airway or full stomach. You don't really have the "deep extubation" option. You want this patient to just gently open their eyes and allow extubation without a lot of *Sturm und Drang*.

- Intracranial case. You don't want the patient to wake up with a horrific bucking jag—that won't help your ICP at all.

- Open eye case. Same argument: you don't want the eye contents under pressure.

- Plastic surgery involving the face. A hematoma here can ruin the reputation of a great surgeon and cut into their over-priced fees.

- Hernia repair. No need to pop those stitches.

- Carotid. Big-time cough at the end of the case could pop those stitches, too, and create a big hematoma right smack dab near the airway.

- God all fishhooks, it's hard to think of a case where a smooth wake up is *not* a good idea!

CONTRAINDICATIONS

- None that I can think of

EQUIPMENT

- Your head screwed on good and tight and your neurons firing on all eight cylinders

THE PHILOSOPHY OF THE SMOOTH LANDING

- Instead of thinking who *could use* a smooth wake up, just go on the assumption that *damn near everyone* could use a smooth wake up. And go from there!

- Because so many patients can benefit from this, do a few smooth wake ups before you *must* do a smooth wake up.

- For example, the next ankle fracture that you do, make the wake up as smooth as silk—no bucking, no thrashing. That way, you'll get the technique down (really, *your* technique, because there is no single way to do this).

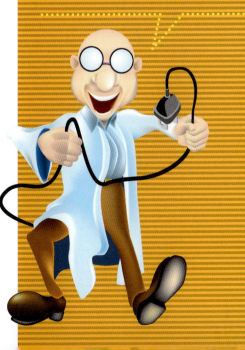

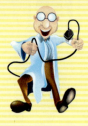

- A smooth emergence can be a little more time-consuming than a "let 'er rip" emergence. But that extra time is well-spent. If you have a smash-'em, crash-'em emergence and then end up reintubating the patient and treating negative pressure pulmonary edema, well, you haven't really saved any time, have you?

- Most importantly, a smooth landing requires planning. That is probably why it is not done more. You really must plan ahead and keep your eyes on the runway far before emergence.

HISTORY AND PHYSICAL FOR A SMOOTH EMERGENCE

- As always, in anesthesia: airway, airway, airway.

- Evaluate how difficult the patient is to intubate and how hard they will be to *reintubate once the procedure is over.*

- Lots of IV fluids, a prone position, surgical swelling in the airway—a hundred things can make an "easy to intubate at the beginning of the case" airway into an "oh my God, I can't see anything it's so swollen up" airway at the end of the case. As you plan your emergence and extubation, always keep your "return ticket" in mind. If you extubate, will you be able to reintubate if somehow you miscalculated.

- Think through the surgical procedure, too. If the patient had a huge cerebral tumor removed, then you can anticipate a lot of cerebral swelling and a fuzzy (at best) neurologic status at the end of the operation. Such a patient will not be able to protect their airway, so a "smooth emergence and extubation" is not even a consideration.

- Unstable hemodynamics, sepsis and shock, massive fluid resuscitation, lung contusions, flail chest—any number of things argue for keeping the patient intubated, so forget about your slick emergence.

TECHNIQUE

Let's talk about what causes *bucking*. Survey says—#1: *pharyngeal/tracheal stimulus.* You would cough, too, if you had a big hunk of plastic in your pharynx, let alone one inch above your carina. The easy way to fix this is with topicalization—our friend lidocaine.

You can instill it at the beginning of a short case or the end of a long case. A numb trachea means less coughing. A handy tool here is the laryngeal tracheal lidocaine, or LTA, in the handy single-use injector. Also, lower the cuff pressure to the minimum to prevent a leak but mostly to minimize uncomfortable pressure on the trachea. Any block to numb the airway will minimize bucking but increase the chance of aspiration. It's a risk/benefit thing.

Richard, what else causes bucking? Survey says—#2: *Stage II*! The discoordinated state we call emergence is a state of confusion and chaos. The patient is confused, does not follow commands, and breathes in an irregular manner. Just think of most of your rushed emergences. Do any of them *really* follow commands? I didn't think so. Now think of the awake ICU patient on the ventilator who is writing on the chalkboard that they want to know when they can go home, and how long until you take this thing out of their mouth! They are out of Stage II because they have eliminated all of the potent anesthetic vapors. Stage II is your *sworn enemy*. And its cause is the sevoflurane (or other vapor of your choice).

Solution: Try to leapfrog over Stage II. If you have enough narcotics on board, you can skate past it. If during Stage II the patient starts to fight, give a little lidocaine or propofol. That will usually (key word: usually) get them to stop coughing but they'll keep breathing. You have just given yourself a little, short-acting TIVA. At the end of this mini-TIVA, the patient will (you hope) be out of the iguana-eyed Stage II and you'll be able to extubate smoothly. If your first round of sedation is not enough and the patient is really out of control, repeat. With any luck (and there is some luck in this), the propofol will wear off just as the vapors wear off, or after they are gone. Nevertheless, the goal is the same—get rid of all of the volatile agent. That means zero end-tidal agent detected. And ideally, you would like spontaneous breathing. This confirms the patient is comfortable and allows you to titrate the narcotics.

Are there other ways to slither through Stage II? Yes. Do the whole case (or the end of the case) with a propofol drip and then slowly dial it down. You slide in with a smooth wake up. Run a dexmedetomidine drip. This reduces your MAC requirements plus constitutes a kind of "magic bullet" of extubation—the patient is sedated, cooperative, yet still breathing.

Hot diggity dog, can't beat that with a stick!

Beta blockers can produce a calming sedative effect and control the blood pressure at the same time. I believe this is a much underutilized technique, mostly because high doses are required to see a clinical calming effect in the patient.

So let us review. The two criteria that will allow a smooth emergence are:

- Out of Stage II, and
- Comfort, allowing the patient to tolerate the tube.

If you accomplish both of these together, you are almost guaranteed a smooth wakeup.

One other option for a smooth wake up is the *deep extubation*. The patient will not be able to protect their airway, so you must make sure you do this on a patient without aspiration risk. To do the deep extubation, get the patient breathing on their own (preferably), completely reverse the muscle relaxant, and make sure they are metabolically optimal for extubation. Put the patient on 100% oxygen (good to "fill the tanks" with oxygen just in case something goes wrong) and keep them on a high percentage of potent inhaled agent. After all, you are extubating "deep." Don't extubate someone "shallow" when the goal is "deep." Suction, then extubate and place the mask. You now turn the inhaled agent off. If you don't want to hold the mask for 15 minutes, just place an LMA. You know those wake ups to be smooth. A word about nausea and vomiting: A nauseous patient may present as anxious at the end of the case and disrupt your smooth emergence, so pretreatment is vital.

GLITCHES

- The main glitch is not planning ahead. Then the patient wakes up like the Apocalypse and you scramble to "make things smooth."
- Don't get tripped up when a long operation turns into a short one (they open, see the cancer is unresectable, and close the patient right up again). In such cases, an anesthesiologist will often pour a ton of muscle relaxant in (expecting a long case) then, oops, case done, and there is no way you can reverse the muscle relaxant. Always be prepared for that! Give just enough relaxant to keep the patient at one twitch—that way, you can reverse

the patient at the end of the case, no matter what the surgeon decides.

- Problem: muscle weakness. Solution: Make sure you follow the twitch monitor like a hawk.
- Problem: narcotics (mixed blessing here). Too much narcotics and your respiratory rate is 0. No one's getting extubated there. Solution: As soon as you are able, get the patient back breathing on their own and titrate until the respiratory rate is about 12. That respiratory rate will keep the patient alive (a worthy goal) but will keep them comfortable and sedated enough to wake up smooth (ideally, keep in mind that no formula is foolproof).
- Problem: metabolic badness. Solution: Keep the patient warm and metabolically hunky-dory.
- Deep extubations, when they work well, work great. But sometimes you won't keep them deep enough, then you extubate when the patient has snuck into Stage II. Now you extubated at the worst possible time and the patient goes into laryngospasm and you're hitting yourself in the head, saying, "Why did I do that?"
- If someone's really thrashing to beat the band, just "put them down" with a slug of propofol. Let some time pass and try again. It's just not worth fighting so hard that you risk patient, staff, or personal injury during an emergence.

TEACHING BY EXAMPLE

The Very Long Case

You are in a long neurology case of 6 hours running on 1.5% isoflurane. If you wait until the end to snap off the vaporizer, you may be able to extubate soon, but not smoothly. So plan your landing in advance, see the runway. Transition the last hour to a propofol drip so all the vapor is gone and a rapid smooth wake up is achieved for a quick neuro-evaluation on the table and not an hour later in the PACU, when the PACU nurse notices their slurred speech.

Tiptoeing Back with Naloxone

Here's one recipe from the trenches.

An anesthesiologist I worked with did a lot of nasal surgery. The patients all woke with blood in the airway and a smooth emergence was essential. The anesthesiologist would always over-narcotize the patients, then just trickle in a little bitty bit of

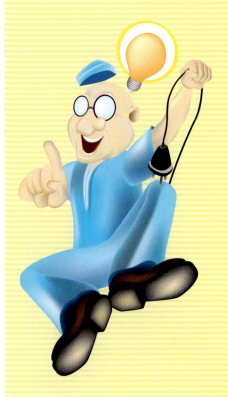

naloxone, 10 μgs at a time, until the patient just opened their eyes.

Zing, out with the tube.

"Don't Blow the Carotid"

The famous vascular surgeon of your institution finishes the carotid endarterectomy, takes off his paper OR gown, shoots his gloves across the room into the trash for two points, and comes over to you. Standing six inches from your face, he says, "Do not let him buck, or the hematoma in his neck will be your fault." He leaves but you know his loyal PA is watching you. While the PA sews up the incision, you extubate the patient deep and easily put in a #4 LMA. The patient is transitioned to spontaneous ventilation. All the gas analyzer reads zero sevoflurane and the respiratory rate is 12. When the drapes come down, you ask the patient to open his eyes, which he does. Then you ask him to open his mouth, which he does, and you take out the LMA. Next week, the surgeon requests you for his case.

PLASTIC SURGERY: AVOID THE BLOODY FACE LIFT

If there is a hematoma, you are sure to be blamed unless you can document consistently low blood pressures and no coughing on emergence. This is a great scenario to use a lot of beta blockers at the conclusion of the case.

ASLEEP FIBEROPTIC WITH LIDOCAINE

When you prep a patient for an awake intubation, you are making a smooth wake up in reverse! Think about it: They are out of Stage II and comfortable—the two key conditions mentioned above. If you topicalize the patient at the beginning of the case, even if you intubate them asleep, you will have great conditions for a smooth emergence for about two hours.

WHAT YOU'RE TRYING TO AVOID

Here's the horror story to make you embrace the need for a smooth wake up.

Big muscular guy. Nose operation for a deviated septum. Has the nose packs in. Wakes up so ferociously, the nose packs shot out and hit the ceiling! Can we say "blood-fountain?" Now a panic-stricken, "Get the tube out!" from the surgeon.

   Extubate.

   Desat.

   Blood everywhere.

   Can't intubate.

   Died.

I am not kidding that this happened, and I am not kidding that you need to know how to manage a smooth emergence.

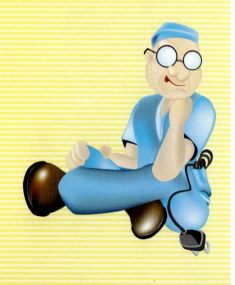

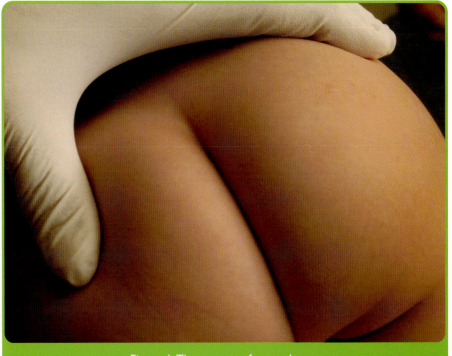

Figure 1. The apogee of smoothness.

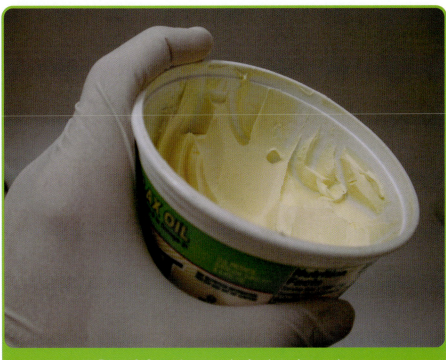

Figure 2. Smoothness in the food-product realm.

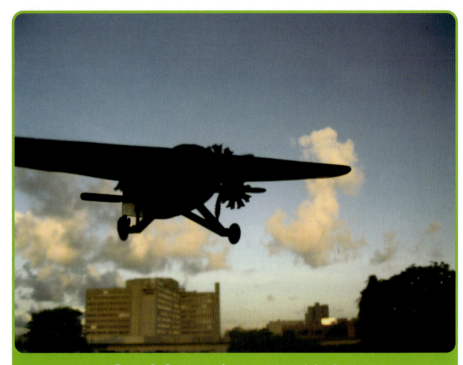

Figure 3. Coming in for a smoooooth landing.

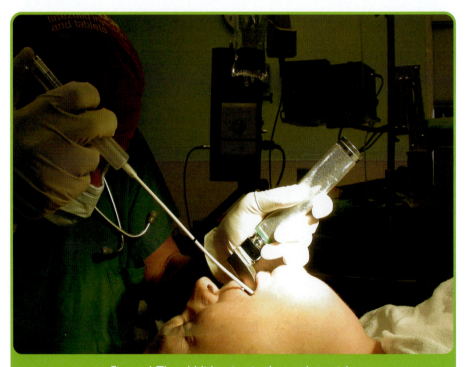

Figure 4. The old lidocaine in the trachea trick.

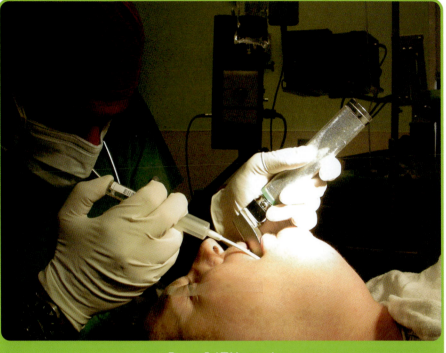

Figure 5. LTA's away!

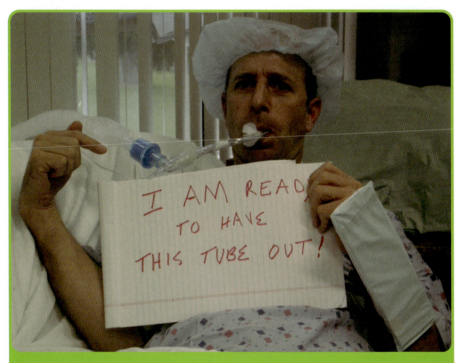

Figure 6. This patient, although burdened with sub-optimal looks, does appear, at first blush, to be somewhat ready for extubation.

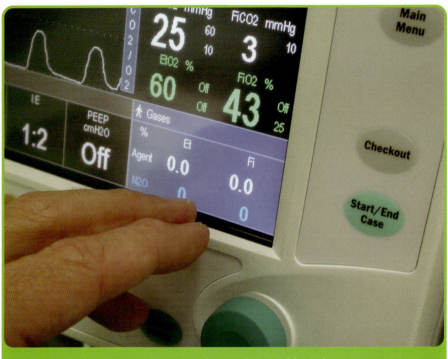

Figure 7. Use thy technology wisely, grasshopper. Note the vapors is gone.

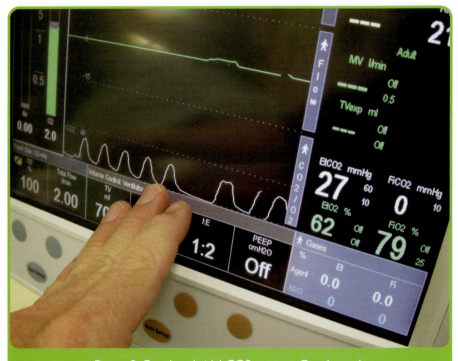

Figure 8. Good end-tidal CO2 pattern. Good, good.

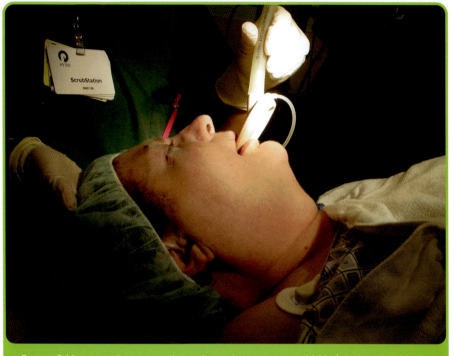

Figure 9. You can always extubate deep then put in an LMA for the ride home.

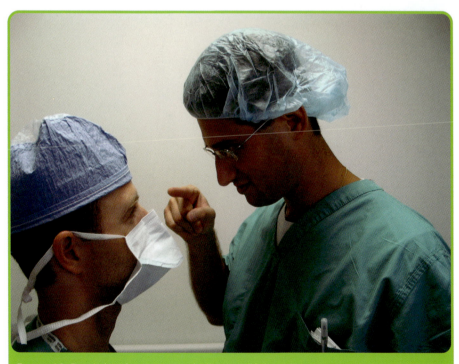

Figure 10. Don't let the surgeons bully you. (If they do, go out and slash their tires in the doctors' parking lot.)

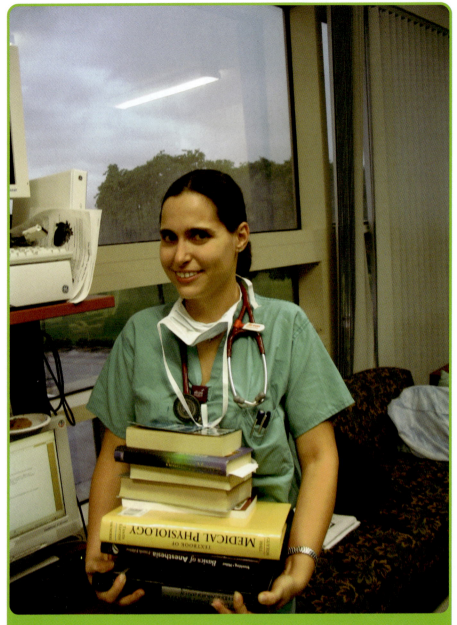

Figure 11. If you don't read, at least carry your books around to build up your arms.

SUGGESTED READING

Aouad MT, Kanazi GE, Siddik-Sayyid SM, et al. Preoperative caudal block prevents emergence agitation in children following sevoflurane anesthesia. Acta Anaesth Scand 2005 Mar;49(3):300–4.
- *Another way of preventing agitation on emergence in children is described.*

Diachun CA, Tunink BP, Brock-Utne JG. Suppression of cough during emergence from general anesthesia: Laryngotracheal lidocaine through a modified endotracheal tube. J Clin Anesth 2001 Sep;13(6): 447–51.
- *The authors use laryngotracheal instillation of topical anesthesia (LITA) through a modified ETT to achieve smooth emergence. Also, an interesting discussion on the suppression of cough reflex by IV lidocaine.*

Estebe JP, Delahaye S, Le Corre P, et al. Alkalinization of intra-cuff lidocaine and use of gel lubrication protect against tracheal tube-induced emergence phenomena. Br J Anaesth 2004 Mar;92(3):361–6.
- *In this study, alkalinized lidocaine is used instead of air to inflate the cuff to reduce the complications associated with emergence.*

Gefke K, Andersen LW, Friesel E. Lidocaine given intravenously as a suppressant of cough and laryngospasm in connection with extubation after tonsillectomy. Acta Anesth Scand 1983:27:111–2.
- *Enough said.*

Guler G, Akin A, Tosun Z, et al. Single-dose dexmedetomidine reduces agitation and provides smooth extubation after pediatric adenotonsillectomy. Pedi Anesth 2005 Sep 15;9:762.
- *A study about the prevention of agitation associated with sevoflurane on emergence in children undergoing adenotonsillectomy by using dexmedetomidine.*

Inomata S, Yaguchi Y, Taguchi M, Toyooka H. End-tidal sevoflurane concentration for tracheal extubation (MACEX) in adults: Comparison with isoflurane. Br J Anaesth 1999;82:852–6.
- *In this article, the values for MACEX for sevoflurane and isoflurane and ED 95 of sevoflurane and isoflurane are measured.*

Kaya S, Turhanoglu, Ozyilmaz MA. Oral ketamine premedication can prevent emergence agitation in children after desflurane anesthesia. Paediatr Anaesth 2004 Jun;14(6):477–82.
- *A study about the prevention of agitation on emergence in children with postoperative ketamine.*

Koga K, Asai T, Vaughan RS, Latto IP. Respiratory complications associated with tracheal extubation. Anaesthesia 1998;53:540–4.
- *This study compares the respiratory complications during deep extubation, awake extubation, and LMA use during emergence, finding that use of LMA after tracheal extubation decreases the incidence of respiratory complications during recovery from anesthesia.*

Loop T, Priebe HJ. Recovery after anesthesia with remifentanil combined with propofol, desflurane, or sevoflurane for otorhinolaryngeal surgery. Anesth Analg 2000 Jul;91(1):123–9.
- *A study about the effects of remifentanil combined with other anesthetic agents on recovery from anesthesia.*

Minogue SC, Ralph J, Lampa MJ. Laryngotracheal topicalization with lidocaine before intubation decreases the incidence of coughing on emergence from general anesthesia. Anesth Analg Oct 2004;99(4): 1253–7.
- *LTA was used in this study to determine the efficacy of endotracheal spraying with lidocaine at the time of intubation to prevent coughing on emergence.*

Nair I, Bailey PM. Use of the laryngeal mask for airway maintenance following tracheal extubation (Letter). Anaesthesia 1995;50:174–5.
- *You get the point.*

Chan PBK. On smooth extubation without coughing and bucking. Can J Anesth 2002;49:324.
- *The author developed his own technique using an infant feeding tube secured with micropore tape to ETT 1 cm above cuff, and instilling 4 ml 2% lidocaine through the infant feeding tube 20 minutes prior to extubation.*

Stix MS, Borromo CJ, Sciortino GJ. Learning to exchange an endotracheal tube for a laryngeal mask prior to emergence. Can J Anesth 2001;48:795–9.
- *This article describes a step-wise method for learning smooth ETT for LMA exchange.*

Takita K, Yamana M, Morimoto Y, Kemmotsu O. The ED(95) of end-tidal sevoflurane concentration for the smooth exchange of the tracheal tube for a laryngeal mask airway is 2.97%. Can J Anaesth 2003 Feb;50(2):184–8.
- *Interesting discussion about MAC required to prevent response to exchange of ETT with LMA compared with MAC required to prevent response to insertion of LMA and MAC required to prevent response to tracheal extubation.*

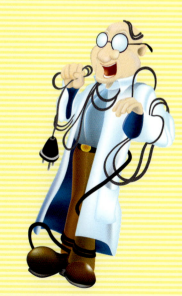

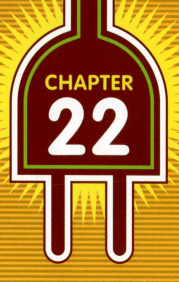

CHAPTER 22

Roomsmanship

Christopher Gallagher and Michael Jarrell

Infinite riches in a little room.

Christopher Marlowe
The Jew of Malta, Act I,
Scene i, 1689

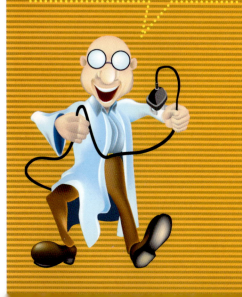

INTRODUCTION

Well, yes, if you work like a dog in the operating room, keep your expenses down, read *Money* magazine or *The Wall street Journal* and invest wisely, you can make infinite riches in that little room.

A lot goes on in that operating room once the lines are in and the case is going. Navigating that room skillfully is an art in itself. Though not strictly *procedures*, there are crucial *maneuvers* to doing a case safely.

These topics are:
- Patient positioning
- Surveillance
- Body mechanics
- Moving a patient to another table, to the lateral position, or to the prone position
- Cleaning up your lines
- Troubleshooting your machine
- Setting up a rapid transfuser
- Professionalism

TECHNIQUE: PATIENT POSITIONING

- Under anesthesia, patients cannot protect themselves against injury, so you must watch them like a hawk.

- Uncover and look, look, look at everything. Occasionally, you may find an arm that has magically been bumped off of the arm board by a surgeon.

- If it looks like it would be uncomfortable on you, then it will certainly be uncomfortable to the patient.

- A great "test" of a position is to put yourself in that same position. If you feel strain, then the patient will feel strain.

- Look for "stealth" problems—a wire from the pulse oximeter sitting right in the ulnar groove, an EKG pad sticking into the patient's ribs, a pool of betadine under the patient's neck, pressure on the eyes, a hyperextended neck.

- No one list can cover every possibility, so view each case and each position for each patient as a unique opportunity for causing harm.

- Go over the patient from stem to stern, making sure each pressure point is padded, no arm is hyperextended, and no shoulder greater than 90°.

- During mask ventilation and intubation at the beginning of the case, you'll often hyperextend the patient's head to improve the airway. Once you've secured the airway, return the neck to the neutral position.

- Legs up in stirrups and thighs hyperflexed? Don't keep the legs in that position forever. Keep the tibia parallel to the floor while in lithotomy and make sure poles are padded to avoid common peroneal nerve damage. For example, during a delivery let the patient's legs extend a little between contractions, don't just keep the legs up and hyperflexed for a long time—femoral or obturator nerve damage may occur.

- Moving the bed? Make sure the fingers are not caught in the hinge of the bed (see picture).

- Head laying flat for a long case? Reach underneath the head and make sure it's well-padded. Make sure the EKG cable isn't sitting underneath the occiput, pressing on the back of the head. If they guy (or gal) didn't have a bald spot before, now they will!

- Where are the stopcocks on your arterial line? Are they sticking into the patient's arm? Reposition them.

- There is no magic to this, just a dogged attention to detail.

- If your BP cuff and IV are on the same arm, run the IV line through the BP cuff so that it won't back up every time the noninvasive cuff goes up.

- A final note: Patients lying on their back will often cross their legs, just before the induction of anesthesia. Make sure that once induction is done, the legs get uncrossed.

TECHNIQUE: SURVEILLANCE

- We're not talking about an undercover CIA or FBI gig, we're talking about scanning the operating room. You should develop a habit of scanning everything in the OR either from right to left or vice versa. Just like on camera, you should pan across your field. What's your field, you may ask? Your cart, your anesthesia machine, your lines and, what else? Oh yeah, the patient.

- As you scan, you should also take note of personnel changes of nursing staff and OR techs who may not be aware of the patient's medical history or recent drama within the OR.

- Speaking of IVs, these little pretties will infiltrate or come out during a case and it may not be recognized until after the case if the anesthesiologist is not vigilant. Take a glance at it every 15 minutes or so. It's also important because you want to be darn sure that your meds actually make it into the patient and not onto the floor in a big puddle. ("I thought that puddle of water was just irrigation fluid from the surgeons" . . . this excuse won't cut it when you're up to your knees in Kim-chee!)

- You will occasionally notice some puddle of fluid (hmmm . . .) be it blood, urine, water, whatever. These present shock hazards not only to you but to your patient as well. Speaking of shock hazards, beware of micro shock. You should never simultaneously touch an electrical device and a saline-filled CVP line or external pacing wires—V-fib may result.

TECHNIQUE: BODY MECHANICS

- How you move *your* body counts, too.
- Take the extra time to take special care of your lower back.
- Not enough people to move a patient? Wait. A few minutes of waiting is better than six months of groaning and pain clinic visits with Dr. Feelgood.
- If you move a patient, lock the bed and get people on both sides lifting. This is all common sense but you'll be amazed how often people ignore this. Remember, your disability insurance will only pay about 60% of your salary if you get disabled from eagerly moving patients with heavy biscuit poisoning.
- Sitting on a crummy chair for a long time can ruin your back. Get the hospital to invest in good chairs. If it comes right down to it, buy a good one yourself. Cheapest "lumbar insurance" you'll ever get.
- When you are doing your charting, don't turn your back on the patient. That automatically makes you "tune the patient out." Rather, aim toward the patient and

glance down to do your writing or computer entry. Frequently glance up.

- Charting can *always* be done later. Saving a patient cannot. So if it comes down to it, do all your charting when the "danger is passed" and the patient is in someone else's hands.

TECHNIQUE: MOVING THE PATIENT

- Be like Winnie the Pooh and think, think, think before you do a move. Think through what will get tangled, what is crucial, and what needs to be reconnected first (hint: oxygen).
- Do a "mental move" before you do the actual move and look for gaps.
- Who will watch this arm? No one? Then get someone.
- This central line will snag? Cap it off, then reconnect once the move is done.
- Don't just "grab the head;" rather, cradle the head, neck, and shoulders as "one unit" and move them "all together."
- Don't forget to disconnect the ETT from the circuit or you may have an extubation to address.
- When you're going lateral decubitus, make sure you have a bean bag (that works) underneath the patient and an axillary roll nearby (a better term for it is a subaxillary roll because you want it below the axilla, not jammed up into the axilla).
- When going prone, arrange your arms so they will be straightened out once the patient is prone. That is, start with your arms crossed—right hand crossed over your left hand, the right hand holding the left side of the patient's head, the left hand holding the right side of the patient's head. Go ahead and perform this maneuver to see what I'm talking about (see picture). Once the patient is all the way over, now your hands are straight—your right hand is going straight ahead and your left hand is going straight ahead. This sounds confusing but works out well. The idea is this: When the patient has just turned prone, you need your hands to be working efficiently and you don't want your hands crossed and klutzy. Remember, half of being good is looking good.
- Keep pressure off the eyes.
- Make sure the neck is not hyperextended or hyperflexed. Apply the old "would this be uncomfortable if this were me" rule.

A move will snag lines, so disconnect everything you can, then reconnect once the move is done. Follow the ABC's when you reconnect—airway, breathing (yes, endotracheal tubes do come out during moves), and circulation. Listen to breath sounds to make sure the tube didn't migrate too deep or come too far out.

In general, however many people you have to help you move, you always end up one short, so get an extra person.

TECHNIQUE: TRANSPORT

- Evil genies lurk in the hallways, making transport a dangerous sport.

- Know your route: Is it to hell and gone far away? Have whatever you might need handy, including drugs, a mask (how will you ventilate if the patient accidentally extubates?) and a full oxygen tank.

- Don't wait for elevators—better to send someone out before you and have the elevator wait for *you*, rather than *you* wait for the elevator.

- If the patient is at all wobbly, don't be in a big rush to leave the room. Better to stay in the room, transfuse another unit of blood, and establish stable hemodynamics before you head off into the wild blue yonder.

- Unstable in the hallway or the elevator is a bad feeling.

- Uncover your lines and get a good look at them when you transport. Lines pull out when blankets are yanked and when patients are moved.

- Beware the bumped stopcock that cuts off your art line.

- Transport monitors fail, die, short-circuit, lose their charge. Don't forget good old fashioned monitors—*your eyes*. Watch the chest rise, look at the patient's color, feel the pulse. No *electronic* monitor doesn't mean no monitor at all. *You* are still the best monitor.

- Transport is so important, we have a whole chapter on it! Chapter 25!

TECHNIQUE: CLEANING UP YOUR LINES

- Time spent cleaning up clutter and rearranging lines is time well spent.

- When things go wrong (and they do), the more clutter you have to wade through, the worse your life. Be a ma-

niac about having clearly labeled, easy to get to, and identifiable lines.

- Don't let lines drape along the floor. It's unsanitary, looks bad, and leads to "line-squishage."

- As often as you can, sneak a peak at your lines, making sure they haven't come disconnected ("Hey look, a giant puddle of blood. I wonder where that came from?").

- Consider taping extra IV line slack with easily removable clear tape.

TECHNIQUE: TROUBLESHOOTING YOUR MACHINE

- The machine is your friend—most of the time.

- When something malfunctions on your machine and you can't troubleshoot it right away, don't allow yourself the luxury of a *Home Improvement*-style machine makeover.

- Do whatever you must do to establish effective ventilation. The simplest trick is to get an oxygen tank and an Ambu-bag, then the entire anesthesia machine is taken out of the equation.

- Common things happen commonly, so hand-ventilate, check the oxygen sensor, and make sure the tube is in the right place.

- Get help if you feel you are getting deeply distracted from patient care. You can always figure out machine stuff after the case.

- Your job is taking care of the patient. Don't forget that!

TECHNIQUE: SETTING UP A RAPID TRANSFUSER

- When blood loss is rapid, don't bother trying to pump in blood by hand—you'll get overwhelmed.

- Also, if blood loss is that rapid, you'll need your hands free to do other things (get blood gases, give calcium, wave and shout at the surgeon to clamp something).

- Do yourself a favor and get familiar with the rapid transfuser at your institution. There are different models but the key is always *familiarity*.

- Before you infuse, make sure your line is a big one (for example, an 8 or 9 Fr introducer in the right IJ or subclavian or

Sevo-Coma

One morning while performing a posterior spinal fusion, the patient began to move so we increased the volatile agent to 8% and forgot to turn it down. Four minutes later, we cut it off after noticing the BIS sensor read 00. And this reading continued to read 00 for over 10 minutes. Beware cranking up on the gas and removing thine hand

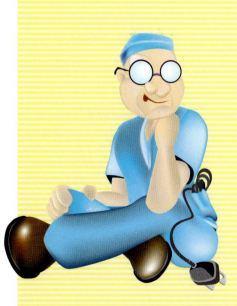

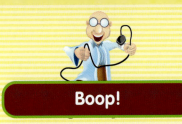

Boop!

This happens when using a rapid infuser. One fine day you will be infusing like thunder, you will clamp the wrong line, and the blood will explode with a soft "boop!" and the spray of blood around the room is virtually instantaneous, with everyone covered in blood and no one laughing. This is an example of bad roomsmanship

O₂, O₂, Wherefore Art thou, O₂?

Once during a trauma case, the wall O₂ supply failed. The anesthesia team then opened the O₂ cylinder in the back of the machine—however, as complacency kills, the team omitted having the anesthesia technician check the cylinder while setting up the room when the cylinder pressure gauge never moved from 1450 psi before starting the days cases. They ultimately moved the patient to another OR to complete the case.

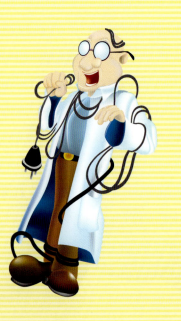

a 14G to 16G peripheral IV), and that it's not kinked or (this is always amusing) turned off.

- Blood under pressure can explode and make for a very colorful room if you clamp in the wrong place.

TECHNIQUE: PROFESSIONALISM

- One of the cornerstones to good roomsmanship is for the anesthesia personnel to have a good night's sleep prior to coming to work. This is one of the few disciplines in medicine where inattention can literally kill in minutes. Just imagine next time you're on that flight to New York and wonder, "Hmmm, how much sleep did my pilot get last night? Hope he wasn't up late watching the game like me!" You should have the same courtesy and respect for your patients.

- While in the OR, always notify the surgeons if you are having issues (e.g., the patient is desaturating, BP dropping, patient coding . . . yes, hard to believe but those numbskulls may actually keep sewing and cutting even if the patient has no *pulse*!) in addition to notifying your attending. Remember, this is *their* patient, too.

- OR conversations: a word or two about this aspect of roomsmanship. While talking to other anesthesia colleagues or your attending, try to keep things on the quiet side, especially if you are commenting on how long this damn closure or operation is taking and that you're starting to decompose while waiting for this to be over. Bottom line: Don't talk too loudly unless you want the surgeons (who may be eavesdropping on your gossiping anyway) to hear all you're saying behind their back.

- Lastly, anyone in the field of anesthesia will become aware—if not already—of the disproportionately high percentage of providers who are substance abusers. You will probably come across one or more persons in the course of your training and practice who have or had substance abuse problems. So for those of you out there who are considering a career in anesthesia and have had a tendency to smoke ganja or indulge in the fine recreational drugs available via your neighborhood friendly drug dealer on the street corner, I recommend reconsidering anesthesia as your path from rags to riches.

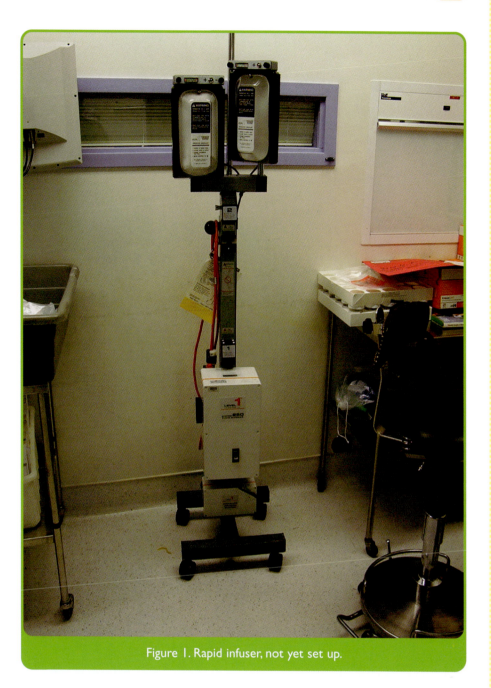

Figure 1. Rapid infuser, not yet set up.

The Achilles Heel of Time

Once, a routine pediatric dental case was scheduled for 2 hours and actually went 10 hours. The patient woke up with a heel ulcer that ultimately resolved but if the patient were old or diabetic, this could have been very costly from a malpractice standpoint. Padding, padding, padding for those pressure points!

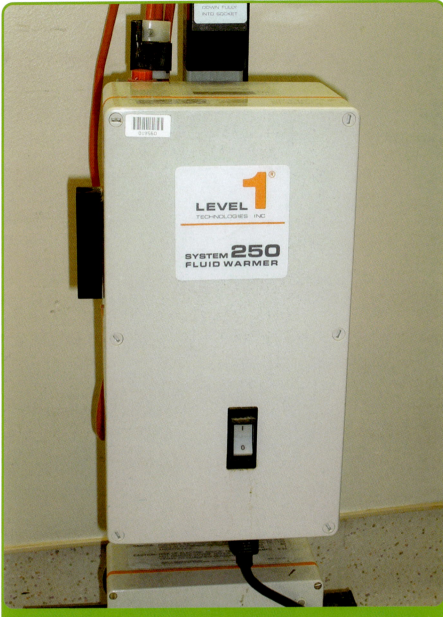

Figure 2. The all important heating unit, trauma patients get cold fast if you don't heat the blood.

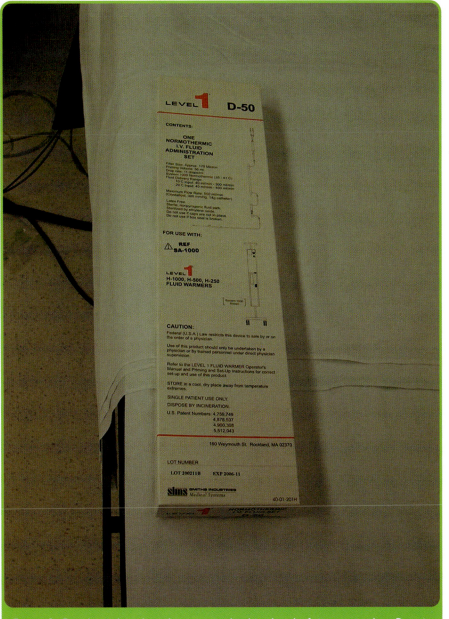

Figure 3. Get the right tubing, be sure to do this ahead of time, not when Bonnie & Clyde show up full of bullet holes.

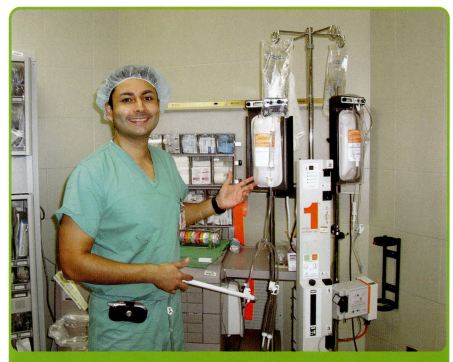

Figure 4. All set up, complete with smiling resident ready to do all the work while the attending drinks coffee.

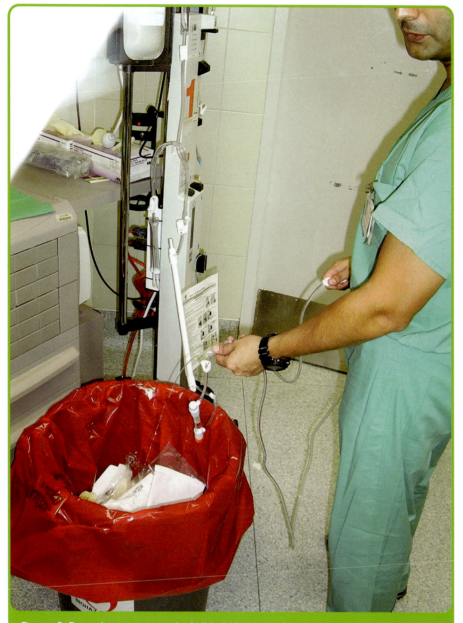

Figure 5. Purge lines getting rid of all bubbles (who knows who might have a PFO).

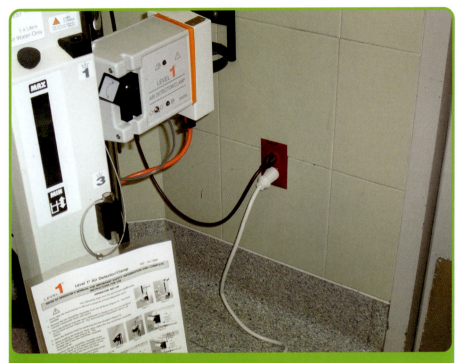

Figure 6. Don't forget to plug in. Just like your toaster at home, the rapid infuse needs electricity.

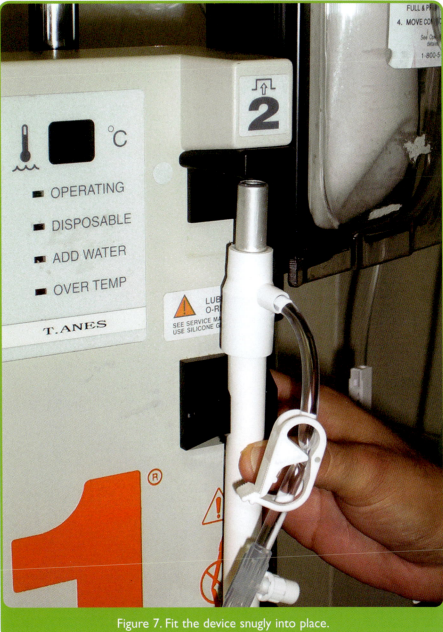

Figure 7. Fit the device snugly into place.

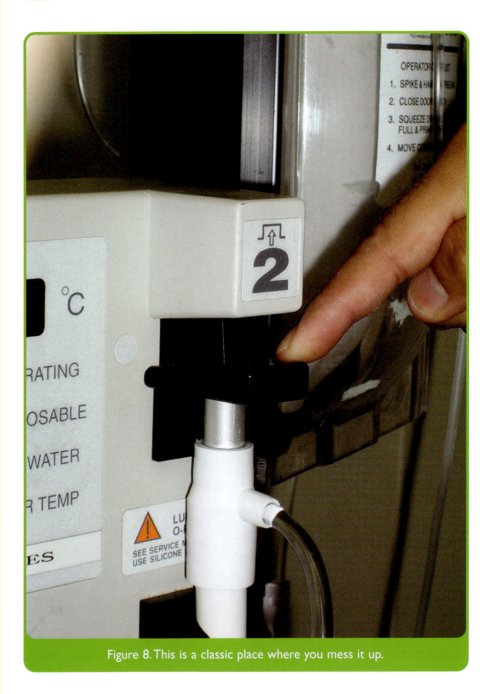

Figure 8. This is a classic place where you mess it up.

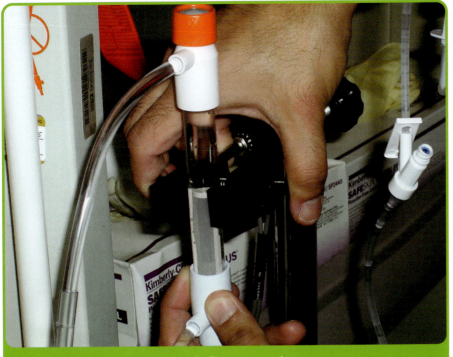

Figure 9. Clamp it in tight.

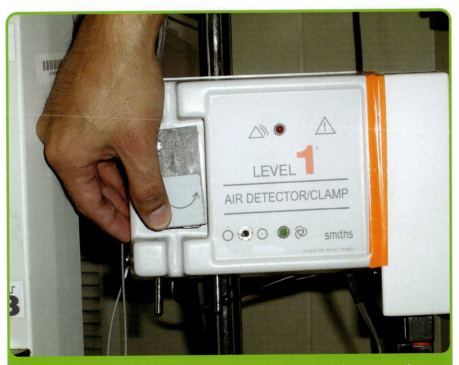

Figure 10. Very important that you're able to detect air. Infusing air under pressure is fatal.

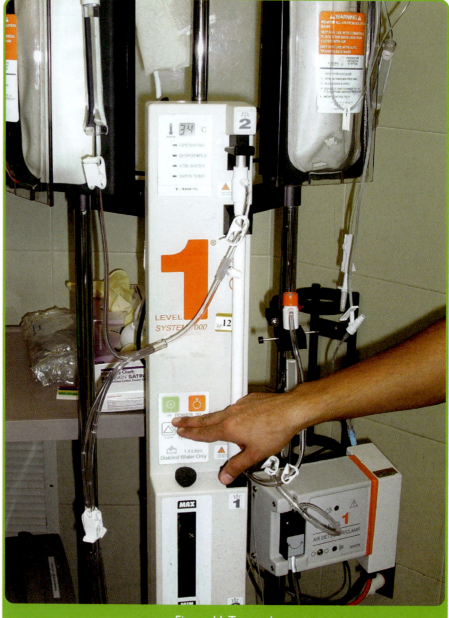

Figure 11. Turn on!

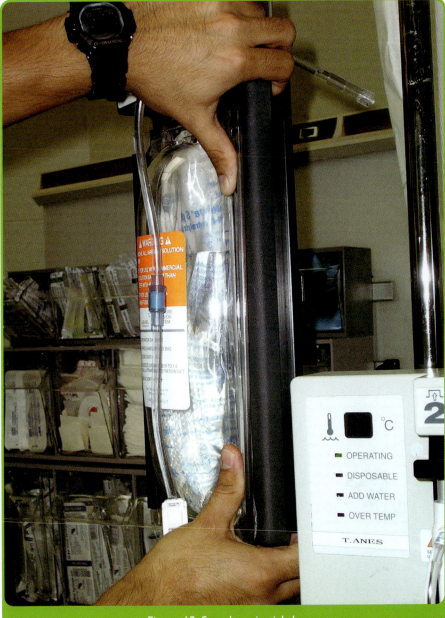

Figure 12. Snap bags in tightly.

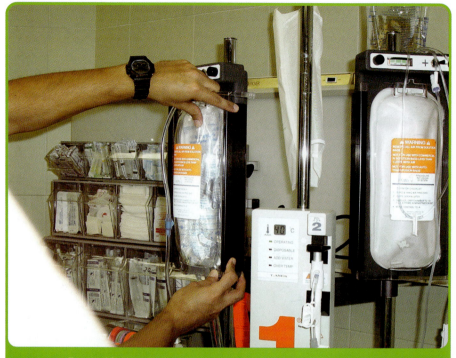

Figure 13. If you don't, then you won't infuse under pressure.

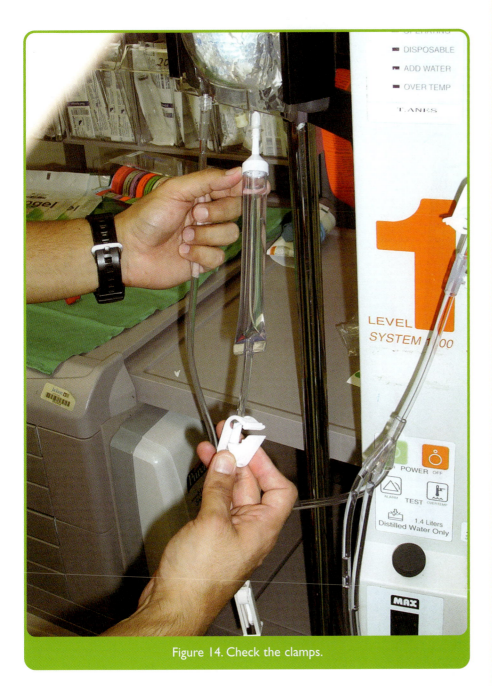

Figure 14. Check the clamps.

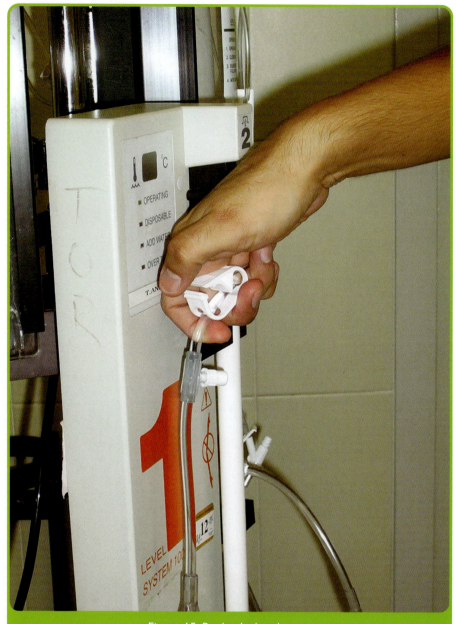

Figure 15. Recheck the clamps.

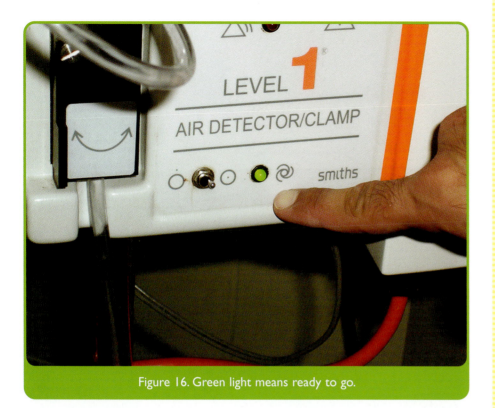

Figure 16. Green light means ready to go.

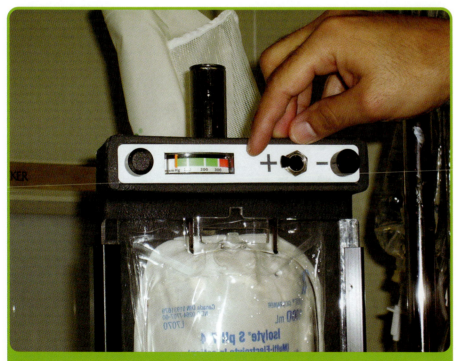

Figure 17. Throw the switch to + and in the fluid goes.

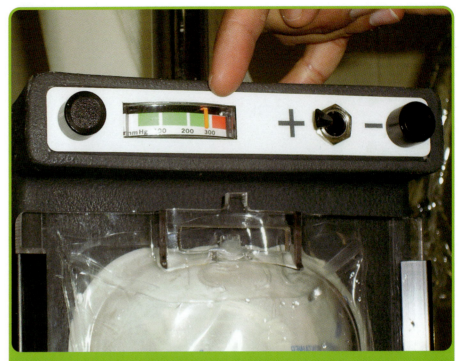

Figure 18. Watch the pressure gauge. Red zone means occlusion or kink somewhere.

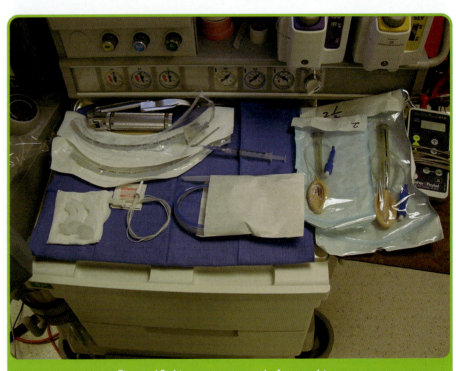

Figure 19. Airway setup ready for anything.

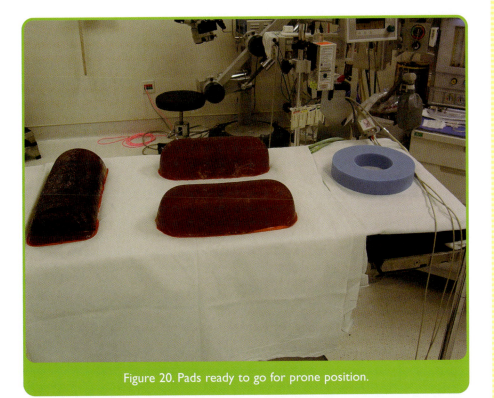

Figure 20. Pads ready to go for prone position.

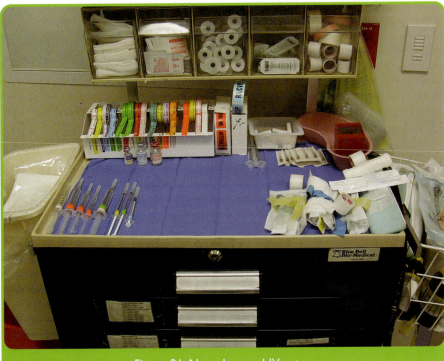

Figure 21. Neat drug and IV setup.

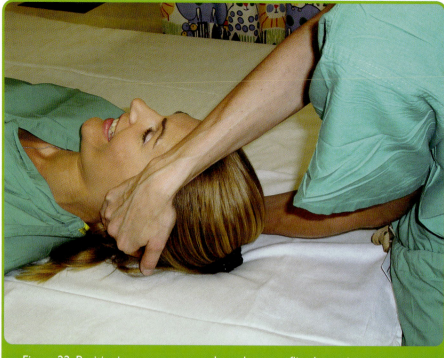

Figure 22. Positioning your arms so that when you flip the patient, your arms will be straight.

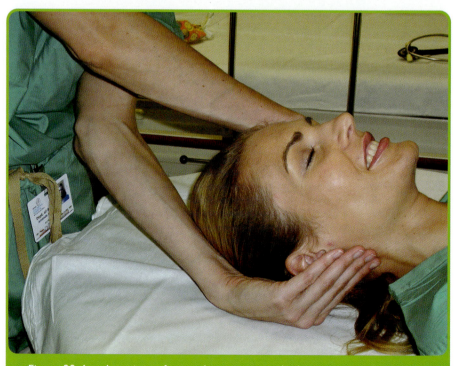

Figure 23. Another view of arms that are crossed when you start but will be straight once you flip.

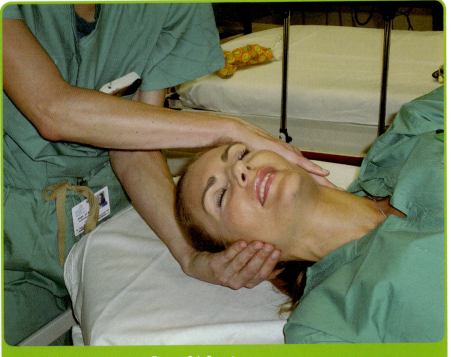

Figure 24. Starting to move.

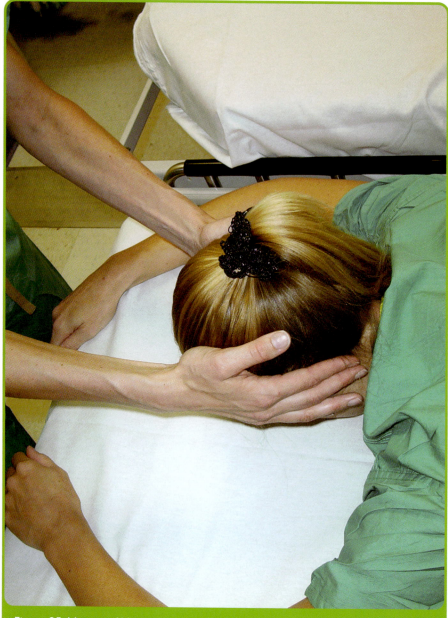

Figure 25. Now, see? Your arms are straight and able to maneuver the head well.

SUGGESTED READING

Domino KB. Risk factors for relapse in health care professionals with substance use disorders. JAMA 2005 Mar 23;293(12):1453–60.

- *A nice article that discusses the increased risk of relapse with substance abuse in health care professionals who used a major opioid or had a coexisting psychiatric illness or a family history of a substance abuse disorder. The presence of more than one of these risk factors and previous relapse further increased the likelihood of relapse. Maybe these folks should consider other specialties.*

Fritzlen T. The AANA Foundation Closed Malpractice Claims Study on nerve injuries during anesthesia care. AANA J 2003 Oct;71(5):347–52.

- *This article gives the experiences of a group of CRNAs in Minnesota and discusses effective strategies for the prevention of nerve injury during anesthesia.*

Helmreich RL. Culture, threat and error: Lessons from aviation. Can J Anesth 2004 Jun;51:R1.

- *A boring article but it highlights some important comparisons of anesthesia simulation to flight simulation. It also expounds on simulation as a method of evaluation of anesthesia providers.*

Howard SK. Simulation study of rested versus sleep-deprived anesthesiologists. Anesthesiology 2003 Jun;98(6):1345–55.

- *This study compared two groups of anesthesia residents with a staggered length of on-call and surprisingly, the clinical performance was the same. However, the group that started their call earlier in the day had impaired psychomotor performance and mood in addition to increased subjective sleepiness compared to their colleagues who started their call later in the day.*

Luck S. The alarming trend of substance abuse in anesthesia providers. J Perianesth Nurs 2004 Oct;19(5):308–11.

- *This article discusses the current alarming trends of addiction in anesthesia providers, treatment options, and reentry into the clinical arena after rehabilitation.*

Prielipp RC. Ulnar nerve injury and perioperative arm positioning. Anesth Clinics N Am 2002 Sep;20(3):351–65.

- *A nice article that discusses anatomical factors, supination versus pronation of arm, and drug and disease process effects on ulnar nerve compression.*

Winfree CJ, Kline DG. Intraoperative positioning nerve injuries. Surg Neurol 2005 Jan;63(1):5–18.

- *This article describes positioning nerve injuries that are generally thought to be preventable yet still occur in patients despite rigorous preventative measures.*

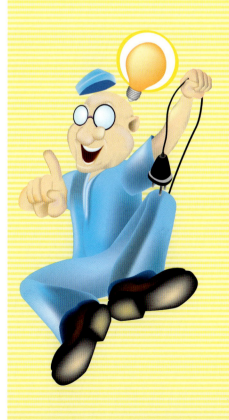

Nasogastric Tube's Away!

Carlos Mijares and Shantanu Srinivasan

INTRODUCTION

Though being one the simplest of procedures, the nasogastric tube (NGT) has the potential of being the one that can make you sweat the most as it is so fraught with troubleshooting and complications. Do not be surprised if it took you less time to get your vascular lines going!

INDICATIONS

- Gastric drainage/decompression for bowel obstruction, improved operating conditions, and full stomach prior to intubation
- Gastric lavage in drug overdose, poisoning, and GI bleed
- Enteral feeding or administration of medications

CONTRAINDICATIONS

- Severe facial trauma—possibility of cribriform plate disruption and nasocranial intubation! An orogastric tube is an alternative in this situation. This is also true for recent sinus surgery.
- Practice caution in coagulopathic patients, those with esophageal varices, and friable mucosa (pregnant women).

COMPLICATIONS

- Aspiration, tissue trauma and pressure necrosis, esophageal perforation and retropharyngeal abscess, endotracheal placement, pneumothorax and intravascular placement (yes, there are case reports of these too!) and every other bad thing you can imagine
- Tube errors in adults can vary from 1.3% to 50%.
- Partially anesthetized and awake patients can gag and vomit. Keep suction handy and wear protective apparel (gloves, gown, and so on).

EQUIPMENT

- Personal protection
- NG/OG tube of appropriate size
- Catheter tip irrigation 60-ml syringe
- Water-soluble lubricant
- Some lidocaine jelly 2% and an atomizer with 4% lidocaine if you are performing it while the patient is awake
- Adhesive tape
- Low-powered suction device or drainage bag
- Stethoscope
- Ice chips or a cup of water (for the awake patient)
- Emesis basin
- pH strips

PROCEDURE

1. Gather the equipment.
2. Wear nonsterile gloves.
3. If the patient is awake, explain the procedure to the patient and show them the equipment—you do not want them to be unpleasantly surprised.
4. In an awake patient, sit the patient up if possible for optimal neck/stomach alignment.
5. Examine the nostrils to see which one is wider.
6. Measure tubing from the bridge of the nose to the earlobe then to a point halfway between the end of the sternum and the navel.
7. If the patient's belly is already prepped, make an estimate to avoid contaminating the field and thus avoiding us gas people from looking clumsy.
8. A quick squirt of lidocaine in the nostril and some on the back of the throat will make this a much more pleasant procedure in an awake patient.
9. Lubricate 2 in. to 4 in. of the tip of the tube with some lubricant jelly.
10. Pass the tube for 8 cm to 9 cm for females and 9 cm to 11 cm for males (this is the approximate length of the

> If there is a possibility of several things going wrong, the one that will cause the most damage will be the one to go wrong.
>
> *Modified Murphy's Law*

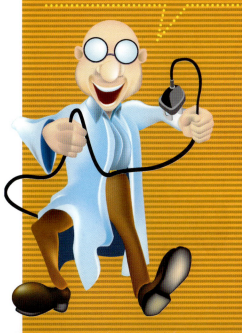

upper cervical vertebra from the anterior nares).

11. Use the natural curvature of the tube to your advantage by making the convexity of the tube approximate the posterior pharynx.

12. Flex the patient's neck.

13. Have the awake patient swallow ice chips or sip water and advance the tube as the patient swallows.

14. Continue to advance the tube into the stomach until the mark is reached.

15. If you have resistance, avoid brute force and gently rotate the tube 180° and advance.

16. If you have trouble advancing despite the above maneuvers, refer to the troubleshooting part of this chapter.

17. Withdraw the tube if the patient coughs, if there is a change in the capnograph in an intubated patient, the ventilator alarms go off (suggesting a breach around the cuff), or the tube coils in the mouth and the patient turns pretty colors.

18. Confirm the position of the tube.

    • This is best done by an x-ray, which is definitely a must if you plan to inject stuff into the tube.

    • If you cannot get an x-ray, *do not* administer anything through the tube until you have one. The next best confirmation test is to aspirate the tube and confirm that you are aspirating gastric content.

    • The contents are typically yellow (exception: GI bleed) and have a pH of less than 6.

    • If you have a higher pH, you might be in the intestine or lungs.

    • Patients with pernicious anemia, on H2 blockers, food in the stomach, medications, or HIV will have unreliable results for pH testing.

    • Auscultation for positive epigastric sounds by insufflating is the least reliable method to confirm tube placement and may be positive even if the tube is in the lungs.

    • Some tubes can be confirmed using an electromagnetic transceiver. This is more effective than aspiration or auscultation but it's usefulness is limited by the fact that it is not available everywhere.

    • Capnography is reliable in detecting the endotracheal placement of an NGT provided the tube does not get kinked

19. Secure the tube with adhesive tape. Make sure to leave some slack so as to not compress the skin and cause ischemic necrosis.

20. Place the tube to drain by gravity or on low intermittent suction, as you deem appropriate.

21. Write a small procedure note and document how you confirmed the placement of the tube.

    • NGT in the right lower lobe
    • NGT in the stomach

TROUBLESHOOTING AND CLINICAL PEARLS

• The most common sites for impaction to the advancement of the NGT are the pyriform sinuses and the arytenoids cartilage. Maneuvers to keep the tube approximated to the posterior/lateral pharyngeal wall facilitate smooth passage. The most common ones are described below.

• Digital assistance using a gloved finger to keep the tube from coiling in the pharynx and to steer it into the esophagus.

• Neck flexion as described earlier is my favorite maneuver and has worked for me when the others have failed. I routinely use it when I place my tubes.

• Forward displacement of larynx (reverse Sellick maneuver)

• Direct laryngoscopy and Magill forceps to facilitate the tube into the esophagus

• Prefreeze the tube to enhance it's natural curvature to your advantage.

• The x-ray is the gold standard and all tubes should be confirmed * with one prior to feeding.

• The presence of a cuffed ETT will not keep the tube from entering the lungs.

• If you must insert a tube in an awake infant, have them suck on a pacifier.

• If a Univent has been used, label the endobronchial blocker as something through which you cannot feed. This is not an urban legend and has actually happened. Rookie ancillary staff on the floor or ICU do not know the Univent and may mistake the endobronchial blocker for a feeding tube.

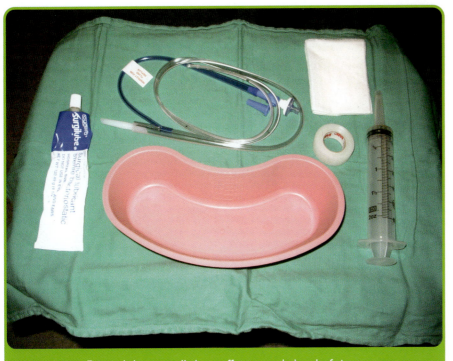

Figure 1. Lay out all the stuff you need ahead of time.

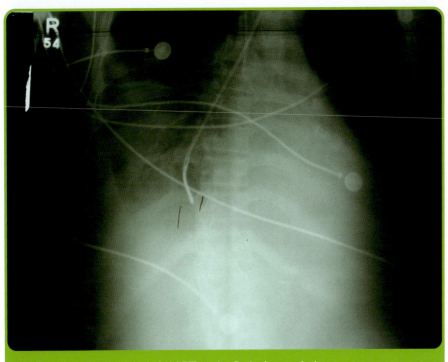

Figure 2. NGT in the Right Lower Lobe

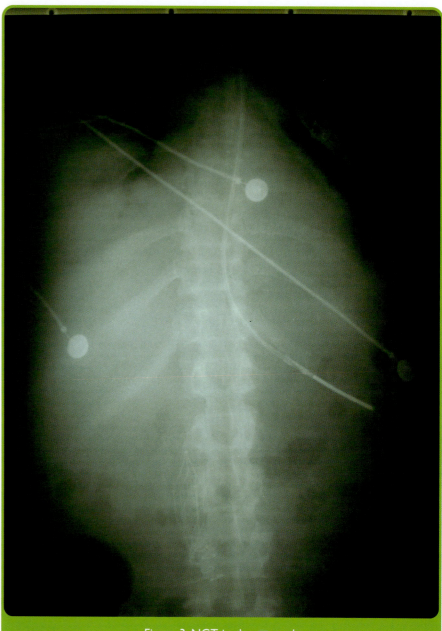

Figure 3. NGT in the stomach

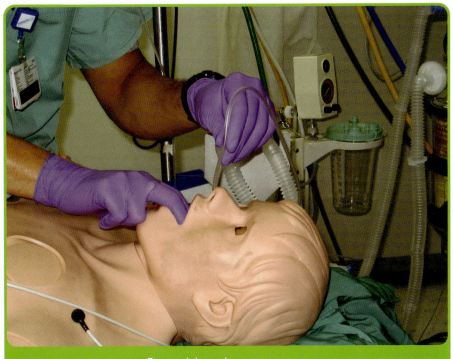

Figure 4. Into the nose you go.

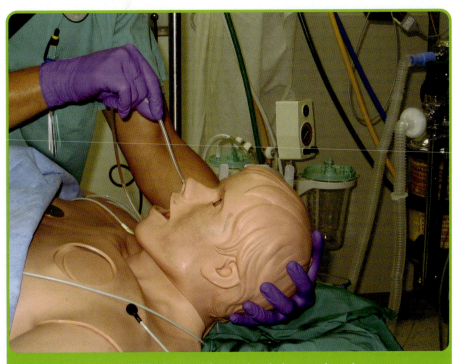

Figure 5. Tilt the head forward to help pass the tube.

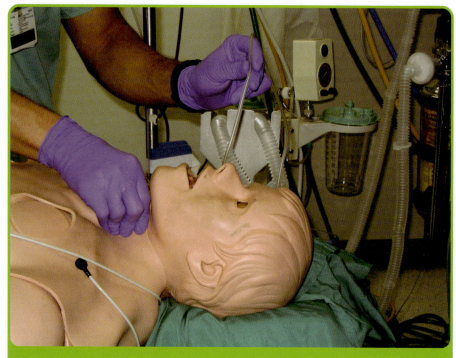

Figure 6. You can compress the neck too, that helps guide the tube the right way.

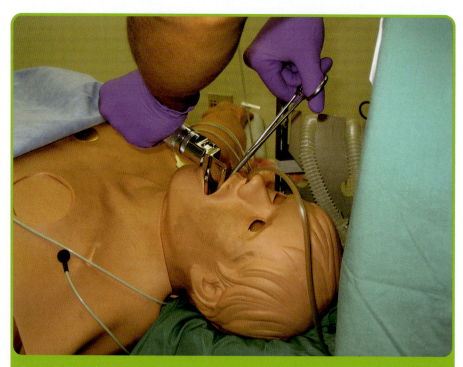

Figure 7. If you're really stuck, use a laryngoscope and Magills forceps to feed the tube down the esophagus.

SUGGESTED READING

Benumof JL, et al. Oro-and nasogastric tube passage in intubated patients: Fibreoptic description of where they go at the laryngeal level and how to make them enter the esophagus. Anesthesiology Jul 1999;91(1):137–43.

- *This is a great article. It describes the mechanics of NGT placement with some really cool fiberoptic images and illustrations.*

Duthorn L, et al. Accidental intravascular placement of a feeding tube. Anesthesiology Jul 1998;89(1);251–3.

- *This is a wild story of how a NGT made its way into the internal jugular and subsequently into the right atrium! Initial aspiration gave an impression of a GI bleed but when 2.1 L of blood was aspirated, things began to look fishy and it so happened that the tube had sneaked into the vasculature at the level of the soft palate. Badness would have happened if air had been injected prior to aspiration—a good idea to steer away from the practice of insufflation and to aspirate instead.*

Mahajan R, et al. Role of neck flexion in facilitating NGT insertion. Anesthesiology 2005;103:446–7.

- *Cross-referenced to other articles that describe troubleshooting maneuvers.*

Pousman RM, et al. Endotracheal tube obstruction after orogastric tube placement. Anesthesiology Nov 1997;87(5):1247–8.

- *Case report of how an OGT neatly coiled around the ETT during repeated attempts to place it and led to the ETT getting kinked. The patient got extubated when the OGT was removed and had to be reintubated!*

Rewari V, et al. Intraoperative detection of tracheobronchial placement of nasogastric tube. Anesth Analg 2005;101:606–15.

- *Another recent article that describes the changes in the capnograph if an NGT is endotracheal. Cross-referenced to other articles on the role of capnography in NGT placement verification.*

Thomas B, et al. Accidental pneumothorax from nasogastric tube. N Eng J Med Oct 24, 1996;334:1325–6.

- *Case report of a pneumothorax caused by a misplaced NGT and the subsequent administration of activated charcoal into the pneumothorax—I guess that would make it a pneumoconiothorax! Luckily, the patient recovered. A strong case to check the x-ray before administering anything through the tube.*
  http://www.joannabriggs.edu.au/protocols/protnasotube.php
  http://www.enw.org/Research-NGT.htm
- Links you to literature on the subject mostly from nursing. Nurses put in a lot of NGTs and are pretty good at it, and it's worth looking at their take on the procedure.

ILLUSTRATIONS

Used with permission from the University of Ottawa, Faculty of Medicine, iMed Office, and the Department of Emergency Medicine.

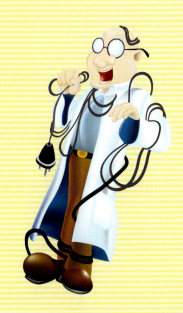

INTRODUCTION

- Positioning of the anesthetized patient is of crucial importance as the unconscious, paralyzed patient has a problem adjusting to a bad position.
- In normal situations, an awake (even a sleepy) individual would feel pain or pressure and would change to a more comfortable position before injuries or damages occur.
- The anesthetized patient *usually* does not move, and it becomes the anesthesiologist's responsibility to find the best position for them.
- Nerve injury was responsible for 16% of the cases in the ASA Closed Claims database, being the second most-frequent category of claim for injury. Claims related to injury of the ulnar nerve were the most frequent, followed by the brachial plexus.

- Nerve injuries unfortunately still occur, despite careful positioning and padding of pressure points. *Not all postoperative nerve injuries are because of a careless anesthesiologist.* Studies suggest that ulnar nerve injuries are not always related to bad patient positioning as they can occur even after appropriate padding and correct positioning; brachial plexus injuries occur in cardiovascular surgical cases requiring median sternotomy.
- The mechanism of nerve injury varies but can be due to stretching to pressure, ischemia, direct trauma, pre-existing neuropathy and other medical conditions, or a combination of these.

In this chapter, we describe the most common surgical positions, their potential effects on the cardiovascular and pulmonary systems, and the possibilities of specific nerve injury of each.

CHAPTER 24

Positioning is Everything

Marco Foramiglio and Gilbert Chidiac

Hold still, you might hurt yourself!

The executioner to Marie Antoinette as he positioned her on the guillotine

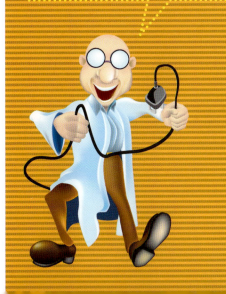

SUPINE POSITION

- Commonly injured nerves in this position are the ulnar nerve and the brachial plexus.
- Minimal effects on the hemodynamics (unless mass effect in abdomen, resulting in caval compression with decreased venous return and hypotension).
- Reduction of lung volumes are due to the change from a standing to a supine position or the use of muscle relaxant, resulting in upper displacement of the diaphragm and loss of skeletal muscle tone of the chest. Effects are offset by positive pressure ventilation.
- Pressure on the ulnar groove and the spiral groove of the humerus must be avoided with elbow padding. Position the arm in a neutral position or in supination. Ulnar nerve injury was more common in men than in women.
- Pressure on the radial groove could injure the radial nerve.
- Hips and knees should be slightly flexed.
- Legs should always be uncrossed.
- Heels should be padded.
- Appropriate use of a pillow under the head minimizes the risk of focal alopecia as well as help in maintaining the stability of the head.

- Keep the head aligned with the axis of the spine.

PRONE POSITION

- Cardiovascular and pulmonary effects are more significant in this position.
- There is pressure on the abdominal wall pushing the diaphragm cephalad, as well as pressure on the aorta and vena cava, which commonly places the patient in hypotension.
- Positioning of the head to one side or another may result in obstruction of jugular venous return on that side with subsequent postoperative neck pain and, rarely, thrombosis.
- Protection of the face—including ears (unfolded), eyes (avoiding pressure on the globe), eyelids, lips, and nose—is of crucial importance to avoid pressure damage. Frequent checks every 15 minutes are important.
- The breasts should be positioned medially and cephalad.
- Arms are placed either on the side or extended alongside the head ("Superman" position). In either case, proper padding is important to avoid pressure on the ulnar nerve.

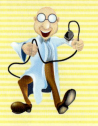

- In this position, the patient may comfortably tolerate arm abduction greater than 90° (although some authors still recommend less than 90° abduction to avoid stretching of the brachial plexus).

- Frequently, patients with shoulder problems cannot move their arms up to 90°; in this case, the arms should be tucked to their sides.

- Firm rolls are placed under the patient's side from the shoulder to the iliac crest to minimize pressure on bony prominences, decrease the compression on the abdomen, facilitate venous return, reduce the pressure on the diaphragm, and allow easier lung movements.

- Proper padding under the inferior iliac spine avoids pressure to that area as well as minimizing the compression of the iliac veins and the inferior vena cava.

- The anesthesiologist must always keep control of the head when moving the patient from supine to prone and vice versa. Careful attention to the endotracheal tube is important to avoid accidental extubation. Disconnection from the anesthesia during the changing of position is always desirable.

- Increasing the FiO_2 to 100% before the changing of positions will buy you time to avoid rapid desaturation in case you have problems with the airway, such as an unanticipated extubation or because your assistant or medical student (who is half awake because they were partying until *very* late last night) forgets to reconnect the tube while you are trying to save the arterial line that was pulled out by the neurosurgical resident during the move.

LATERAL DECUBITUS

- Surgical procedures such as thoracotomies and hip surgeries are positioned this way.

- Significant changes on lung physiology occur in this position. The dependent lung receives more blood simply because of gravity. The upper lung is better ventilated because it is less compressed by the abdominal content than the dependent lung. This creates a ventilation-perfusion mismatch and, consequently, unexpected hypoxemia.

- Pressure on the abdomen can result in pressure on the vena cava, decreased venous return, and subsequent hypotension (especially with the kidney rest elevated).

- Appropriate padding under the head should be used and the usual care of avoiding pressure to the eyes, ears, and soft tissues taken. Attention to avoid pressure to the dependent eye and ear is essential. Also, you do not want to give your patient a corneal abrasion caused by contact of the eye with the "soft innocent" foam. If the patient's ear becomes ischemic and falls off because of prolonged pressure, you might get your medical license revoked like Mike Tyson had his boxing license revoked after biting Holyfield's ear off during the memorable "bite fight."

- The head should be aligned with the axis of the spine. Positioning incorrectly could result in neck pain and possible stretching of the brachial plexus.

- A chest roll (commonly and erroneously called an axillary roll) should be placed under the chest (and *not* under the axilla) to avoid compression on the brachial plexus. To make sure the plexus is free from pressure, your hand should move freely under the axilla.

- The upper arm is placed on a padded support in front of the patient's face. Proper position is necessary to avoid injury of the brachial plexus.

- A pulse oximeter placed on the down arm can help in the detection of pressure on the neurovascular axillary structures.

- A pillow is placed between the knees to avoid pressure on the bony prominences. The lower leg is positioned with flexion. Legs should be positioned with the dependent knee flexed and the nondependent knee less flexed. Remember, padding the pressure points between the knees prevents injury or compression of the saphenous nerves.

LITHOTOMY

- This position is used frequently in gynecologic and urologic procedures.

- Suspend the legs flexed at the hips and perpendicular to the torso.

- Simultaneous elevation of the legs while the person is in the supine position reduces torsion on the pelvis and lower back.

- Stretching of the hamstring muscle group beyond a comfortable range may stretch the sciatic nerve.

- Injury to the peroneal nerve is possible if it is compressed between the head of the fibula and the "candy bar"; padding of the fibular head decreases the risk of injury. Also, injury to the saphenous nerve can occur if pressure is applied to the medial aspect of the leg. Compartment syndrome of the lower extremity (requiring fasciotomy) has been reported in this position.

- Another disastrous injury may occur if the fingers are caught in the gap as the foot of the bed is being rolled to a vertical position.

- Three risk factors have been associated with neuropathies after surgery in this position: very thin body habitus, cigarette smoking, and prolonged surgery.

- Correct position:
  - The legs flexed at the hips perpendicular to the torso.
  - The legs are suspended away from any pressure from the support.
  - The supports are padded in case of contact with the legs.

SITTING POSITION

- Offers surgical advantages for craniotomies of the posterior fossa

- Prevents excessive flexion of the neck to avoid spinal cord ischemia and obstruction of carotid and vertebral arteries

- Support of the arms at the elbows is essential to prevent overstretching of the brachial plexus by the weight of the arms hanging down.

- Padding under the buttocks and the sciatic notch prevent the possible pressure ischemia of the sciatic nerve.

- Although large series of safety records exist about this position, concerns still exist—especially when it comes to a venous air embolism. Other complications are arterial air embolism (through a potent foramen ovale, vascular instability, airway obstruction, neurological complications, and macroglossia).

- Caution is advised in patients with atherosclerotic cardiovascular disease, severe hypertension, cervical stenosis, and right-to-left intracardiac shunts.

- "The sitting position in neurosurgery: A critical appraisal" is an excellent review article that covers this subject from A to Z. Written by J.M. Porter et al., you will find it in the 1999 *British Journal of Anesthesia* 82(1):117–128.

CASE REPORT

This was a 72-year-old man who underwent a 12-hour spine instrumentation surgery in the prone position. Blood loss was evaluated at 2500 ml but because the patient was a Jehovah's Witness, no blood was given. His hematocrit at the end of the case was 23%. The patient recovered from anesthesia well; however, he was complaining of not being able to see. *Postoperative blindness* following prone position surgery is a well-known complication—it could be related to direct compression on the ocular globe (not in this case though, as this patient had his head in a Mayfield) and to factors such as low hematocrit, hypotension, and other risk factors such as diabetes, anemia, atherosclerosis, and advanced age. A prolonged surgical time has also been shown to be a factor for this ischemic optic neuropathy (ION). *Always work with a fast surgeon!*

REMEMBER

Padding, padding, padding . . . and still nerve injuries unfortunately occur. *Not all postoperative nerve injuries are because of a careless anesthesiologist.* Patients at risk include skinny patients, diabetics, and patients with preexisting neuropathies.

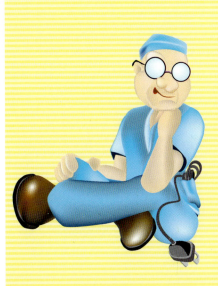

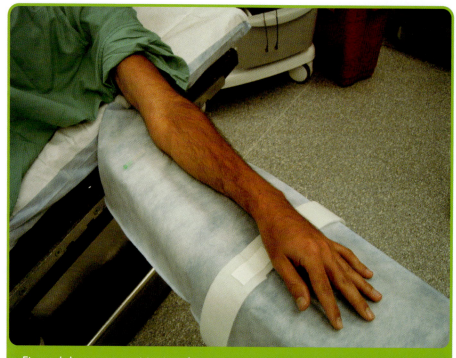

Figure 1. Incorrect positioning: the arm in pronation could result in pressure of the ulnar nerve in the ulnar groove

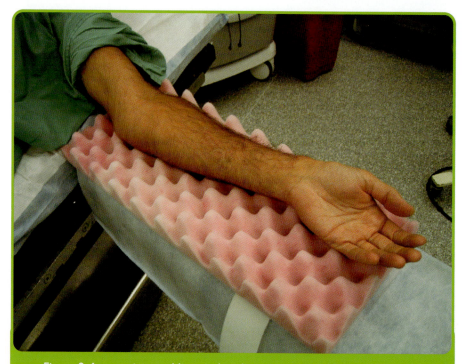

Figure 2. Appropriate padding at the ulnar groove and placing the arm in supination minimize injury to ulnar nerve

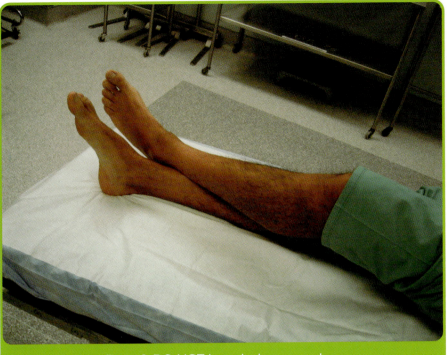

Figure 3. DO NOT keep the legs crossed. . . .

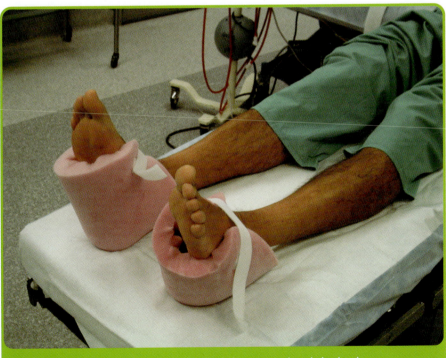

Figure 4. The great Chidiac's legs . . . and pad the heels.

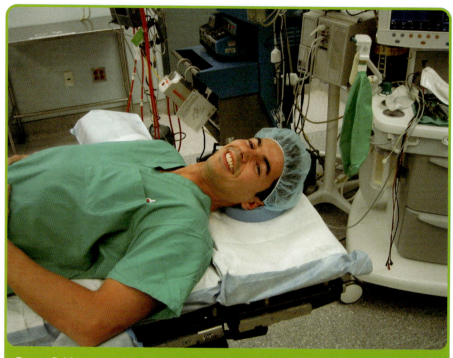

Figure 5. Maintaining the head in neutral position avoids neck pain and stretching of brachial plexus.

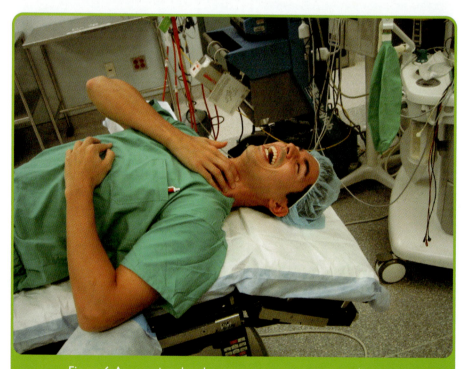

Figure 6. Appropriate head support prevents pressure alopecia.

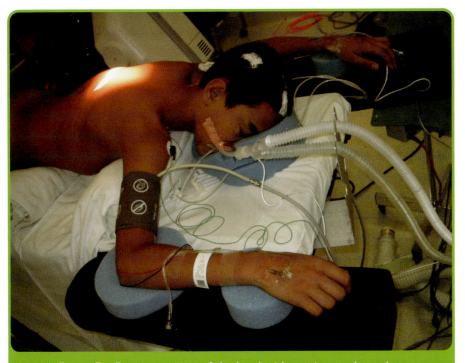

Figure 7. • Proper position of the head with caution to dependent
eye (avoid pressure)
• Padding on the ulnar nerve
• Padding on the knees
• Support under chest iliac region.

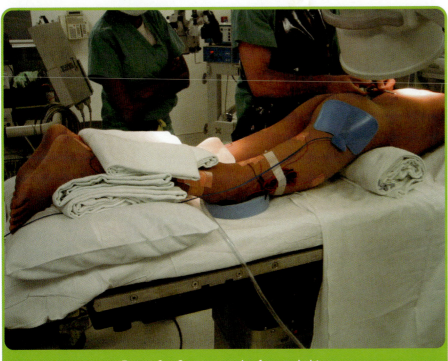

Figure 8. • Support at the feet and shins
• Padding on the knees
• Support at the iliac region

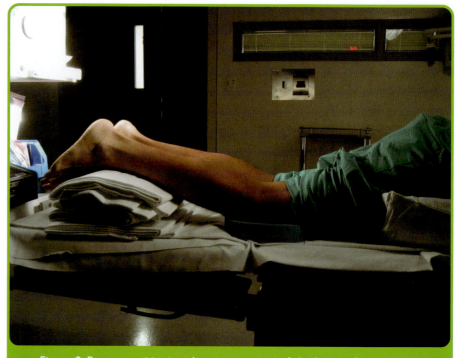

Figure 9. Proper positioning showing support of the legs to favor venous drainage, knee support and support of pressure points at the hips.

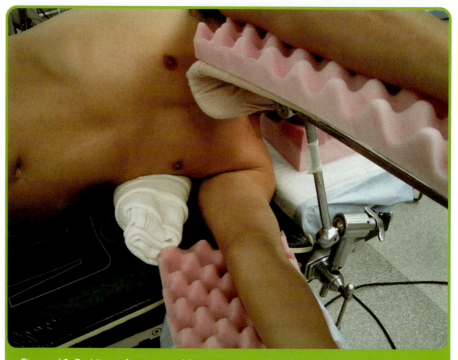

Figure 10. Padding of upper and lower arms and a chest roll prevent injuries to ulnar nerves and brachial plexus.

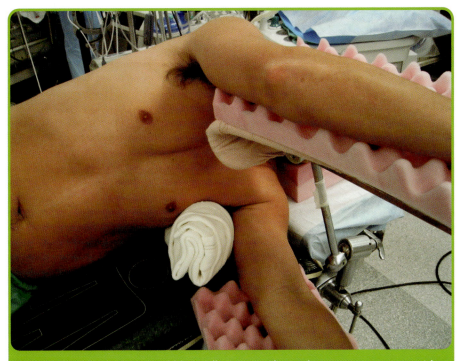

Figure 11. Upper arm should be well positioned on a bar or arm support with appropriate padding.

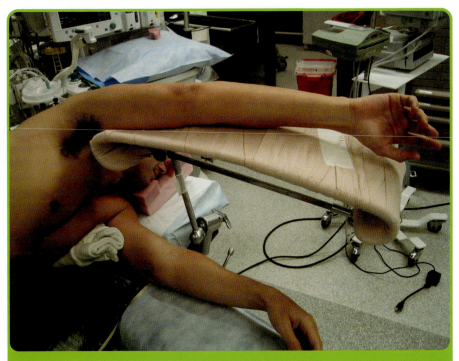

Figure 12. Incorrect position:
1. The upper arm is very badly positioned with the inside of the arm- rest almost touching the axilla, possibly putting pressure onto the brachial plexus. The arm should rest freely on the support that should be well padded to prevent ulnar nerve injury.
2. The lower arm rests on an unpadded arm-board in pronation placing at risk the ulnar nerve
3. The chest roll is too far up the axilla placing the brachial plexus at risk of compression.

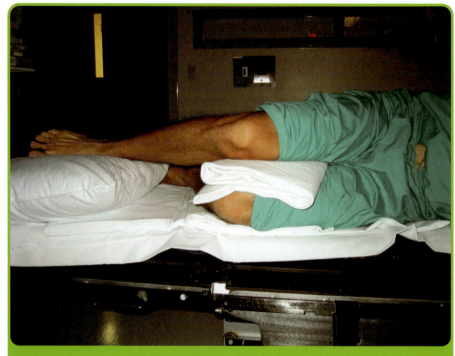

Figure 13. Pad the knees, so's is how they don't cause knee squishage. Pad the ankles so's is how you don't get ankle squishage.

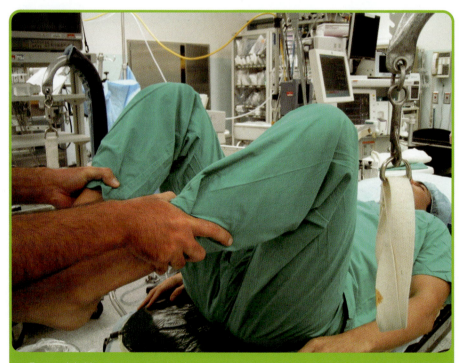

Figure 14. Always position both extremities together as doing each separately could result in. . . .

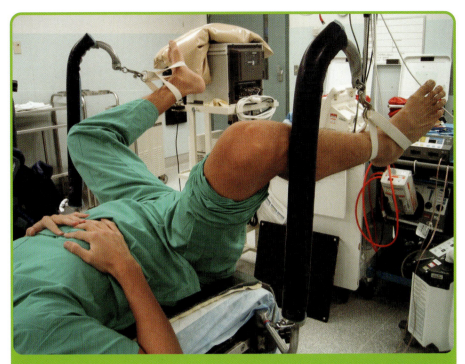

Figure 15. Incorrect position: the right leg is in contact with the vertical suport (AKA the "candy bar") resulting in pressure on the peroneal nerve.

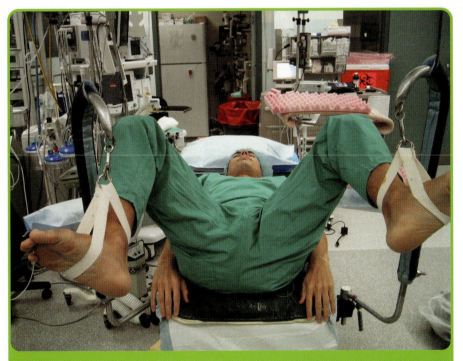

Figure 16. Correct position:
The legs flexed at the hips perpendicular to the torso.
The legs are suspended away from any pressure from the support.
The supports are padded in case of contact with the legs

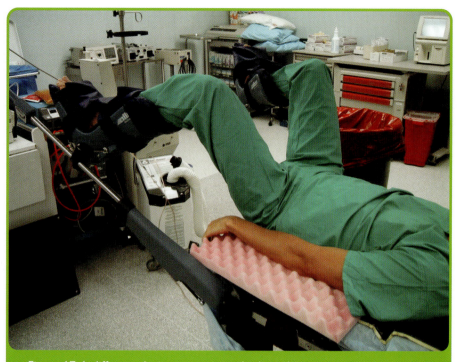

Figure 17. A different device to support the legs; this one present less risk of injury to the personeal or saphenous nerves as the vertical bars have been substituted with horizontal ones.

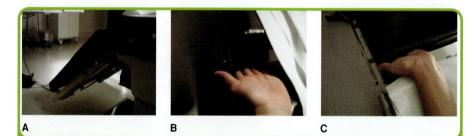

Figure 18. Patients' fingers could be caught and mashed when the "foot" portion of the operating table is raised at the end of the procedure to put the patient's legs back on the table.

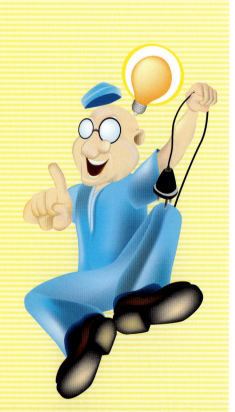

SUGGESTED READING

ASA Task Force on Prevention of Perioperative Peripheral Neuropathies. Practice advisory for the prevention of perioperative peripheral neuropathies. Anesthesiology 2000;92:1168–82.
- *After so many claims, the ASA decided to review and come up with recommendations.*

Faust RJ, Cucchiara R, Bechtle P. Patient positioning. Section III: Anesthesia Management. *Miller's Anesthesia*, 6th edition. Oxford: Elsevier Science, 2005:1151–68.
- *Miller is Miller: It is The Book of anesthesiology for any subject. This chapter is no different. It gives a good and practical overview on this topic.*

Martin JT. The prone position: Anesthesiologic considerations. In Martin JT (ed):

Positioning in Anesthesia and Surgery, 2nd edition. Philadelphia: WB Saunders, 1987.
- *The title is self-explanatory.*

Prielipp RC, Morell RC, Butterworth J. Ulnar nerve injury and perioperative arm positioning.
- *This article presents an excellent review of the most commonly injured nerve. It provides details and an explanation of the mechanism of injury, anatomy, and recommendations for proper position to prevent injury of the ulnar nerve.*

Winfree CJ, Kline, DG. Intraoperative positioning nerve injuries. Surg Neuro 2005;63:5–18.
- *This article explains the mechanism of nerve injuries and describes the possible nerve injury in each position, along with the diagnosis and therapy.*

Transportation Made Somewhat Less Deadly

**Ricardo Irizarry
and David Sinclair**

INTRODUCTION

- Transporting sick patients is an important part of our jobs.
- We transport patients to and from operating rooms, intensive care units, diagnostic/interventional suites, and patient care wards.
- Frequently, we transport critically ill patients, hemodynamically unstable patients, and intubated patients.
- You must have a reasonable understanding of your patient's underlying disease process to anticipate (and hopefully prevent) troubles during transport.
- Having the right equipment is *extremely* important.
- Having the right equipment that *functions* is *even more important*.
- Minimize your lines and tubing for transport—cap off IVs you don't need, tape down as much IV tubing as you can, and sort out all monitoring lines, cables, and leads.
- Bring help.

We're halfway there, what could go wrong?

Titanic passenger

BACKGROUND

- Adverse effects may occur in up to 70% of transports, and critically ill patients are at an increased risk of morbidity and mortality during intrahospital transport.
- These events include changes in heart rate, arrhythmias, arterial hypertension or hypotension, increased intracranial pressure, respiratory derangements, hypercapnea, hypocapnea, hypoxemia, and cardiac arrest.
- Mishaps occurring during transportation may be due to the patient's underlying illness or to equipment malfunction.
- Most problems are related to *equipment failure*—ECG lead disconnection, monitor power failure (happens *all* the time), IV disconnection, drug infusion disconnection, and ventilator disconnection.
- In one study by Smith et al., most mishaps were noted at the destination site and *not* during the actual transport!

PROCESS

- Pre-transport communication and coordination is important.
- The team at the receiving location (ICU, patient care ward, PACU, Interventional Radiology suite) must have the report ahead of time to properly prepare to assume care for the patient.
- Communication ensures continuity of care, and before transport, the receiving location must confirm that it is ready to receive the patient.

- Transportation involves disconnecting the patient from existing monitors and connecting them to an equivalent set of portable monitors.
- Sometimes the patient must be physically moved onto another bed—a challenge when a patient has many lines and monitors or is morbidly obese.
- Remember to pad patients appropriately, keep patients warm (especially the very young and very old), raise guardrails, and have circumferential padding on cribs (small children tend to bounce around).
- Think one step ahead—if you need an elevator, have someone run ahead of you to hold the elevator *before* transporting the patient. The elevator waits for *you*, not the other way around!
- Always rely on the ABCs of ACLS in the event of a mishap during transportation: airway, breathing, circulation.
- Have appropriate equipment to manage the airway, support ventilation, and support circulation.
- Monitoring during transport must be equal to or better than that prior to transport.
- Upon arrival, a report of any mishaps occurring during transport is given to the receiving team.

PEOPLE

- A minimum of two people are required to transport a critically ill or intubated patient.

The Prone Patient

Patients undergoing prone procedures in the OR are turned supine at the conclusion of surgery, prior to transportation. The process of turning them supine can be a harrowing experience. As in any transport, organization is absolutely paramount. First, disconnect all superfluous connections—IVs, drips, cables, and monitors. Second, make sure you have plenty of help. Next, have the stretcher in the room properly aligned with the OR table. Remember, leave the patient connected to a circuit on 100% oxygen in the few minutes prior to transport—this will give you added time while the patient is apneic during turning. At the last minute, disconnect the remaining IV, pulse oximeter, and circuit. Make sure the arms are tucked at their sides and gently log-roll the patient onto the stretcher. Immediately reconnect the circuit once the patient is supine and ventilate the patient. Check for breath sounds and reconnect the pulse oximeter. Whew!

Paralysis and Sedation

Once the decision has been made to leave a patient intubated for transport, it follows that the patient should be sedated and paralyzed. Practitioners usually have a good reason for not pulling the tube, and if you do not want the tube out in a controlled setting such as an OR or ICU—for whatever the reason—then you probably do not want the tube out en route anywhere, either. To *guarantee* that tube stays in, you should paralyze the patient. Why not? The only thing you lose by paralyzing the patient is the worry of having the patient wake up and pull the tube out! You have a peripheral nerve stimulator—use it! Titrate muscle relaxant to ensure the patient is too weak to pull the tube out, and then make sure the patient is adequately sedated to prevent unpleasant recall.

- The more hands you have to help, the better off you will be.
- Usually, a nurse will accompany you for a routine transport, e.g., transporting an extubated patient after an uneventful surgery to the post-anesthesia care unit.
- Consider enlisting the services of a respiratory therapist, a second nurse, or a second physician to accompany unstable patients.

EQUIPMENT

- A blood pressure monitor, pulse oximeter, and continuous electrocardiography are considered standard transport monitors.
- An oxygen source to last the expected length of transportation plus a 30-minute reserve is recommended.* *Make sure the oxygen tank has enough oxygen to get you to your destination.* For example, at 475 psi an oxygen tank has 165 L of gas. At a flow rate of 4 L/min, this will last about 40 minutes.
- Note that in adults and children, the default oxygen concentration for transport is 100%. However, this is *not* true for neonates, patients with single ventricle physiology, or those dependent on a right-to-left shunt to maintain systemic perfusion!
- Airway management equipment: a laryngoscope blade, a tongue depressor, an oral airway, a nasal airway, a cuffed endotracheal tube, stylette, syringe, and face mask
- A means of delivering positive pressure ventilation: a bag-valve ventilator (i.e., AMBU-bag) or a Mapelson circuit are most commonly used
- In specific patients, capnometry, continuous blood pressure measurement, intracranial pressure measurement, cardiac output, and filling pressures may be necessary for safe transport.
- Basic drugs to help secure the airway: an induction agent (propofol, etomidate, or ketamine) and a muscle relaxant (succinylcholine, rocuronium)
- Sedative/hypnotic drugs or opioids may be individualized to the patient.
- Basic resuscitation drugs, including epinephrine and atropine, and anti-arrhythmic agents are useful in the event of cardiac arrest or arrhythmia.

- Alternatively, particularly for stable patients, the transport team may rely on the availability of drugs from supply depots (i.e., "crash carts") located along the transport route or at the destination.
- A good, functioning IV that can serve as a volume line (in an emergency, certain drugs can be administered intramuscularly, via the endotracheal tube, or intraosseous, but IVs are preferable).
- A fluid bag for the IV
- Consider a transport ventilator for the intubated patient with poor lung compliance, ARDS, or otherwise requiring ventilation parameters (e.g., inverse I:E ratios) that are difficult to reproduce with manual ventilatory assist devices such as AMBU-bags.
- If a transport ventilator is to be used, a respiratory therapist *must* be present and the ventilator *must* have alarms to signal a disconnection, high peak airway pressures, or insufficient oxygen, and *must* have a backup battery power supply.

THE MECHANICS: MOVING THE PATIENT FROM THE OR TABLE TO A STRETCHER

- Avoid "spaghetti" at all costs.
- Make your life easy: disconnect *everything* you don't need.
- One good IV is all you should need *most* of the time.
- Occasionally, you will need a second IV to serve as a continuous infusion line for drips (e.g., vasopressors).
- Discontinue any drip or infusion that is not absolutely necessary for transport (insulin drips, KCl, diazepam, morphine, and so on).
- Discontinue all monitors that are not absolutely essential for transport.
- Keep the pulse oximeter on until the very last moment prior to moving the patient. It should be the *last* monitor you disconnect.
- After disconnecting an IV, tape the residual IV tubing to the patient. Leave a tab on the end of the tape to allow for easy removal.
- Leave a stopcock on the end of any residual IV tubing so that, in an emergency, drugs or fluid may be easily administered.

- Transport the IV bags (remember: usually one, at most two) to a portable IV pole or onto the stretcher *first*.
- If automated pumps for continuous infusions must accompany the patient, firmly attach them either to the portable IV pole or to a built-in IV pole on the stretcher *before* moving the patient.
- Make sure the pumps have enough battery power to last the length of the transportation route—keep the pumps plugged into an AC outlet *as long as possible* to avoid draining the battery life!
- Make sure *anything* draining *any part* of the patient stays with the patient (nasogastric tube, Foley catheter, chest tube, Jackson-Pratt drain, and so on).
- Change over from the OR monitors to the transport monitors—start with the ECG leads; next, change over the arterial line; and last, the pulse oximeter. Keep the patient monitored on the OR monitors until you are switched over to the corresponding transport monitor.
- Now you're ready! You have your airway and resuscitative equipment, you have an oxygen source, and you have properly functioning monitors that have adequate battery life.
- Next, ask the patient to move onto the stretcher if they are able. If the patient is unable to move, the patient must be moved manually.
- If the patient is mechanically ventilated, keep 100% oxygen in the few minutes prior to transport and detach the patient from the circuit at the last possible moment prior to moving them (just *after* disconnecting the pulse oximeter).
- If the patient is to remain intubated for transport, make sure they are adequately sedated and paralyzed for transport.
- Log-roll the patient onto the stretcher, keeping the neck midline.
- Make sure all remaining IV tubing and monitor lines or cables are free and clear.
- Once successfully transported onto the stretcher, *first* reconnect the circuit.
- *After* reconnecting the circuit, connect the pulse oximeter.
- If the patient is still intubated, check for breath sounds to make sure the endotracheal tube did not move during transport.

THE LONG ROAD AHEAD

- Now that the patient is on the stretcher, and assuming the ABCs are established, start a secondary assessment of the patient.
- Check for positioning and adequate blankets to keep the patient warm.
- Make sure the guardrails are up and that proper padding is available.
- You're off! Hopefully, your destination is a nearby PACU with an extubated, healthy, stable patient in your hands. In that case, all you need is an oxygen source, a standard face mask, and a nurse to accompany you.
- However, for the critically ill patient, a long journey to the ICU (or worse, a diagnostic/interventional radiology suite) awaits!
- For the intubated patient, ventilation must be preserved—change over to either a manual ventilation device (AMBU-bag, Mapelson circuit) or a transport ventilator.
- Check your vital signs on the transport monitor prior to leaving the OR.
- Make sure your airway equipment and all necessary drugs are on the stretcher with the patient.
- Turn *off* the ventilator on the anesthesia machine, and turn *off* the anesthetic gases!
- Make sure all lines are free and clear prior to transport. Make sure the wheels on the bed are unlocked (duh!) and that the hallway is clear. The elevator, if needed, should be waiting for you.
- You should be at the head of the bed, managing the airway and monitoring the patient.
- Have someone else help you steer at the foot of the bed.
- Remember to paralyze and sedate a critically ill, intubated patient prior to transport!

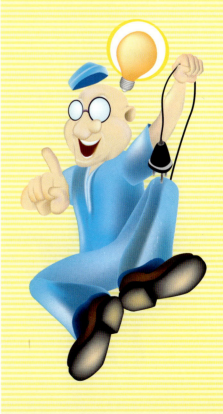

TRANSPORT PITFALLS

- *Never* take your eyes off the patient or the monitor.
- If any monitor stops working en route, *always* fall back on the ABCs—airway, breathing, circulation.
- If all monitors fail, you know the patient is being adequately ventilated if they have a symmetric chest rise, bilateral breath sounds, and fogging in the endotracheal tube.
- To assess adequate circulation, check a pulse! A carotid pulse tells you the patient is perfusing their brain!
- If a monitor fails mid-route, check the ABCs. Assuming the patient is stable, you must assess the necessity for the monitor relative to your point on the transportation route.
- How badly do you need the monitor? Are you closer to your destination or your origin? Can another monitor aid you temporarily?
- For example, if the ECG no longer works, do you have a nice, steady waveform on your pulse oximeter? If so, it is telling you a great deal about the patient's hemodynamic state! Do you need to turn around? Should you forge ahead to your destination? Should you send someone for another monitor mid-route?
- What about IV failure? If the IV infiltrates en route, the first thing to do is *stop* any more fluid from flowing into the IV! Disconnect the tubing and pull the catheter!
- Now what? Do you place another IV? Do wait until you arrive at your destination?

- In an emergency, drugs can be given intramuscularly, via the endotracheal tube, or even via a proximal tibial intraosseous needle.
- All these decisions are made on an individual basis after clinically assessing patient and establishing the ABCs.
- What about oxygen? If your oxygen source fails (I *told* you to check it!), what are your other options? Some manual bag-valve devices automatically inflate with room air in the event of oxygen failure—21% oxygen is better than nothing!
- If all else fails, breathe into the endotracheal tube—16% oxygen is better than nothing!
- Always, always, always call for help! It is better to err on the side of caution when issues of patient safety are concerned.

THE DROP-OFF

- You made it!
- Now you must safely transfer the patient from your temporary transport monitors back to monitors that are more permanent at your destination.
- For the intubated patient, change over from a transport ventilator or manual ventilatory device to the more permanent ventilator.
- Hang all IVs and check lines for any air that may have been inadvertently entrained during transport.
- Give a report to the receiving team; notify them of any changes during transport or any mishaps that may have occurred.
- Take a deep breath and relax—your job is done!

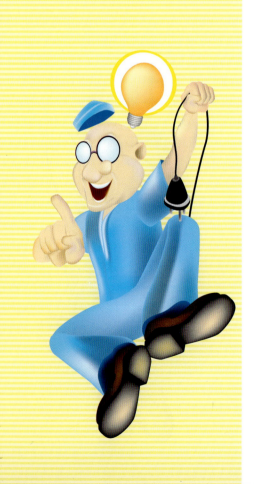

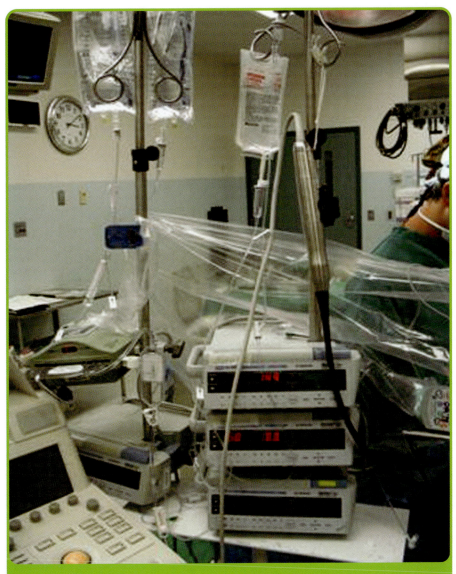

Figure 1. All of these cables, wires, and tubes need to be sorted prior to transport. Note the two unused pumps that should be set aside prior to moving the patient in order to avoid clutter.

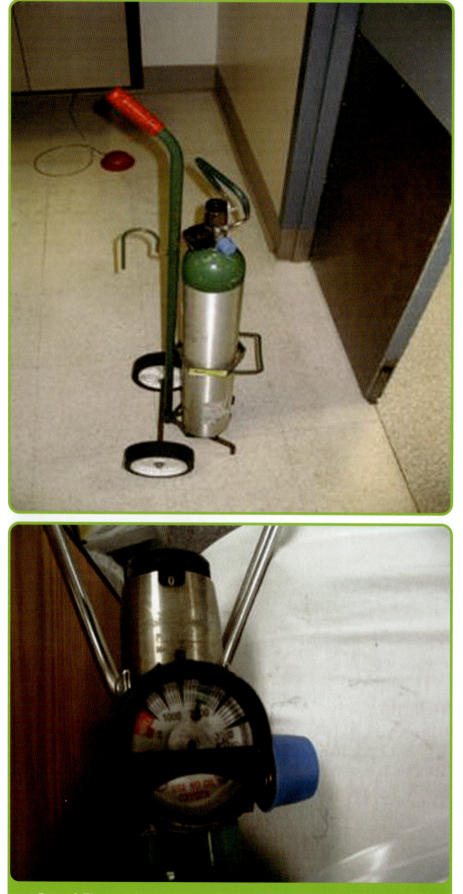

Figure 2. The portable oxygen source. Always make sure you have enough pressure in the cylinder to provide you with 30 minutes of oxygen MORE than you need!

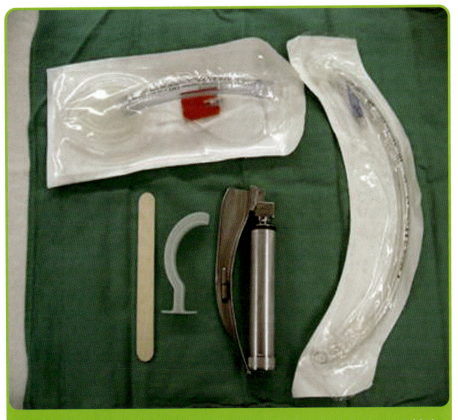

Figure 3. The tools of the trade: the laryngoscope blade, oral airway, tongue blade, and endotracheal tube. Don't forget the laryngeal mask airway (LMA) for backup!

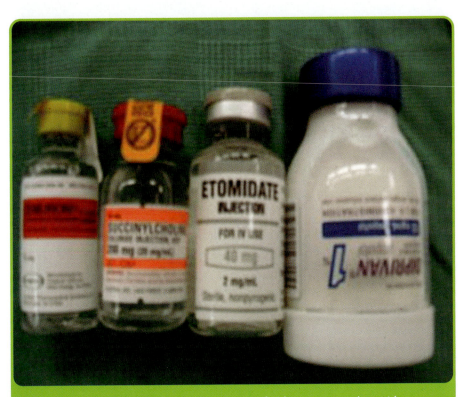

Figure 4. The bare essentials: your choice of induction agent (etomidate or propofol) and a muscle relaxant (rocuronium or succinylcholine) to facilitate intubation of the trachea.

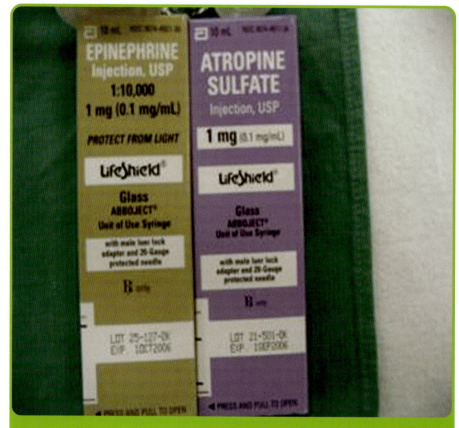

Figure 5. Two basic drugs for resuscitation.

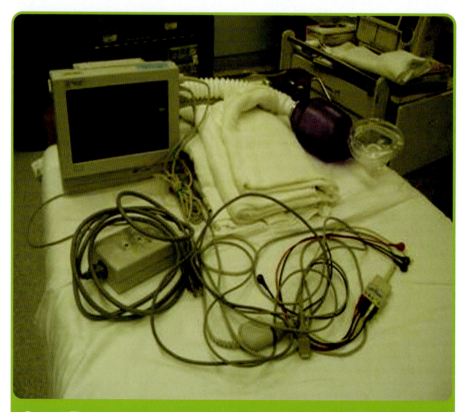

Figure 6. The transport monitor. Complete with continuous ECG monitor, pulse oximeter, and arterial line monitor. Note the manual bag-valve ventilator with attached face mask to deliver positive pressure ventilation.

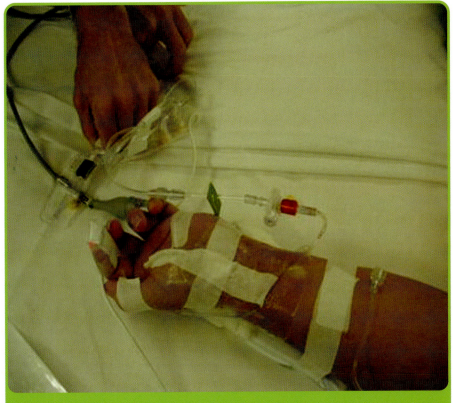

Figure 7. An arterial line is disconnected from its native transducer and reconnected to a portable transducer that will, in turn, be connected to the transport monitor.

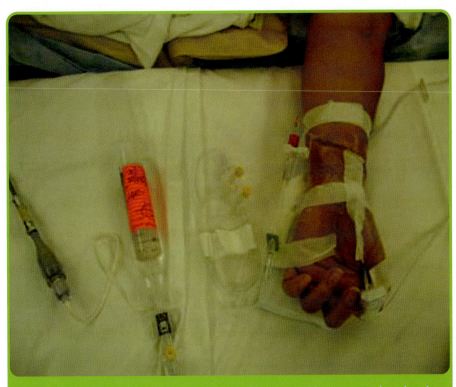

Figure 8. Stepwise transfer of the patient. The arterial line is transduced and displayed on the transport monitor. Note the patient still has a pulse oximeter in place (index finger) that is attached to the original monitor in the OR.

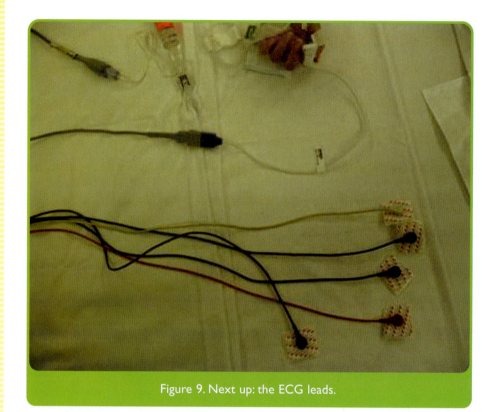

Figure 9. Next up: the ECG leads.

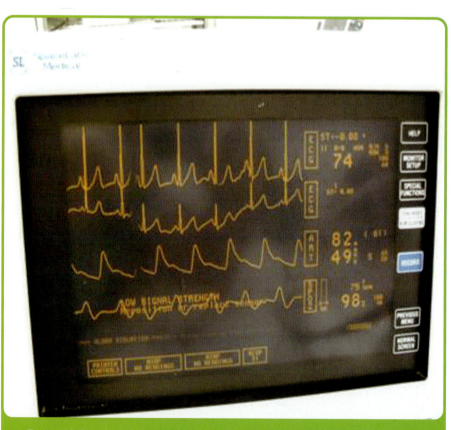

Figure 10. The finished product. The patient has been safely transferred and monitored. Note the continuous ECG, pulse oximeter, and arterial line waveform.

SUGGESTED READING

Beckman U, Gillies DM, Berenholtz SM, et al. Incidents relating to the intra-hospital transfer of critically ill patients. Intensive Care Med 2004;30:1579–85.

- *Of the 191 incidents analyzed, 39% were equipment related and 61% were patient/staff related.*

Dockery WK, Futterman C, Keller SR, et al. A comparison of manual and mechanical ventilation during pediatric transport. Crit Care Med 1999;27:802–6.

- *The manually ventilated cohort had a greater fluctuation of end-tidal carbon dioxide in transit and had a significantly lower end-tidal carbon dioxide at destination versus the cohort on mechanical ventilation. No significant changes in hemodynamic measurements were noted between the two groups.*

Fioritto BA, Mirza F, Doran TM, et al. Intraosseous access in the setting of pediatric critical care transport. Pedi Crit Care Med 2005;6:50–3.

- *Don't panic! If all IVs come out, this is a viable option. The IO route delivers drugs as quickly as central access and faster than peripheral access.*

Hurst JM, Davis K Jr, Johnson DJ, et al. Cost and complications during in-hospital transport of critically ill patients: A prospective cohort study. J Trauma 1992;33:582–5.

- *The controls were stationary ICU patients and the test group was a cohort of patients matched for age and APACHE II score. No differences found.*

Insel J, Weissman C, Kemper M, et al. Cardiovascular changes during transport of critically ill and postoperative patients. Crit Care Med 1986;14:539–42.

- *A comparison of patients transported from the OR to the ICU with ICU patients transported elsewhere for diagnostic tests. The postoperative patients had a higher incidence of transport hypotension, hypertension, and arrhythmias.*

Smith I, Fleming S, Cerinaianu A. Mishaps during transport from the intensive care unit. Crit Care Med 1990;18:278–81.

- *In 125 transports, most of the reported mishaps were equipment-related and were not noted during the actual transport!*

Warren J, Fromm RE Jr, et al. Guidelines for inter- and intrahospital transport of critically ill patients. Crit Care Med 2004;32:256–62.

- *These are the current guidelines from the American College of Critical Care Medicine regarding inter- and intrahospital patient transport. A good resource!*

Waydhas C. Intrahospital transport of critically ill patients. Crit Care 1999;3:R83–9.

- *A good review of the literature—interestingly enough, patient age, duration of transport, APACHE II score, and personnel accompanying the patient did not correlate with an increased complication risk.*

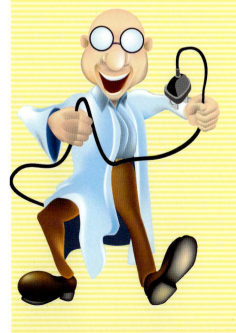

PART 6

THE REGIONAL LANDSCAPE

Armed and Dangerous: The Arm Block

**Howard Palte
and Ady Bermudez**

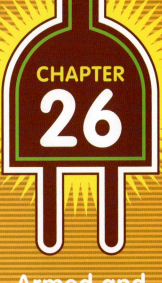

Come on, whaddaya say? I'll fight ya with one hand tied behind my back!

The Cowardly Lion
The Wizard of Oz, 1939

INTRODUCTION

We don't actually attempt to *tie* someone's hand behind their back, but we do try to take one arm out of commission for a while with our arm blocks.

Upper extremity blocks can be divided as follows:

- brachial plexus blocks
- peripheral nerve blocks at the elbow and wrist

Indication, anatomy, techniques, and complications will all suffer intense scrutiny in this chapter. By the end, you may be able to do one of these blocks, well, with one hand tied behind *your* back!

BRACHIAL PLEXUS BLOCKS

Four approaches to brachial plexus blocks have evolved over the years—interscalene block, axillary block, supraclavicular block, and infraclavicular block. We will focus on interscalene and axillary blocks, which are the ones most commonly used.

INTERSCALENE BLOCK

Indications

- Shoulder and upper arm surgery
- Postoperative analgesia
- Plexus is blocked at level of roots
- May miss C8 and T1

Anatomy

- The fascia surrounding the brachial plexus originates from the muscular fascia of the anterior and middle scalene muscles. The brachial plexus is therefore found between these two muscles in the interscalene groove.
- The interscalene groove is at the level of the cricoid cartilage.

Technique

- Paresthesia or nerve stimulator use
- Patient supine with head rotated away from side of block (30° to 45°)
- Locate interscalene groove (between anterior and middle scalene muscles). For real experts with fingers like a safecracker, this groove is palpated without any problem at all. For regular folk who don't do this all the time, this groove can be damned hard to feel. Plus, if you press hard enough, you can make *anything* feel like a groove. Best advice? Tag along with someone who really does this on a daily basis and figure out how *they* figure it out.
- Prepare and drape
- Local for skin wheal
- A 22G, 1.5-in. needle is placed perpendicular to skin, advancing slowly in a medial-caudal direction
- Aspirate constantly (vascularized area). The neck is a *very* crowded place, with all kinds of things squished in there. Caution is the watchword.
- Once paresthesia (in shoulder, arm, or hand) or nerve stimulation has occurred, 30 cc to 50 cc of local anesthetic is introduced. Remember to aspirate. Which dose is a test dose? *Every damn dose is a* test dose. Anytime you inject this potentially deadly stuff, ask yourself, "If that last bolus just went intravascular, just how bad off would I (and by extension, the patient) be?"

Complications

- Dyspnea, diaphragmatic paresis (phrenic nerve). No big deal if your patient is healthy as a horse but if your patient has COPD and is hanging on by an alveolus, then this diaphragmatic paralysis might push them into respiratory failure. In case anyone asks, the endotracheal tube you placed is called the "plastic endotracheal regional supplementation block."
- Horner's Syndrome (Stellate ganglion)
- Intra-arterial injection (vertebral artery). The seizure happens in about a nanosecond because you deliver a whopping dose right smack dab into the brain. Your reaction to this intravertebral artery injection is called the "anesthesia provider Pampers changing maneuver."
- Hoarseness (recurrent laryngeal nerve)

- Epidural, subarachnoid, or subdural injections. Because these blocks are so high, respiratory depression occurs pretty quickly, so keep all your resuscitative goodies nearby.
- Pneumothorax
- A great way to get an "anatomy primer" is to pay close attention the next time your ENT surgeon does a radical neck procedure. Once the skin is out of the way (pesky stuff, too bad we're not transparent), get up close and personal with the neck and see all the places your needle *should* go and all the bad places your needle *can* go. I kid thee not—this is a great refresher. With all our diagrams, websites, computer animations, and the like, seeing the real thing is still a tremendous help, and the "free lesson with each radical neck dissection" is there for the asking.

AXILLARY BLOCK

Indications

- Hand and forearm surgery
- Elbow surgery

Anatomy

- In the axilla, the plexus forms three cords (medial, lateral, and posterior) that surround the axillary artery.
- The cords form the median (found superior to the artery), radial (found posterior to the artery), ulnar (found inferior to the artery), and musculocutaneous nerves.
- The musculocutaneous nerve must be blocked at the coracobrachialis muscle because it has already exited the sheath at this level.

Technique

- There are three techniques: transarterial, paresthesia, or with a nerve stimulator.

Transarterial

- Patient should be supine with the arm in 90° abduction and elbow flexed, kind of like giving the Boy Scout oath.
- Identify arterial artery by palpation (do this as high as possible in the axilla). You may mark the site.
- Prepare the area with cleansing solution.
- Prepare your needle with an IV extension set to connect to your local anesthetic syringe.

- Again, locate the artery with the index and middle finger of your nondominant hand.
- Raise a skin wheal between your fingers where you should be feeling a pulse.
- Insert a 22G, 1.5-in. needle at a 45° angle to the skin.
- Aspirate as you insert.
- You may feel a pop or snap as you traverse the sheath
- Continue inserting until you aspirate pulsating bright red blood. At this point, you continue slowly until it stops (you are now posterior to the axillary artery).
- Begin injecting local anesthetics.
- Aspirate a few times to make sure you are not intravascular.
- A total of 40 cc to 50 cc of local anesthetics are injected. Some inject the entire amount either posterior or anterior. Others choose to inject half posterior and half anterior.

Paresthesia

- Preparation is identical.
- A 25G, 1.5-in. needle is used to locate the nerves that will be innervating the surgical site.
- Once paresthesia is elicited (a feeling of pins and needles), 10 cc of local anesthetic is injected in each region.

Nerve Stimulator

- Preparation is identical.
- An insulated needle is used to evoke a motor response of the stimulated nerve: median, ulnar, radial, or musculocutaneous (see individual nerve blocks).
- A quantity of 10 cc of local anesthetic is injected for each response elicited.

Complications

- This technique is relatively safe if one is careful not to inject intravascularly. Keep talking to the patient and if they say anything weird is happening, even something as vague as, "I feel funny," then stop. Because you need the patient to talk to you, make sure you don't oversedate the patient before you perform this block. They could "doze through" the premonitory symptoms of an intravascular injection and your first clue would be a seizure.
- Rare complications include infection and hematoma.

INDIVIDUAL NERVE BLOCKS

It is important to recall the motor response elicited by individual nerves when using a nerve stimulator. Here we will be going over such responses as well as the different anatomical locations where you can block those nerves.

Musculocutaneous

- This nerve derives from the lateral cord. It is frequently missed when an axillary approach to a brachial plexus block is used.

- The musculocutaneous nerve pierces the coracobrachialis muscle and continues anterior to the humerus between the brachialis and biceps.

- Sensory innervation of the lateral aspect of the forearm via lateral cutaneous nerve of forearm. Motor innervation to flexor region of the arm.

- The nerve may be blocked by using a 22G, 1.5-in. needle, inserting it into the belly of the coracobrachialis, and injecting 5 cc to 10 cc of local anesthetic.

- When innervating the musculocutaneous nerve, an elbow flexion will be elicited.

Median

- This nerve is formed by the medial and lateral cords.

- In the arm, this nerve runs medial to the brachial artery. It remains medial in the antecubital fossa and continues its course until it reaches the wrist, at which point it lies behind the palmaris longus tendon.

- Sensory innervation to the thumb, index, middle, and half ring finger. Motor innervation to the flexor region of the forearm and thenar muscles in hand.

- The median nerve can therefore be blocked in the aforementioned locations given the anatomy.

Elbow

- In a supinate arm, find the brachial artery (medial to biceps tendon) and inject 5 cc of local anesthetic medial to the artery once paresthesia or motor stimulation is elicited.

Wrist

- In a supinate hand, ask the patient to flex their wrist, at which time the tendon of the palmaris longus is easily visible in most patients.

- The nerve runs between the palmaris longus and the flexor carpi radialis (lateral to palmaris longus).

- With a 25G needle, inject 5 cc of local anesthetic into this area.

- Motor stimulation will cause wrist flexion and second and third finger flexion and pronation because this nerve provides innervation to the wrist flexors and to the lumbrical muscles of the second and third fingers.

Ulnar

- Derives from the medial cord

- The nerve runs medial to the brachial artery in the arm then moves medially to go under the arcuate ligament of the medial epicondyle. It continues down the arm and is found medial to the ulnar artery at the wrist.

- Lateral to flexor carpi ulnaris tendon.

- Sensory innervation of pinky and medial half of ring finger. Motor innervation to intrinsic muscles of hand. I love how, even as doctors, we still say "pinky."

- These above mentioned areas are the locations where we will be blocking the ulnar nerve.

Elbow

- Patient's arm should be flexed at the elbow at an angle of slightly more than 90°.

- Palpate between the olecranon and the medial epicondyle to find the ulnar nerve.

- Using a 22G, 1.5-in. needle, inject 2 cc to 4 cc of local anesthetic in this location.

Wrist

- Palpate the ulnar artery and find the flexor carpi ulnaris tendon (it is medial to the artery and lateral to the tendon).

- Insert a 22G, 1-in. needle.

- Aspirate.

- Inject 2 cc to 4 cc of local anesthetic in this location.

- Motor stimulation will cause flexion of fourth and fifth finger as well as flexion at the wrist.

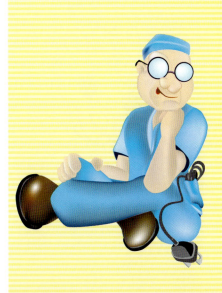

Radial

- Derives from the posterior cord
- Runs in posterior region of arm, moves laterally at elbow and branches to superficial and deep nerves. The superficial nerve remains close to the radial artery at distal areas of the forearm.
- Sensory innervation is dorsum of hand on lateral aspect. Motor innervation to extensor of elbow, wrist, and fingers.

Elbow

- Locate the biceps tendon at the antecubital fossa.
- Using a 22G, 1.5-in. needle, inject 4 cc to 5 cc of local anesthetic lateral to the tendon aiming toward the lateral epicondyle.

Wrist

- Locate the radial styloid process and palpate the radial artery.
- You will find the radial nerve lateral to radial artery and 1 in. proximal to the styloid process.
- Using a 22G, 1-in. needle, inject 2 cc to 3 cc of local anesthetic at this point.
- Aspirate.
- Motor stimulation will cause extension of the elbow, extension of the wrist, or extension of the fingers. This depends on the location of the nerve stimulation.

INDIVIDUAL DIGIT BLOCKS

- Each finger has a sensory innervation that is derived from four digital nerves found at the base of each finger, each in one corner.
- Using a 25G, 5/8-in. needle, inject 2 cc of local anesthetic at each corner.
- No epinephrine. (A somewhat off-color mnemonic for where not to use epinephrine is "fingers, nose, toes, and hose," with the last term referring in somewhat jocular fashion to the male organ of generation. Pretend you didn't read it here but do remember the lesson.)

Intercostobrachial and Medial Brachial Cutaneous Nerve

- The intercostobrachial nerve is not found in the brachial plexus sheath. This nerve, along with the medial brachial cutaneous nerve (which exits the sheath before the axillary region), must be blocked for tourniquet use.
- These nerves innervate the skin of the upper arm where the tourniquet is placed.

- Using a 22G, 1–in. needle, 5 cc of local anesthetic is injected starting in the medial aspect of the upper arm. Fan the anesthetic anterior and posterior.

BIER BLOCK (INTRAVENOUS REGIONAL ANESTHESIA)

Indications

- Surgical procedures from elbow to hand
- Procedures less than 1 hour

Technique

- Place an 18G IV on the dorsum of the hand.
- If a double tourniquet system is used, verify that proximal and distal tourniquets are working.
- Place tourniquet on the upper arm.
- Exsanguinate the extremity by lifting the arm and then placing an elastic bandage from distal to proximal.
- Inflate the proximal tourniquet.
- Remove the elastic bandage.
- Inject 45 cc to 55 cc of local anesthetic via the 18G IV.
- Remove the IV.
- During the procedure, the patient may complain of tourniquet pain. At this point, inflate the distal tourniquet and then deflate the proximal.

Complications

- Shorter than expected procedure—need to leave tourniquet inflated for at least 15 min.
- Equipment failure—may cause system circulation of IV anesthetic and the complications that may bring. Remember the ABCs.

COOL EXTRA TIP WITH THE BIER BLOCK

- When you need a big peripheral line and can't get one, you can do a kind of "fake Bier block" to make a big vein appear.
- Do the standard things for a Bier block using a small IV (say, a 20G).
- Inject 60 cc of just saline with the tourniquet still up.
- Shazam! Big veins will pop up all over the place and now you can put in a big IV!

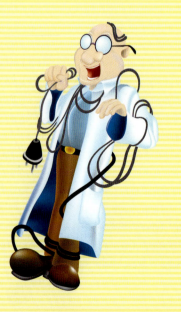

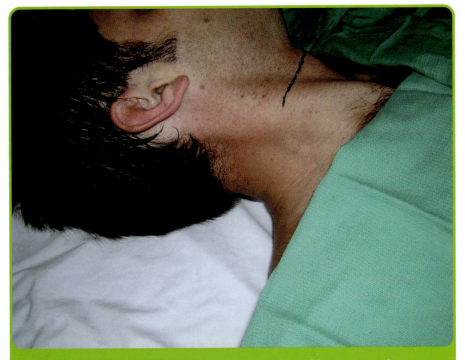

Figure 1. We're going for the interscalene block here. Use a pen to draw your landmarks. Here we go across from the thyroid cartilage. No kidding, use the pen to get oriented. It makes you think through your landmarks and get it right the first time, rather than just plunging the needle in and floundering around.

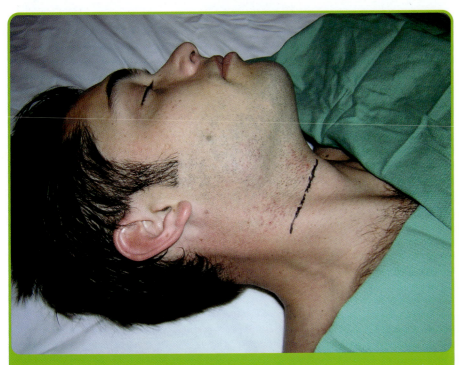

Figure 2. Periodically ask the patient to open their eyes. It creeps you out when they have them closed like this. This might be my sixth sense talking here, but, I think I might be seeing dead people. Creepy.

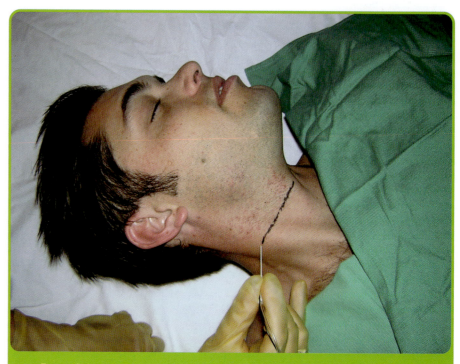

Figure 3. In goes the needle, that should make the bastard open his eyes.

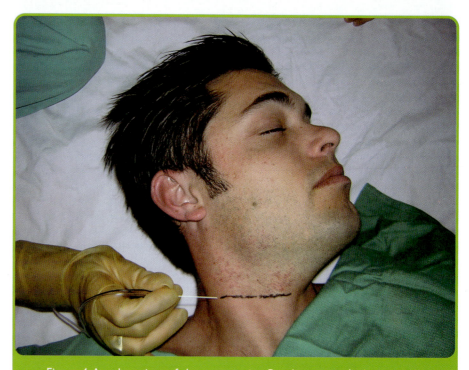

Figure 4. Another view of the entry point. Boy, he sure isn't doing much.

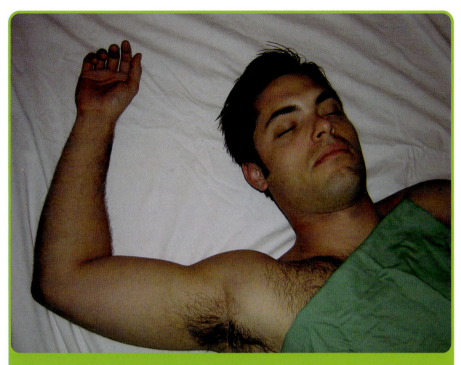

Figure 5. For an axillary block, move the arm up (funny, the arm seems a little stiff here). This looks like a salute. Hey, open your eyes! Damnation, call 911! This guy is dead!

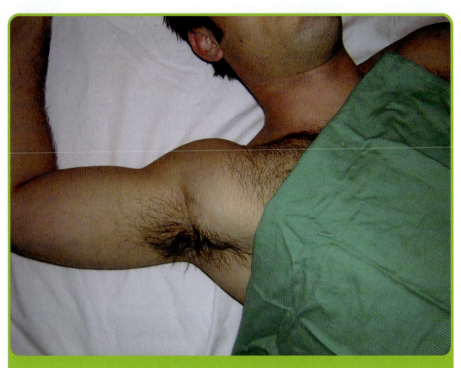

Figure 6. Just kidding! He coughed, he's not really dead, just playing possum. Now then, where were we?

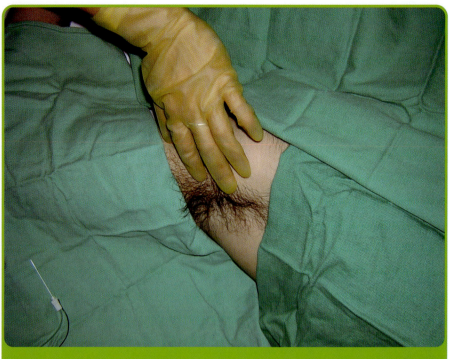

Figure 7. Prep, drape, palpate the axillary artery.

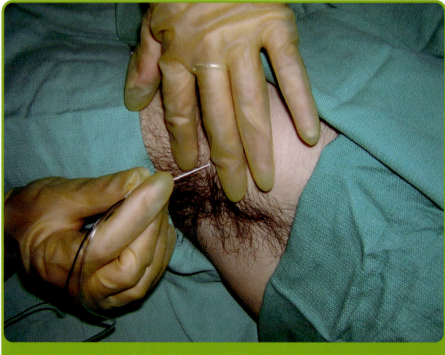

Figure 8. Little local then in you go.

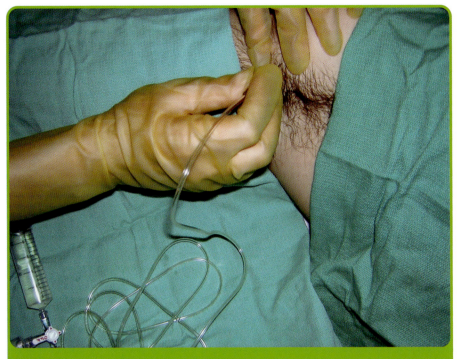

Figure 9. Note the tubing. You don't want the needle directly attached to a big old syringe or you'll be a clumsy oaf.

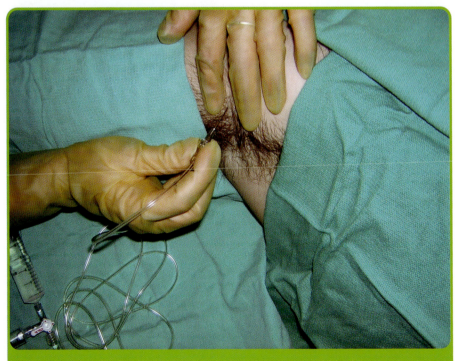

Figure 10. Needle going for a trans-arterial block.

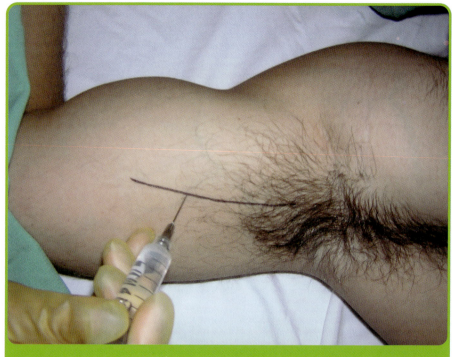

Figure 11. Now we're going for the musculocutaneous nerve.

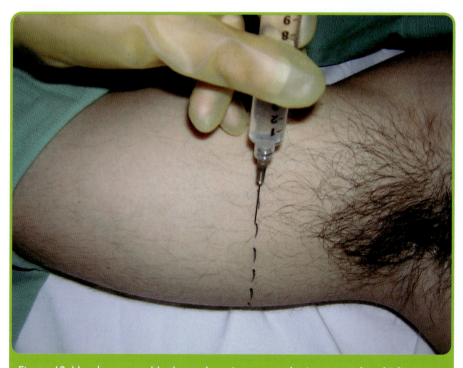

Figure 12. Here's an easy block, a sub-q ring to get the intercostobrachialis nerve.

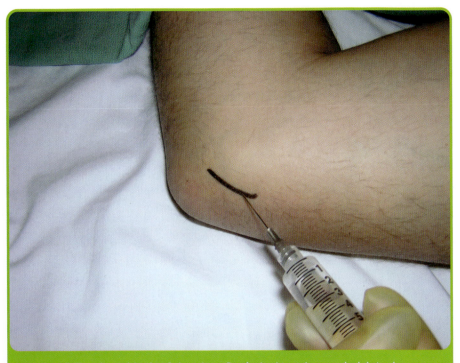

Figure 13. Touch up block of the ulnar. *Don't do this right smack dab in the groove itself at the elbow.* You'll squash the nerve in that tight space.

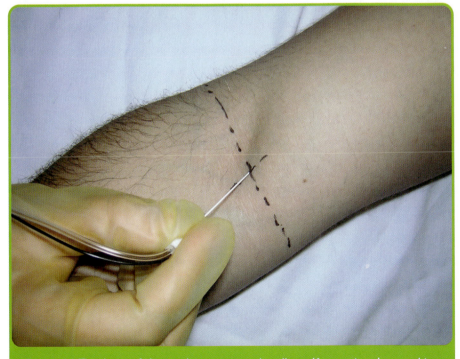

Figure 14. Touch up of the median nerve at the elbow. Keep using that marking pen to keep the landmarks straight.

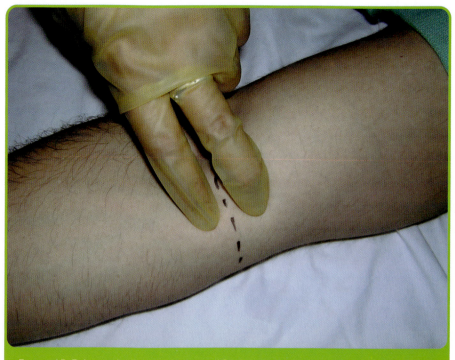

Figure 15. Palpate the brachial artery. (God put arteries near most of the things we block to serve as guide posts.)

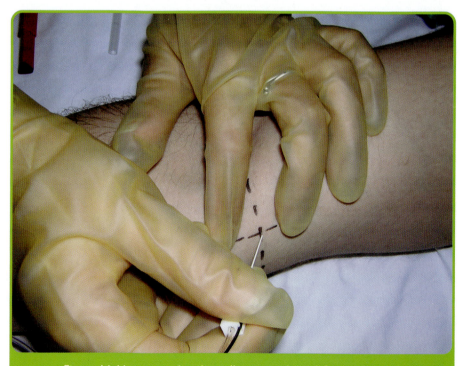

Figure 16. Use an insulated needle on touch ups? Sure, why not?

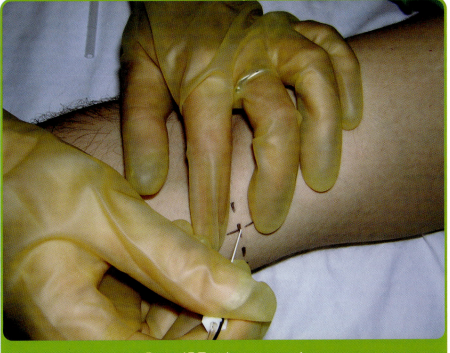

Figure 17. Twitch, away we go!

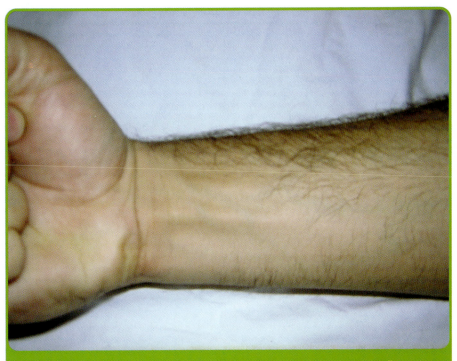

Figure 18. Palmaris longus tendon. This is your "God-given guide post" for the median nerve touch up at the wrist. (Sorry, can't have arteries everywhere!)

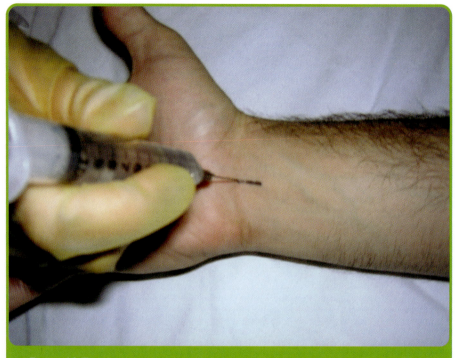

Figure 19. Touch up at the wrist for the median nerve. Some might say "Real doctors don't need touch-ups", but we don't buy into that.

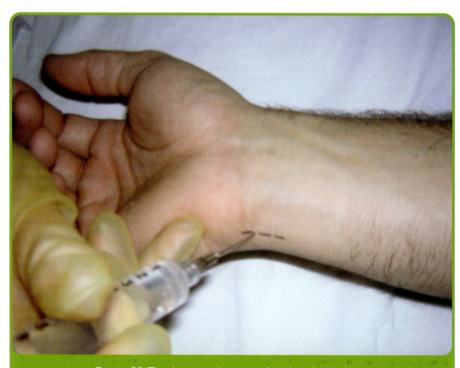

Figure 20. Touch up at the wrist for the ulnar nerve.

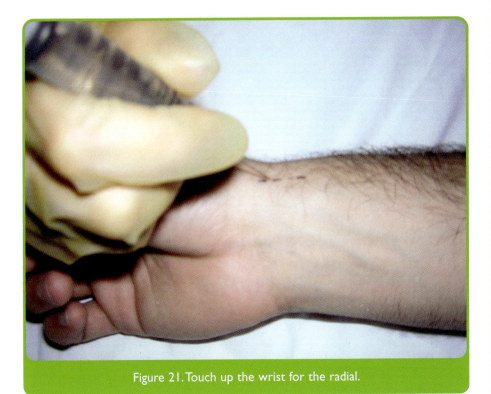

Figure 21. Touch up the wrist for the radial.

SUGGESTED READING

Hahn MB, McQuillan PM, Sheplock GJ. *Regional Anesthesia: An Atlas of Anatomy and Techniques*. St. Louis, MO: Mosby, 1996.
- Raj PP. *Textbook of Regional Anesthesia*. London: Churchill Livingston, 2002.

Rodriguez J, et al. A comparison of four stimulation patterns in axillary block. Reg Anesth Pain Med Jul-Aug 2005; 30(4):324–8.

- Tetzlaff JE. Peripheral nerve blocks. In: Morgan GE, Mikhail MS. *Clinical Anesthesiology*, 2nd edition. Stamford, CT: Appleton and Lange, 1996:245–71.

Wedel DJ. Nerve blocks. In: Miller RD, Cucchiara RF. *Anesthesia*, 5th edition. Philadelphia: Churchill Livingstone, 2000:1520–48.
- Winnie AP. *Plexus Anesthesia: Perivascular Techniques of Brachial Plexus Block*, 2nd edition. Philadelphia: Saunders, 1990.

Lego-Land: Lower Extremity Nerve Blocks

Howard Palte and Sarah Kafi

They also serve who only stand and wait.

John Milton
On His Blindness, 1652

INTRODUCTION

You won't have to stand and wait *that* long if you put these lower extremity nerve blocks in correctly. But these are big nerves (especially the sciatic), requiring pretty hefty doses of local anesthetics, so while you are standing and waiting for them to set up, make sure the local anesthetic didn't go astray.

FEMORAL NERVE BLOCK

Anatomy of the Femoral Nerve
- Formed within the psoas major muscle
- Posterior divisions of L2, L3, and L4
- Emerges from lateral border of psoas muscle
  - Descends in the groove between psoas and iliacus muscles
- Passes under inguinal ligament lateral to femoral artery
- Divides into anterior and posterior divisions
  - Anterior branches mainly cutaneous
  - Posterior branches mainly motor

Innervation
- Anterior compartments of thigh
- Skin of anterior thigh from inguinal ligament to knee
- Medial leg to big toe (saphenous branch)

Clinical Applications
- Surgical procedures limited to anterior thigh
- Knee arthroscopy
- Surgical repair of mid-femoral shaft fractures. (A medical note on such fractures: You can hide a ton of blood in the thigh after a femur fracture, so keep your eyes peeled for signs of hypovolemia. Don't let your enthusiasm for the block blind you to everything else that is happening with the patient!)
- In conjunction with other peripheral blocks

Technique
- Place patient supine.
- Draw a line between the anterior superior iliac spine (ASIS) and the pubic tubercle.
- Mark the femoral artery.
- Advance a 22G, 4-cm needle lateral to artery after anesthetizing the skin.
- Paresthesia or motor response verifies correct needle placement.
- Inject 20 ml of local anesthetic.

Nerve Stimulation: Correct Placement
- Want to identify the posterior branch
- Will see patellar ascension with quadriceps contraction

Common Problems
- Nerve stimulation
  - Anterior branch usually identified first
  - Will see contraction of sartorius muscle on medial thigh
    - Redirect needle laterally and deeper to find posterior branch

Complications
- Intravascular injection
- Hematoma
- Nerve damage

Relative Contraindication
- Femoral vascular grafts

LATERAL FEMORAL CUTANEOUS NERVE BLOCK

Anatomy
- L2 and L3
- Emerges from lateral border of psoas muscle just caudad to ilioinguinal nerve
- Descends under iliac fascia
- Enters thigh deep into inguinal ligament
  - 1 cm to 2 cm medial to ASIS
- Divides into anterior and posterior braches 7 cm to 10 cm below ASIS

Innervation
- Anterior branch
  - Anterolateral thigh to knee
- Posterior branch
  - Skin of lateral thigh from hip to mid-thigh

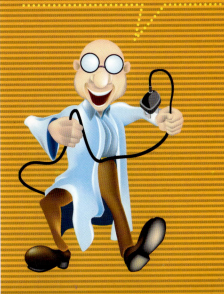

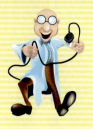

Clinical Applications

- Skin graft harvesting
- In conjunction with other blocks of the lower extremity

Technique

- Find ASIS.
- Mark point 2 cm medial and 2 cm caudad to ASIS.
- Anesthetize the skin.
- Use a 22G, 4-cm needle.
- Keep the needle perpendicular.
- The first "pop" felt is the needle going through fascia lata.
- Move needle in a fanlike pattern medially to laterally while injecting anesthetic.
- Inject 10 ml to 15 ml total, above and below fascia.

Alternative Technique: Belt-and-Suspenders Method

- Block nerve as stated above.
- Also, block nerve medial and posterior to ASIS.
  - Inject 10 ml of anesthetic solution.

Complications

- Neuritis or nerve trauma

THE "3-IN-1" BLOCK

- This is simply a modified high-volume femoral nerve block.
- Blocks lateral femoral cutaneous, obturator and femoral nerves

Technique

- Find ASIS.
- Mark a point 2 cm medial and 2 cm caudad to ASIS.
- Anesthetize the skin.
- Use a 22G, 4-cm needle.
- Angle the needle proximally.
- The first "pop" felt is the needle going through fascia lata.
- Local should spread proximally up the femoral sheath toward the lumbar plexus.

Complications

- Failure to block the obturator nerve

OBTURATOR NERVE BLOCK

Anatomy

- L3 and L4, sometimes with L2
- Deep into obturator canal
- When it leaves the canal, it divides into anterior and posterior branches.

Innervation

- Anterior branch—supplies anterior adductor muscles, skin to lower medial thigh, articular branch to hip
- Posterior branch—deep adductor muscles and articular branch to knee

Clinical Applications

- Knee surgery
- Diagnosis of extent of adductor spasm

Technique

- Place patient supine.
- Find the pubic tubercle.
- Mark 2 cm lateral and 2 cm caudad.
- Anesthetize the skin.
- Advance a 22G, 8- to 10-cm needle perpendicular to the skin and slightly medial.
- After going 2 cm to 4 cm, the needle will encounter the inferior pubic ramus.
- Walk the needle lateral and caudad until it passes into the obturator canal.
- The obturator nerve is 2 cm to 3 cm deeper than the pubic ramus.
- Inject 10 cm to 15 cm of local anesthetic.
- Nerve stimulator—contraction of adductor muscles of medial thigh

Alternative Technique: Interadductor Approach

- Mark skin 2 cm medially to femoral artery and immediately below inguinal ligament.
- Insert a needle behind the adductor tendon, close to the pubic insertion.
- Direct the needle laterally toward mark in the skin.
- You should see the contraction of adductor muscles of medial thigh.

Side Effects and Complications

- Hematoma
- Nerve damage
- Intravascular injection
- Inadequate blockade

SCIATIC NERVE BLOCK

Anatomy

- L4, L5. S1, S2, and S3
- Passes through the sacrosciatic foramen under the piriformis muscle
- Lies between the ischial tuberosity and greater trochanter
- Becomes superficial at lower border of gluteus maximus
- Descends down posterior thigh to the popliteal fossa

Innervation

- Skin of posterior thigh and all of leg and foot except for medial leg and foot (supplied by saphenous nerve)

Clinical Applications

- Blocked in conjunction with femoral or saphenous nerve for surgery below the knee that doesn't require a tourniquet
- Postoperative pain relief

Technique: Classic Approach of Labat

- Posterior approach
- Position patient on side, flexing hip and knee of leg to be blocked.
- Draw a line from the prominence of the greater trochanter with the posterior superior iliac spine (PSIS).
- From the midpoint of this line, draw a 4 cm perpendicular line caudally.
- These lines are called Labat's lines, named after the famous physician, Dr. Lines.
- Make a skin wheal.
- Insert a 22G, 3.5-in. needle perpendicular to the skin.
- Nerve located 4 cm to 6 cm deep
- Nerve stimulator—dorsiflexion or plantar flexion of the foot
- Inject 20 ml of local anesthetic.

Complications

- Partial blockade
  - May miss the posterior cutaneous nerve of the thigh, which separates from the sciatic nerve more proximally. The patient will complain of tourniquet pain.
  - Inadequate block of one sciatic component (either peroneal or tibial)
- Intraneural injection

POPLITEAL BLOCK

Anatomy

- Sciatic nerve divides into common peroneal and tibial nerves high in the popliteal fossa.
- Proximal borders of popliteal fossa
  - Medially—semitendinosus and semi-membranosus tendons
  - Laterally—biceps femoris tendon
- The tibial nerve continues deep into the gastrocnemius muscle.
- The common peroneal nerve leaves the popliteal fossa by passing between the head and neck of the fibula.

Clinical Applications

- Foot and ankle procedures

Technique

- Prone
- Outline popliteal fossa proximal to the flexion crease of the knee.
- Identify the midline of the crease.
- After anesthetizing the skin, insert the needle 2 in. proximal to the crease.
- Inject 20 ml to 30 ml of anesthetic.
- Common peroneal block: 5 ml
  - At the junction of head and neck of fibula, just below the knee
- Saphenous nerve: 5 ml to 10 ml
  - Inject just below the medial surface of the tibial condyle.

Complications

- Intravascular or intraneural injections

ANKLE BLOCK

Anatomy

- Five nerves supply sensation to the foot.
  - Four are terminal branches of the sciatic nerve: superficial peroneal, deep peroneal, posterior tibial, and sural.
  - One nerve is a terminal branch of the femoral nerve: saphenous.

Clinical Applications

- Surgery of the foot not requiring a tourniquet

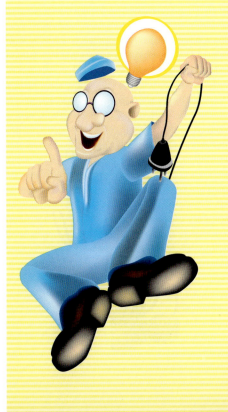

Technique

- Superficial peroneal, deep peroneal, and saphenous nerves
  - Draw a line from the medial malleolus to the lateral malleolus across the dorsum of the foot.
  - Have patient dorsiflex their big toe to identify the extensor hallucis longus tendon.
  - Find the tendon of the extensor digitorum longus.
  - The anterior tibial artery lies between these two tendons.
  - Just lateral to the artery is where you should make a skin wheal.
  - Use a 25G, 3-cm needle.
  - Advance the needle perpendicular to the skin.
  - Inject 5 ml of local anesthetic deep to the extensor retinaculum. This blocks the deep peroneal nerve
  - Then direct the needle laterally. Inject 5 ml subcutaneously. This blocks the superficial peroneal nerve.
  - Then direct the needle medially. Inject 5 ml subcutaneously. This blocks the saphenous nerve.
- Posterior tibial nerve
  - Position patient supine or prone.
  - Palpate posterior tibial artery.
  - Use a 25G, 3-cm needle.
  - Anesthetize the skin posterolaterally to the artery at the level of the medial malleolus.
  - Insert the needle and inject 5 ml of local anesthetic. You should get anesthesia of the heel, sole, and plantar aspect of toes.
- Sural nerve
  - Locate the space between the Achilles tendon and the lateral malleolus.
  - Anesthetize the skin.
  - Use a 25G, 3-cm needle.
  - Insert lateral to the tendon and direct toward the lateral malleolus.
  - Inject 5 ml to 10 ml of local anesthetic subcutaneously as you move the needle toward the malleolus.

Complications

- Paresthesias
- Requires a few injections to block the ankle

INTRAVENOUS REGIONAL ANESTHESIA OF THE LOWER EXTREMITY

Clinical Applications

- Foot, ankle, and knee surgery lasting up to one hour
- Treatment for complex regional pain syndrome
- Knee arthroscopy

Technique

- Obtain venous access on the dorsum of the foot or in the saphenous vein.
- Place a pneumatic double-cuffed tourniquet around the thigh, padding the thigh underneath the cuff.
- Elevate the limb for several minutes, then exsanguinate with an Esmarch bandage.
- Inflate the proximal tourniquet to 100 mmHg above the limb occlusion pressure. This is a minimum of 300 mmHg.
- Inject lidocaine 0.25% to a maximum of 3 mg/kg slowly.
  - Can use 40 ml of lidocaine 0.5% for knee arthroscopy
- Place a single cuff around the calf.
- Re-exsanguinate the foot before inflation of the calf tourniquet.
  - Allows for anesthesia to be concentrated around the knee
- Recommended inflation time is 20 min to 90 min.
- At the end of surgery, deflate the calf cuff first, then deflate the proximal cuff.
  - Allows for residual lidocaine to enter the foot

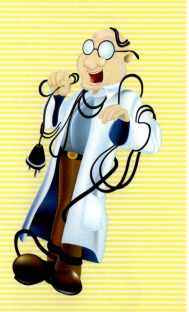

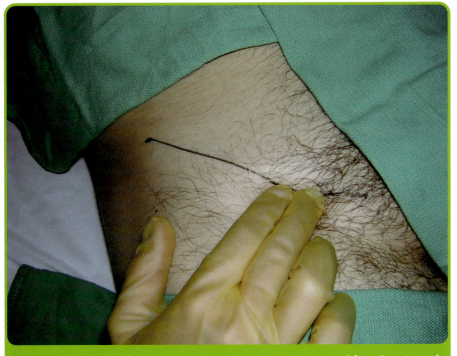

Figure 1. Palpate the femoral artery, an ever-present anatomical friend in time of topographical need.

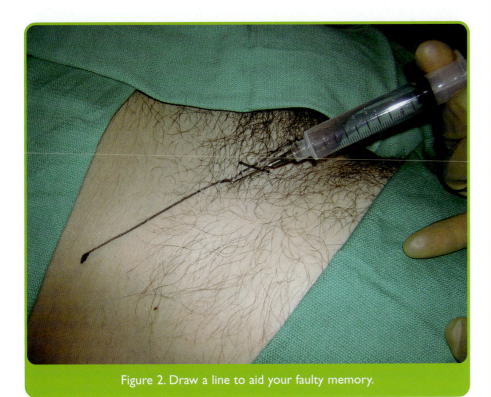

Figure 2. Draw a line to aid your faulty memory.

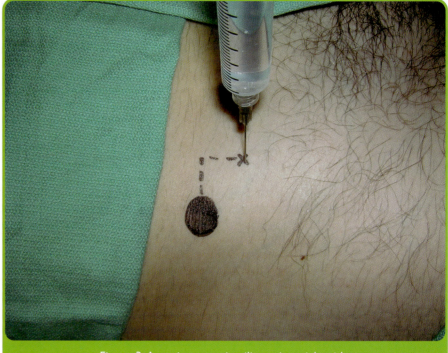

Figure 3. Anterior superior iliac spine, right side

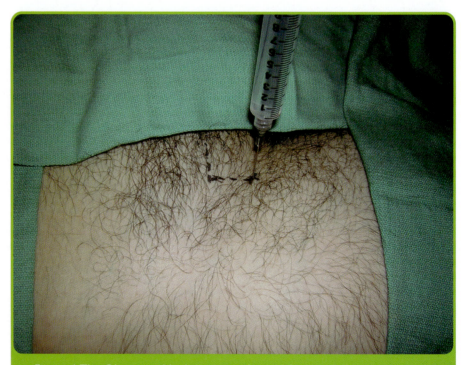

Figure 4. The Obturator block is not performed frequently. It is a technically difficult block and is very uncomfortable for the patient to suffer through.

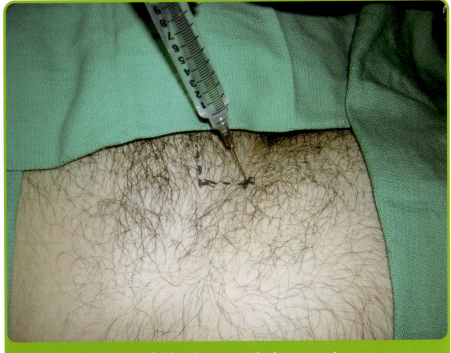

Figure 5. More lines to guide the wayward.

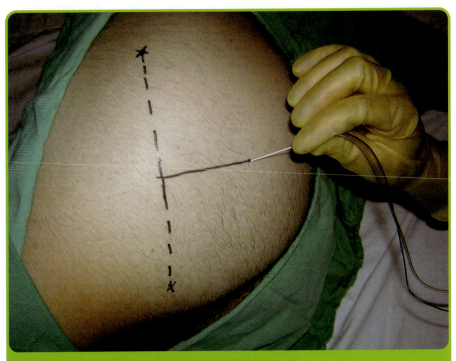

Figure 6. Greater trochanter (upper star), sciatic nerve (center line), posterior superior iliac spine (PSIS, lower star).

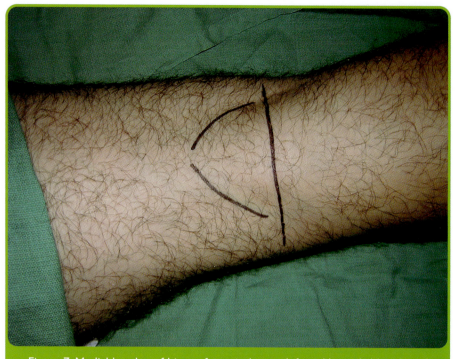

Figure 7. Medial border of biceps femoris (upper, left arch), medial border of semitendonosis (lower, left arch), and flexion crease of knee (vertical line).

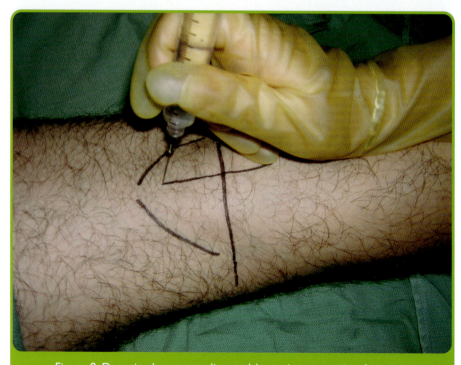

Figure 8. Draw in that center line and *boom*, instant regional expert.

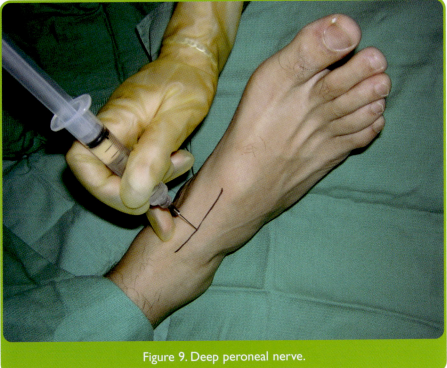

Figure 9. Deep peroneal nerve.

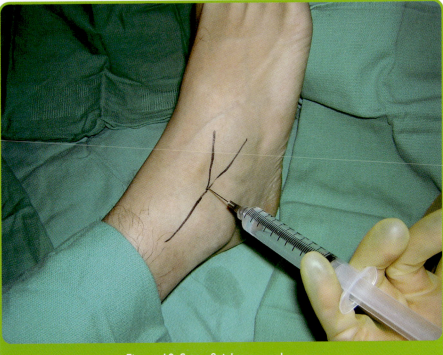

Figure 10. Superficial peroneal nerve.

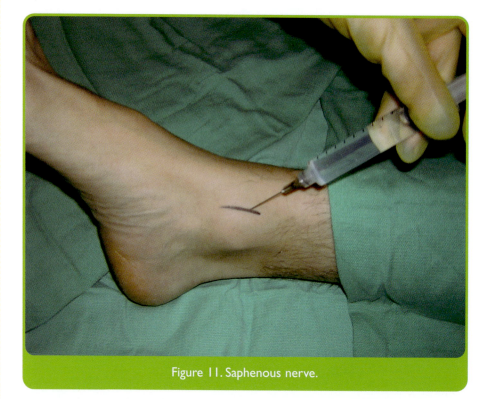

Figure 11. Saphenous nerve.

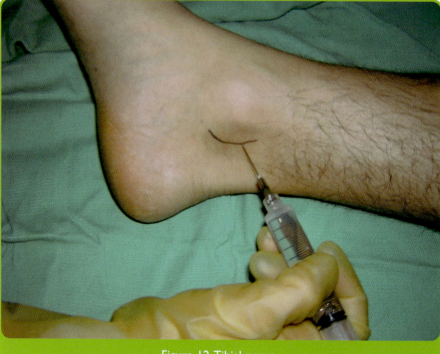

Figure 12. Tibial nerve.

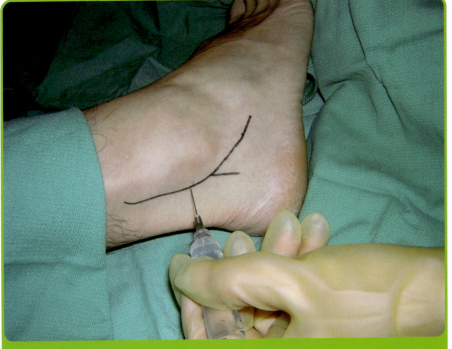

Figure 13. Sural nerve.

SUGGESTED READING

Chang PC, Lang SA, Yip RW. Reevaluation of the sciatic nerve block. Regional Anesth 1993;18:18–23.
- *Worth reading.*

Enneking FK, Chan V, Greger J, et al. Lower-extremity peripheral nerve blockade: Essentials of our current understanding. Regional Anesth Pain Manag 2005;30:4–35.
- *Great review and great pictures!*

Hadzic A, Volka JD, Kuroda MM, et al. The practice of peripheral nerve blocks in the United States: A national survey. Regional Anesth Pain Med 1998;23:241–6.
- *Anything with Dr. Birnbach's name on it must be great.*

Lang SA, Yip RW, Chang P, Gerard M. The femoral 3-in-1 block revisited. J Clin Anesth 1993;5:292–6.
- *This article is a good review of the 3-in-1 block.*

Miller R. *Miller's Anesthesia*, 6th edition. Philadelphia: Churchill Livingstone, 2005:1695–1704.
- *This is the bible of anesthesia.*

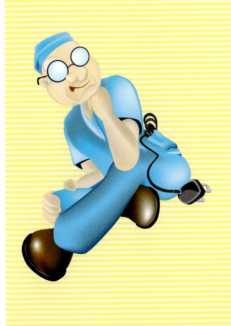

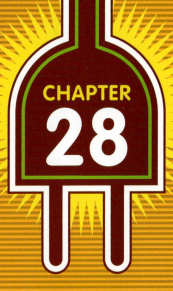

A Sympathetic Ear and a Sympathetic Block

Emilio Alarcon and David Lindley

The social smile, the sympathetic ear.

Thomas Grey
The Alliance of Education and Government, 1748

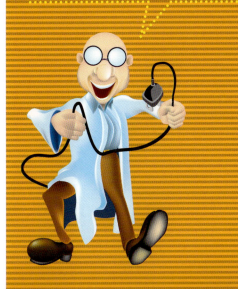

INTRODUCTION

And to accompany that sympathetic ear, now the sympathetic block. These blocks are the mainstay of pain therapy, plus they can help in cases of vascular mishaps. For example, a stellate ganglion block may help restore blood flow to an ischemic hand. Here are the major sympathetic blocks:

- Sympathetic blocks
  - Stellate ganglion
  - Celiac plexus
  - Superior hypogastric plexus
  - Ganglion impar
  - Lumbar sympathetic ganglia
- Transforaminal nerve block
- Medial branch nerve block
- Lumbar epidural steroid injection
- Sacroiliac joint lateral branch nerve block

STELLATE GANGLION BLOCK (OR INFERIOR CERVICAL SYMPATHETIC BLOCK, OR CERVICOTHORACIC GANGLION BLOCK)

Indications

Pain Syndromes

- Sympathetically mediated pain (Complex Regional Pain Syndrome Type I and II)
- Intractable angina
- Herpes zoster
- Phantom limb pain
- Neoplasm
- Postradiation neuritis
- Paget's disease
- Vascular headaches

Vasculopathies of the Head, Neck, or Upper Extremities

- Raynaud's Syndrome
- Scleroderma
- CREST syndrome
- Frostbite
- Obliterative vascular disease
- Occlusive vascular disease
- Embolic vascular disease
- Vasospasm
- Trauma
- Revascularization (i.e., s/p vascular reconstruction or limb reimplantation)

Other Cool Things You Might Do a Block For

- Hyperhidrosis

Complications

The complications of stellate ganglion blocks are related to proximal structures (see picture). Complications include those caused by a needle and those caused by the local anesthetic injection. Those caused by the needle include vascular injury resulting in hemothorax, hematoma, and internal jugular vein or carotid artery trauma. Neural injury may occur to Cranial Nerve X or the brachial plexus roots, all of which are in the proximity of the block. In addition to hemothorax as listed, damage to the lung or thoracic duct may cause hemothorax or chylothorax, respectively. Needle trauma to the esophagus may result in perforation of this structure. Finally, insertion of the needle through the skin and into the soft tissues, neuraxial regions, or bone may result in abscess, meningitis, or osteitis/osteomyelitis, respectively.

Those complications caused by local anesthetic injection include intravascular injection and subsequent seizure or cardiac arrest. Accidental epidural or intrathecal injection may result in a high neuraxial block requiring endotracheal intubation. Intraneural injection of the brachial plexus or Cranial Nerve X will result in damage to these nerves. Local anesthetic spread to the recurrent laryngeal nerve may result in aspiration or hoarseness and spread to the phrenic nerve, which may result in ipsilateral elevated hemidiaphragm and possible respiratory distress.

In lieu of the above possible complications, this block should only be performed in an area with proper resuscitative equipment and practitioners skilled in resuscitative maneuvers.

Signs of a Successful Block

Pain relief may be expected for the duration of action of the local anesthetic; however, relief in excess of the duration of action of the local anesthetic often occurs.

A successful block will also exhibit the following signs with an onset of about

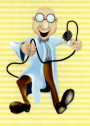

10 minutes and a duration of about 4 hours to 12 hours: nasal stuffiness, warmth and redness of the arm and face with a temperature increase of greater than two degrees Celsius in these areas, hoarseness of the voice, enophthalmos, injected conjunctiva, ptosis, miosis, and dysphagia.

Landmarks

- Cricoid cartilage (used to identify the level of C6)
- Chassaignac's tubercle (anterior tubercle of the transverse process of C6; may be palpated 3 cm cephalad to the sternoclavicular joint at the medial border of the sternocleidomastoid muscle, approximately 2 cm later to the lateral edge of the cricoid cartilage)
- C7 is located approximately 2 cm distal to Chassaignac's tubercle

Procedure

The sympathetic fibers from the T1 to T8 spinal cord segments ascend to pass through three cervical sympathetic ganglia: superior, middle, and inferior. Most fibers pass through a fusion of two ganglia known as the stellate ganglion. In up to 8% of patients, the inferior cervical ganglion and the first thoracic sympathetic ganglion fuse to form the stellate ganglion. However, in approximately 20% of patients, the first thoracic sympathetic ganglion may itself form the stellate ganglion.

The procedure may be performed at C6 or C7. Traditionally, it is performed at C6, which has the advantages of Chassaignac's tubercle for assistance in palpatory landmarks and is in less proximity to the cupula of the lung and to the vertebral artery. The disadvantages of the C6 target include a further distance from the usual position of the stellate ganglion at C7, although the anatomy tends to vary greatly. Performing the procedure at C7 has the advantage of being closer to the usual location of the stellate ganglion and the disadvantages of being closer to the cupula of the lung and to the vertebral artery.

Position the patient supine and prep the neck. Identify the target using landmarks and fluoroscopic guidance (see pictures). Inject subcutaneous local anesthetic. Using fluoroscopic guidance, insert a 25G needle down onto the anterior tubercle of the tranverse process of C6 or C7. Confirm the negative aspiration of blood. Inject a radiographic contrast medium such as iohexol to confirm the proper location (see picture). Inject a local anesthetic solution and remove the needle. Observe the

patient for signs of a successful block and for complications as listed above.

Equipment

- 5 ml to 20 ml of dilute local anesthetic solutions (i.e., lidocaine 0.5% or bupivacaine 0.25%) may be used. Larger volumes are recommended when upper extremity sympathectomy is the goal. Obviously, larger volumes result in higher incidence of certain local anesthetic complications.
- 22G, 5-cm needle
- Syringes
- Prep solution

CELIAC PLEXUS BLOCK

The celiac plexus is the largest plexus of the sympathetic nervous system. The celiac plexus receives fibers from the greater, lesser, and least splanchnic nerves (visceral afferent and efferent fibers from T5 to T12 paravertebral sympathetic ganglia) and, to a lesser extent, vagal nerve fibers. Although the celiac plexus is most commonly located anterior to the L1 vertebral body, this actually varies from T12 to L2. The celiac plexus is a paired structure with many interconnecting fibers between the left and right sides. These fibers surround the celiac artery; therefore, many consider the celiac artery the best landmark for celiac plexus block.

Percutaneous Methods to Block T5 to T12 Paravertebral Sympathetic Ganglia

- Splanchnic nerve block, retrocrural (posterior) approach
- Celiac plexus block
  - Posterior retrocrural approach, inject at posterolateral aspect of body of L1
  - Posterior anterocrural approaches
  - Transcrural (antecrural) approach
    - Transaortic approach
    - Anterior approach
  - Note: Retrocrural splanchnic nerve block and retrocrural celiac plexus blocks rely on the spread of injectate to respective fibers.
  - Note: Anterior approaches have less neurologic and psoas compartment complications and allow supine positioning, which is better tolerated for some patients. Disadvantages of anterior approaches include the risk of stomach, intestine, liver, or pancreas puncture.

- Guidance may be fluoroscopic, ultrasound, or CT. CT guidance is optimal for avoiding organ puncture and documenting contrast spread.
- Bilateral approaches versus unilateral (single-needle) approaches: Single-needle approaches rely on the bilateral spread of injectate. Bilateral injectate spread above and below the celiac artery is necessary to achieve a reliable, long-lasting effect.

Indications

- Postoperative biliary procedure pain
- Benign chronic abdominal processes
- Primary or metastatic cancer of the upper abdominal viscera
- Pancreatitis and other upper abdominal visceral pain syndromes

Complications

- Neurologic complications arising from inhibition of compensatory vascular reflexes leading to orthostatic hypotension (posterior approaches)
- Psoas compartment complications (posterior approaches)
- Renal puncture (posterior approaches)
- Complications arising from intolerance of prone positioning (posterior approaches)
- Retroperitoneal hematoma (posterior approaches)
- Aortic injury (left posterior approach)
- Stomach, intestine, liver, or pancreas puncture (anterior approaches)
- Diarrhea due to sympathetic block of the bowel (anterior approaches)
- Failure of block effect (especially if adequate bilateral and longitudinal spread is not achieved)
- Paraplegia from injury to lumbar plexus or spasm of lumbar segmental arteries supplying the spinal cord (rare)

Procedure

As discussed above, CT guidance is usually the safest method to perform a celiac plexus blockade. Below, a patient is diagrammed for a posterior (retrocrural) celiac plexus block.

The insertion site is identified 5 cm to 7 cm lateral to the L1 vertebrae. The needle is inserted at approximately a 45° angle to the skin and advanced with intermittent CT confirmation of its proper course. The technique is to contact the anterolateral aspect of the body of L1 and subsequently "walk" the needle off the anterior edge. Care must be taken to avoid the aorta

when approaching from the left and the kidneys when approaching from either side. Approximately 20 ml may be injected on each side. If performing a neurolytic block with alcohol, it is prudent to first inject 10 ml of local anesthetic solution to avoid the severe burning pain experienced with alcohol injection. Phenol may be used without prior local anesthetic injection.

LUMBAR SYMPATHETIC GANGLION BLOCK

GANGLION IMPAR BLOCK (OR GANGLION OF WALTHER BLOCK, OR SACROCOCCYGEAL GANGLION BLOCK)

The paired paravertebral sympathetic chains typically end in a fused, single, midline, retroperitoneal ganglion located just anterior to the sacrococcygeal junction. This structure is referred to as the ganglion impar, as impar means "unpaired."

Indications

- Sympathetically mediated perineal pain
- Visceral pelvic pain
- Rectal pain s/p abdominoperineal resection
- Hyperhidrosis of buttocks and perineum
- Radiation proctitis

Complications

- Rectal tear, infection, bleeding

Signs of a Successful Block

Procedure

The ganglion impar block may be performed in the lateral recumbent position or the prone position. In the lateral decubitus position, the hips are slightly flexed. In the prone position, pillows are placed under the hips. Needle insertion may be through the anococcygeal ligament or through the sacrococcygeal ligament. This author prefers needle insertion through the sacrococcygeal ligament because the ganglion impar lies directly below the sacrococcygeal junction, a loss of resistance technique may be employed, and it may carry a lower risk of rectal penetration and therefore infection.

Position the patient prone with two pillows under the hips. Prepare the sacral and coccygeal area. Identify the sacrococcygeal junction via palpation and fluoroscopy. A rectal exam under fluoroscopy may be performed to identify this junction and

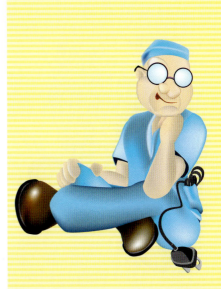

confirm location of the sacrococcygeal ligament. Inject a subcutaneous local anesthetic. Using fluoroscopic guidance and loss-of-resistance technique, insert a 25G needle through the sacrococcygeal ligament. Confirm the negative aspiration of blood. Inject a radiographic contrast medium such as iohexol to confirm proper location (see picture). Inject 4 ml to 10 ml of local anesthetic solution and remove the needle. Observe the patient for signs of a successful block and for complications as listed above.

INVASIVE PROCEDURES FOR CANCER PAIN

Between 70% and 90% of all cancer pain can be controlled with oral medication but for those patients with unrelieved pain, invasive procedures have an important role. Recent surveys show that (a) cancer pain is both underdiagnosed and underrated, and (b) physicians unfamiliar with current pain treatment modalities are more likely to support assisted suicide for their patients. Appropriate use of invasive measures in the 10% to 30% of patients—most often, those with advanced disease—who fail oral therapy can relieve nearly all cancer pain.

It is important to emphasize that regional techniques such as nerve blocks for cancer pain management are intended to be analgesic "adjuvants" and not definitive treatment. These procedures should allow patients to lower drug dosages and thereby reduce side effects, or to experience better pain relief from current dosages to improve their quality of life. Neither the primary physician nor the pain specialist should promise permanent relief because the patient's disease may progress and spread. Twycross reported that most patients referred for cancer-related symptom management have at least two anatomically distinct pain sites, and more than 40% have four or more sites. It is unreasonable to expect one regional block to eliminate pain from multiple sites. On the contrary, medical care of the suffering pain patient requires a multimodal, multispecialty approach combining psychotherapy, social support, and pain management to provide the best possible quality of life or quality of dying.

Application of Invasive Measures to the 10% to 30% of Patients Who Fail Oral Therapy Can Relieve Nearly All Cancer Pain

Invasive techniques for managing cancer pain often employ neurolytic substances

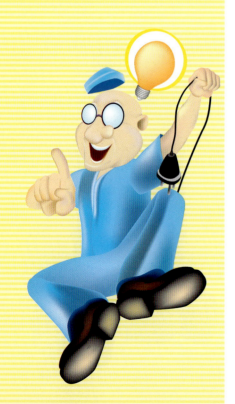

like ethanol or phenol. A thorough knowledge of relevant anatomy and the mechanism of action by which the agent destroys neural tissue are essential to minimize irreversible complications. Several points must be addressed before one proceeds with a neurolytic block. Only physicians with extensive experience and skill should perform these blocks. As stated above, nerve blocks should be regarded as part of a multimodal approach to pain and not as a stand-alone pain "cure." Patients should be thoroughly informed about likely sensory deficits and possible complications. In most cases, neurolytic blocks should first be simulated with local anesthetic to allow the patient to experience the sensory changes that may occur. The patient should be followed for several days after the diagnostic block. Finally, close monitoring and planned opioid reduction should follow a successful neurolytic block to prepare for somnolence and respiratory depression when the respiratory stimulation of pain is removed.

Neurolytic Agents

Ethanol (Alcohol)

Ethanol has been used extensively for neurolytic procedures in concentrations from 3% to 100%. It acts by destroying nerves and producing Wallerian degeneration without disruption of the Schwann cell sheath. Thus, axonal regeneration can and will occur, sometimes resulting in neuroma formation. However, if cell body destruction occurs, regeneration is not possible. Recent studies have shown that ethanol destroys nervous tissue by extraction of cholesterol and other lipids and by protein precipitation. Topical application of alcohol to exposed nerves results in both axon and Schwann cell destruction.

Studies in the early part of this century demonstrated that an approximately 50% alcohol solution is required for analgesia when performing major nerve blocks. Labat showed that 33% alcohol can produce analgesia without motor paralysis when applied to peripheral nerves. When alcohol is applied to autonomic nerves and ganglia, all effector organ input is blocked. Permanent blocks occur when postsynaptic nerves in the ganglia are affected. A blockade limited to the rami or preganglionic fibers produces only temporary analgesia followed by the return of sensation in three to six months. Subarachnoid injection of 100% alcohol produces damage to the dorsal roots, Lissauer's tract, and posterior columns. Wallerian degeneration follows nerve destruction. Almost 90% of injected alcohol is removed by the cerebrospinal fluid (CSF) within 10 minutes after subarachnoid injection.

Clinically, alcohol in a concentration of 33% to 100% is hypobaric (specific gravity, s.g. = 0.8) relative to CSF (s.g. = 1.1), so target sites in the spinal cord should be above the site of injection to allow the alcohol to float upward. The effective duration of intrathecal alcohol analgesia is about six months. Complete, prolonged analgesia can be achieved if cell bodies are destroyed along with axons in peripheral and autonomic nervous tissue. High concentrations of alcohol (90% to 100%) sometimes produce a chemical neuritis under clinical conditions, probably owing to residual partial neural destruction of some tissues. Injection of alcohol into peripheral nerves or ganglia not surrounded by fluid requires no special positioning.

Phenol

Studies by Mandl in 1950 reported that 6% phenol applied to cervical ganglia in animals produced local necrosis in 24 hours, complete degeneration by 45 days, and regeneration in 75 days. Thus, sensory recovery after phenol is faster than after alcohol. Like alcohol, phenol has been administered for subarachnoid, peripheral nerve, and ganglion neurolysis.

In the subarachnoid space, phenol is hyperbaric with respect to CSF. The target site should be below the site of injection to allow the phenol to migrate downward. Concentrations of 5% to 10% produce nonspecific neural destruction similar to alcohol. Some studies suggest that larger-diameter fibers are damaged to a greater extent than smaller diameter fibers. Extensive fibrosis and thickening of the arachnoid can also occur. Phenol destroys axons along the dorsal roots and posterior columns without disrupting cell bodies.

When 3% to 6% phenol is applied to peripheral nerves, both acute and chronic damage to axons and myelin occurs. In addition, protein coagulation and necrosis ultimately result in axonal and Wallerian degeneration. Phenol is injected in a range of concentrations from 3% to 15%. Suggestions that phenol may be more destructive to vascular than neural tissue have not been borne out clinically. Lema et al. reported that autopsy samples of patients who had received 3.4 g of phenol interpleurally showed little evidence of vascular, organ, or even neural histological destruction.

Invasive Techniques

To be considered invasive, a procedure must violate the integument of the body; thus, all needle and scalpel procedures are invasive. Moreover, patient-controlled analgesia using intravenous, subcutaneous, or epidural sites may be considered invasive in this sense. Invasive procedures can be categorized according to three general targets: autonomic nervous system, peripheral nerve, and neuraxis.

Autonomic Nervous System Blocks

The autonomic nervous system is largely responsible for visceral nociception. A diagnostic local anesthetic block of a sympathetic nerve or plexus establishes the relative contribution of autonomic and visceral pain and can simulate the effect of a neurolytic nerve block.

Stellate Ganglion Block

The stellate ganglion lies anterior to the lateral process of the C7 vertebra. Autonomic pathways to the ipsilateral head and upper extremity are interrupted by a block of this ganglion. Because of the proximity of other vital structures, many clinicians are reluctant to perform neurolytic blocks in this area. However, serial blocks with neurolytic agents in dilute concentrations (3% to 6% phenol) after encouraging a diagnostic local anesthetic block have been recommended. Potential complications include injection into the vertebral artery, phrenic and superior laryngeal nerve blocks, and—rarely—intrathecal injection.

Celiac Plexus Block

The celiac plexus lies on the anterolateral surface of the aorta at the T12 to L2 vertebral level. Blockade of this plexus reduces visceral pain from abdominal organs and has gained widespread acceptance for the treatment of pancreatic cancer pain. The incidence of pain relief has been reported to be more than 84% or patients, although occasionally repeat blocks are required. Possible complications include transient hypotension; intrathecal, epidural, or intrapsoas injection; injection into the aorta or vena cava, puncture of the kidney, intestine, or lung; anterior spinal artery syndrome; paraplegia; and death.

Hypogastric Plexus Block

The hypogastric plexus lies anterior to the L5 to S1 vertebrae and controls autonomic activity to the pelvis and lower limbs. A block of these nerves has been described to reduce pain associated with pelvic malignancy. Injury to sacral nerves, bladder or bowel perforation, intravascular injection, and urinary or fecal incontinence are potential complications.

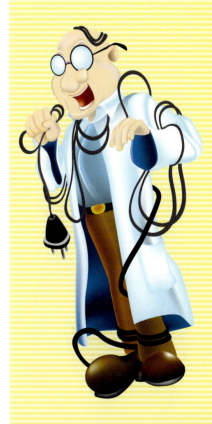

Ganglion Impar Block

Intractable perineal pain presents problems to the pain practitioner because somatic, visceral, and autonomic nerves controlling excretory and sexual functions converge in the pelvis. Blockade of the ganglion impar (also called the ganglion of Walther or sacrococcygeal ganglion) provides pain relief without significant somatovisceral dysfunction for many patients with advanced cancer. The only unpaired autonomic ganglion, the ganglion impar lies anterior to the sacrococcygeal junction and can be blocked with 5 cc to 10 cc of solution administered through a needle penetrating the anococcygeal ligament or directly passing through the sacrococcygeal (calcified) ligament. Patients experiencing significant rectal discomfort or pain after abdominoperineal resection of rectal cancer often benefit from this technique.

Interpleural Analgesia

Interpleural analgesia has been successfully used for minor surgical anesthesia and in the management of certain chronic pain states such as pancreatic pain and post-thoracotomy pain syndrome. It has also been used to alleviate acute exacerbations of pain in advanced stages of various cancers.

The mechanism of action of interpleural analgesia appears to be a somatic nerve block, but an autonomic block has also been suggested. Diffusion of local anesthetic into the brachial plexus and cervical sympathetic ganglion can relieve upper extremity pain while also producing a Horner's syndrome. The success of this block depends on the correct positioning of the patient such that the solution gravitates to the appropriate paravertebral area. Possible complications include tension pneumothorax, pleural infection, and local anesthetic systemic toxicity from rapid tissue absorption. Interpleural administration of phenol has also been successful in the long-term relief of cancer pain.

Peripheral Nerve Blocks

Neurolytic blockade of peripheral nerves can be effective as an analgesic adjuvant to oral therapy, but the long-term benefits of this approach are controversial. One concern is the transient nature of the neurolysis and possible neuritis or deafferentation pain experienced as the block "wears off." This problem is generally avoided by selecting patients likely to succumb before development of the neuropathic pain (i.e., within four to six months).

Intraspinal Therapies

Intraspinal administration of opioids is frequently used to treat pain not controlled with oral medications. Opioids can be delivered by the spinal or epidural routes to provide analgesia, generally at a lower dose than for systemic administration and without the motor, sensory, or sympathetic block associated with intraspinal local anesthetic administration.

Combinations of opioids plus local anesthetics given spinally produce effective analgesia with relatively few side effects. Spinal opioids can be delivered by intermittent bolus injection or by continuous infusion. Morphine is most commonly given, although hydromorphone, fentanyl, sufentanil, and oxymorphone have also been successfully used. Opioids in combination with clonidine are often effective in patients with advanced disease. However, sedation and hypotension associated with clonidine can limit titration.

Three systems used for chronic intraspinal opioid administration include percutaneous tunneled epidural or spinal catheters, tunneled catheters connected to subcutaneously implanted injection ports, and implanted infusion pump systems. Implantable pumps are more convenient to manage and less likely to become infected, and become cost-effective when life expectancy exceeds six months. Tolerance to chronic intraspinal administration of opioids is managed by increasing doses, changing to another opioid, or substituting local anesthetic for a short period. Other opioid side effects include pruritus, urinary retention, somnolence, myoclonus, catheter infection, and—rarely—respiratory depression.

Neurosurgical Procedures

With the development of the multidisciplinary approach to pain management and an ever-growing range of available pharmacologic agents, few patients require surgical intervention to interrupt central or peripheral nociceptive pathways.

The most commonly performed surgical procedure for cancer pain relief is anterolateral cordotomy, which ablates the spinothalamic tract. This procedure can be done by an open technique, which has significant morbidity; potential complications include hemiparesis, urinary retention, and sexual impotence. Percutaneous cordotomy has largely replaced the open method and is usually performed under local

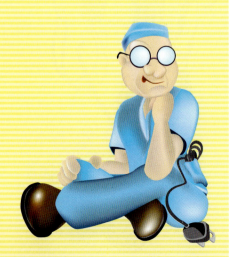

anesthesia by advancing a thermal coagulation probe with fluoroscopic guidance. It is usually ineffective in neuropathic pain because it does not reverse central sensitization, and has only limited use in visceral pain. Immediate pain relief is achieved in the majority of patients, but pain recurs in roughly half of these by six to twelve months. Many patients in whom pain recurs also develop paresthesias or dysesthesias.

Placement of an Omaya reservoir under the scalp, connected to a catheter whose tip lies within the lateral cerebral ventricle, may provide satisfactory analgesia with relatively few side effects. Other less often used procedures include rhizotomy, dorsal root entry zone (DREZ) lesioning, commissurotomy, and dorsal root ganglionectomy.

CONCLUSION

For a minority of patients with pain due to cancer, oral drug therapy titrated according to the World Health Organization analgesic ladder fails to control pain adequately. In these patients—who often have an advanced stage of disease—more aggressive intervention is required. In a field replete with clinical anecdotes and uncontrolled case series, there is an urgent need for clinical trials and outcomes assessment to generate firm evidence on the risks, benefits, costs, and failures of such intervention. However, few would question that aggressive intervention is often appropriate. Invasive pain therapies must be provided with skill and caution, and are best offered within a multidisciplinary framework of care.

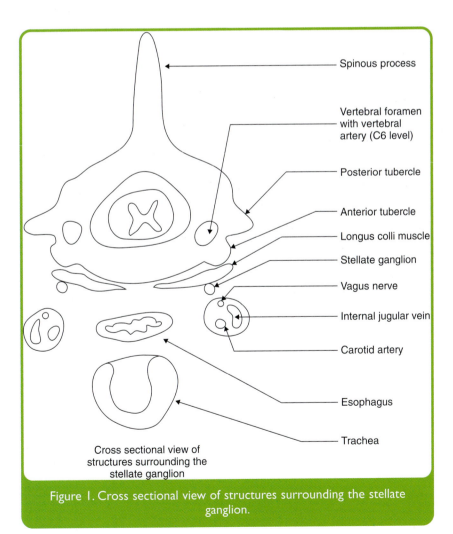

Cross sectional view of structures surrounding the stellate ganglion

Figure 1. Cross sectional view of structures surrounding the stellate ganglion.

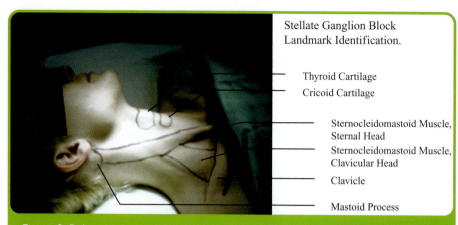

Stellate Ganglion Block
Landmark Identification.

— Thyroid Cartilage
— Cricoid Cartilage

— Sternocleidomastoid Muscle,
Sternal Head
— Sternocleidomastoid Muscle,
Clavicular Head

— Clavicle

— Mastoid Process

Figure 2. Believe it or not, these are not marks, these are actually tattoos placed during a drunken weekend spree after a regional anesthesia workshop.

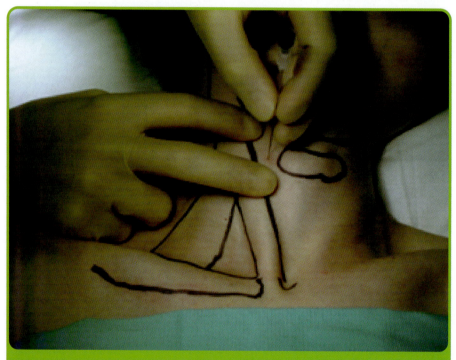

Figure 3. Stellate ganglion block with needle insertion at C6. The sternocleidomastoid muscle is retracted laterally. Needle insertion is approximately 2 cm lateral to the lateral border of the cricoid cartilage. Fluoroscopic needle guidance to the anterior tubercle is additionally recommended.

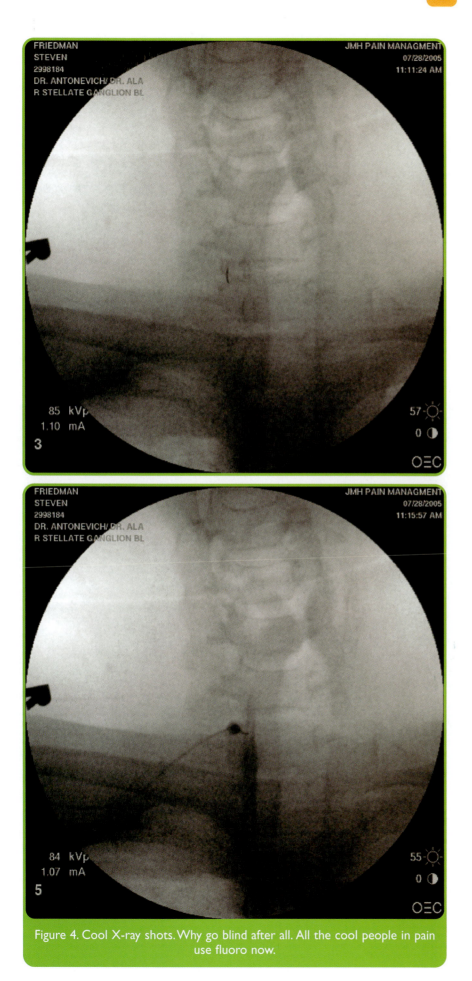

Figure 4. Cool X-ray shots. Why go blind after all. All the cool people in pain use fluoro now.

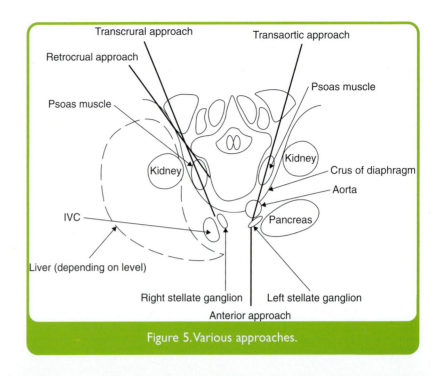

Figure 5. Various approaches.

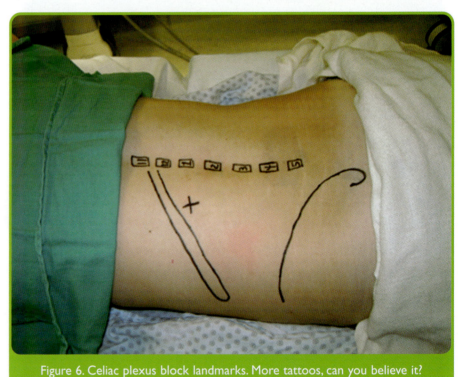

Figure 6. Celiac plexus block landmarks. More tattoos, can you believe it?

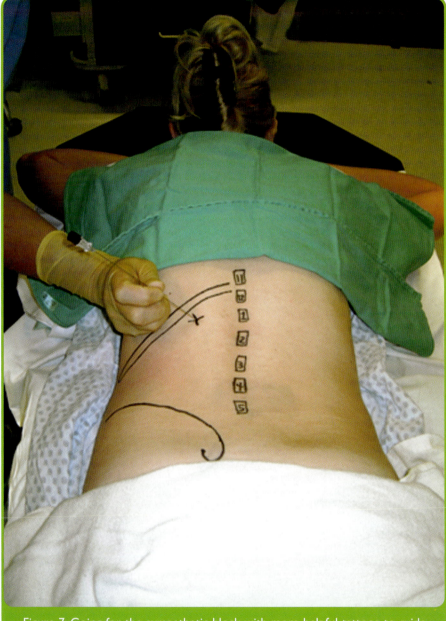

Figure 7. Going for the sympathetic block with more helpful tattoos to guide the way.

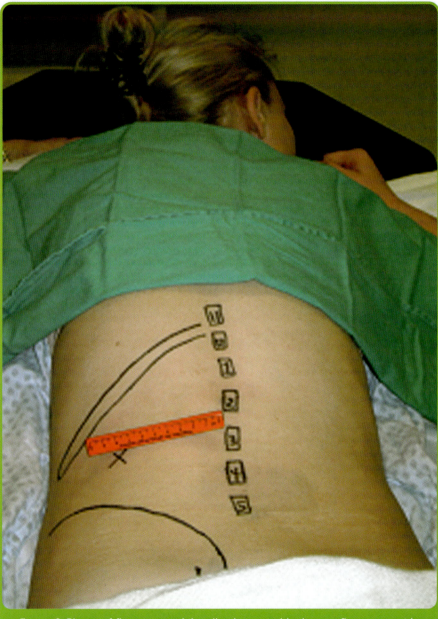

Figure 8. Photo of fluoroscopy. Like all other pain blocks, use fluoro to guide the way.

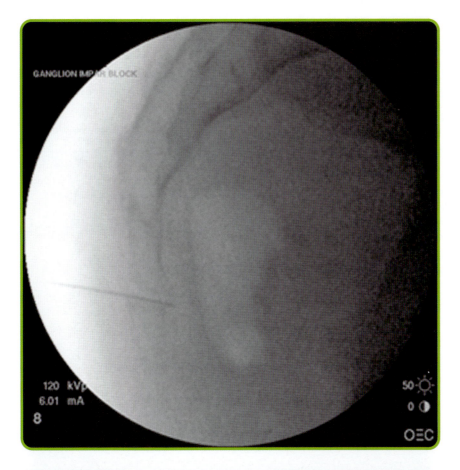

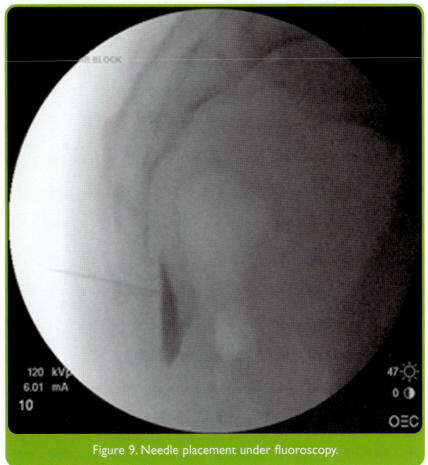

Figure 9. Needle placement under fluoroscopy.

SUGGESTED READING

Benzon, Raja, Molloy, Liu, Fishman. *Essentials of Pain Medicine and Regional Anesthesia*, 2nd edition. Philadelphia: Elsevier Churchill, Livingstone, 2005.

Brown DL, Bulley CK, Quiel EL, et al. Anesth Analg 1987;66: 869–73.

Cleeland CR, Gonin R, Hatfield AK, et al. N Eng J Med 1994; 330:552–96.

Cousins MJ, Bridenbaugh PO. *Neural Blockade in Clinical Anesthesia and Management*, 3rd edition. New York: Lippincott-Raven, 1998.

Eisenberg F, Carr DB, Chalmers TC, et al. Anesth Analg 1995;80:290.

Lema MJ, Myers DP, De Leon-Cassasolo OA, et al. Regional Anesth 1992;17: 166–70.

Plancarte R, De Leon-Cassasolo OA, El-Helaly M, et al. Regional Anesth 1997;22:562–8.

Plummer JL, Cherry DA, Cousins MJ, et al. Pain 1991;44:215–20.

Saberski L, Ligham D. Neuroablative techniques for cancer pain management. Tech Regional Anesth Pain Manage 1997;1(1):53–8.

Zech DFJ, Grond S, Lynch J, et al. Pain 1995;63:65–76.

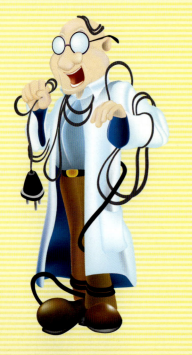

Ophthalmic Anesthesia: More than Meets the Eye

Steven Gayer

INTRODUCTION

Ophthalmic anesthesia is mostly eye block + monitored anesthesia care (MAC). MAC is important because angina, arrhythmias, hypertension, apnea, hypoxia, hypercarbia, confusion, seizures, and more can occur. Personnel with airway and resuscitation skills must be immediately available.

Most anesthesiologists skip the block and default to the ophthalmologist, claiming anesthetizing eyes is too risky. When was the last time you went to do an urgent C-section and told the obstetrician, "This patient's too risky, can you do the block?"

Real anesthesiologists know how to block eyes.

PHILOSOPHY

- Surgeons do retrobulbar blocks (RBB) because that's what they were taught way back when in residency and the onset of anesthesia is almost immediate.
- Anesthesiologists perform peribulbar blocks (PBB) because they are generally safer because Brainstem anesthesia is much less likely, the odds of skewering the back of the eye are far less, and damage to other key orbital structures is rare.
- The fact that more volume and time are needed is immaterial to the anesthesiologist who blocks patients awaiting surgery ahead of time in a holding area.

INDICATIONS

- Ophthalmologist's needs for an akinetic, anesthetized eye: corneal transplant, retina surgery, glaucoma surgery, enucleation, any procedure of long duration
- Patient's need or desire for an akinetic, anesthetized eye: hypernervousness, painful eye, and so on
- Anesthesiologist's need for a good day in the OR in the face of 10 to 20 eye surgery patients or a patient with a difficult airway, crippled ventilatory status, or feeble cardiovascular function that would otherwise need an awake intubation or postoperative ventilation or an ICU bed after general anesthesia

CONTRAINDICATIONS

- Most are relative contraindications
- Severe bleeding diathesis, real bad infection, marked bony orbit deformation, actual honest-truth allergy to local anesthetics

- If a patient will not be able to lie relatively still during surgery, the best option is to use general anesthesia or postpone elective surgery until such time that the patient can repose tranquilly and be done via regional anesthesia and MAC.

BEWARE (NOT OF THE FLOOR BUT OF THE PATIENT)

- Patients with longer-than-normal or deeply recessed eyes are at greater risk of having their globes skewered by a needle. Some patients have abnormal outpouched areas in the side or back of the eye.
- Recessed eyes are noted by looking at the patient (interesting notion). Nearsighted people and those that had prior scleral buckle surgery have longer eyes. Eye length and shape are determined by ultrasound.

THE *MOST IMPORTANT* PREOPERATIVE TEST OF EYE PATIENTS

- U/A? No.
- CBC? No.
- EKG? No.
- Ultrasound of the eye? Bingo!

An ultrasound is a prerequisite for the ophthalmologist to determine the appropriate lens implant to insert and is done on every patient scheduled for *cataract* surgery. Due to the outpatient nature of cataract surgery, this information is rarely placed on patients' surgical charts. Be aware: it exists. If one intends to perform an eye block, ask the ophthalmologist for the ultrasound data. Confirm that the eye length is normal (less than 26 mm) and

Why settle for a Big MAC when you can do the Combo?

Anonymous Anesthesiology Resident

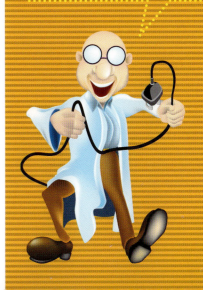

Value-Added Anesthesiologist

Most anesthesiologists work in group practices. If you can do something no one else can do, you become a "value-added member."

When you volunteer to block that 400-lb Pickwickian open-globe-eye-injury patient with a nightmarish airway and angina, your group will love you. Ask for a raise or early partnership.

Brain Stew

On the other hand, Green Day described what it is like to experience a poor eye block in their song, "Brain Stew:"

My eyes feel like they're gonna bleed

Dried up and bulging out my skull

My mouth is dry

My face is numb

So the adage, "see one, do one, teach one," is inappropriate. Study the technique, read the texts, and watch others block prior to picking up a needle.

that the shape of the eye is normal. Write this down on the chart somewhere. Even if you just scrawl, "US OK per Ophth" or "US wnl," it indicates that you took eye length and shape into account before blocking the eye.

EQUIPMENT

- Patient hooked up to pulse oximeter, rhythm monitor, blood-pressure cuff, and O_2 by nasal cannula
- Clearly marked indicator of side-of-anesthesia and surgery on the patient
- No patient cap. Caps just obscure that clearly marked indicator of side-of-anesthesia and surgery.

  RN or other assistant to confirm patient ID, consent, side-of-anesthesia, and to hold the patient's hand, eyelid open as needed, and so on
- Amp of atropine and syringe nearby, just in case of severe oculocardiac reflex
- Resuscitation stuff nearby as a precaution
- Syringe of local anesthetic. A few units of hyaluronidase is always nice. Some prefer their hyaluronidase derived from sheep testicles rather than the bovine stuff—we don't think it matters. We don't bother adding epi because tachycardia from absorbed epi isn't always a good thing for elderly patients.
- Label on the syringe. We know of one poor soul who accidentally injected a syringe of unlabeled pentothal. Bad day.
- Needle. Long or short? The commonly used 1.5-in. (38-mm) needle can reach the apex of the orbit in one of five patients, so a shorter needle, less than or equal to 1.25 in. (31 mm), is more prudent. Sharp or dull? More difficult to puncture an eye with a dull needle but they cause more damage if the globe is penetrated. Sharp needles are less painful.
- Topical drops. Optional prior to block.
- Antiseptic prep.
- Some gauze to wipe the shmutz away and keep the eye shut if needed.
- An occulo-occlusive device. This is a fancy term for Pinky-Ball to put light pressure on the globe and encourage the local to diffuse posteriorly. We usually just use digital pressure and skip the occulo-occluder

TECHNIQUE

- Confirm you have the correct patient in front of you.
- Check the ultrasound data, if available.
- Make sure that you are about to block the proper side.
- Provide apropos sedation.
- Wipe the lower eyelid with alcohol if that makes you happy.
- Apologize to the patient for making their eye sting from the alcohol wipe.
- Next time, consider giving a few anesthetic drops before searing someone's eye with alcohol.
- Style point: Tetracaine drops sting; proparacaine drops do not. If one is using anesthetic drops to prevent stinging from the prep, use one that doesn't sting!
- Examine the surface anatomy to assess if there is significant recession of the eye (increases the risk of puncture).
- With the patient's eyes in neutral gaze, draw a plumb line down from the lateral border of the pupil to the bony ridge of the orbit. Alternatively, identify the same spot at the junction of the lateral one-third and medial two-thirds of the orbital rim. This is the traditional injection point.
- We are not traditionalists, so we shift our needle entry point further laterally toward the inferotemporal corner of the orbit. The further laterally you move the injection point, the less likely you are to have postoperative strabismus from trauma to the inferior rectus muscle.
- Place a finger on the orbital rim and ballot the globe, creating a space between bone and globe. This is where the needle will go. Remember that the eye's equatorial margin may extend into that space somewhere below your fingertip. Be careful! Don't puncture the eye!
- Orient the needle bevel towards the globe. This maneuver lessens the chance of globe puncture by creating another millimeter or so of distance from the eye.
- Angle the needle essentially parallel with the globe. Enter the orbit close to the rim while pressuring the eye cephalad and away from the oncoming needle. A few things to avoid: The floor of the orbit (pain, bleeding), the eye (duh), the apex of the orbit (nerve and muscle trauma, brainstem anesthesia), and intravascular injection (seizures).
- Fix the needle hub between two fingers while abutting the back of your hand

against the patient's cheek. This provides stability and helps ensure that the needle will not impale the patient's brain should they decide they no longer want to participate in today's activities.

- Look for evidence of blood in the needle hub prior to injecting local anesthetic. Alternatively, consider aspirating the syringe to determine if the needle tip is in a blood vessel.

- Consider wiggling the needle 2 mm to 3 mm in a plane parallel to the eye or ask the patient to gaze left or right to assure that the needle is not in the eye. The only thing worse than puncturing the eye is penetrating the eye and injecting local anesthetic.

- Inject slowly. Watch the eye. Look for the Good, the Bad, & the Ugly:

  - The Good: Observe the lid droop slightly (sign of sympathetic block), the globe shift forward, or the pupil to begin to dilate.

  - The Bad: Arterial hemorrhage. Soft, mushy eye equals a punctured eye. Milky floaters in the pupil mean local anesthetic is precipitating in an eye that has been punctured and injected. This is usually associated with a terrible postoperative visual outcome. A rock-hard eye may have excessive intrinsic or extrinsic pressure on it that may compromise perfusion and jeopardize vision.

  - The Ugly: Local anesthetic can dissect under the conjunctiva. This is self-resolving and usually meaningless. A small bleed may result in a lower lid shiner; this too is self-resolving, although it may take a few weeks. It is usually not otherwise significant.

- Remove the needle, examine the eye for evidence of bleeding, close the lid, and assess globe pressure while gently encouraging backward flow of local anesthetic by intermittent digital pressure.

- Ask the patient to gaze left, right, up, down. Assess that onset of akinesia is occurring. Place a drop of anesthetic or Betadine on the eye to confirm that analgesia is present.

- Betadine must be in place for at least 3 minutes. Many times, it seems as though an OR prep is placed and rinsed off in under 60 seconds; therefore, we are in the habit of dripping or swabbing Betadine on or around the eye after a block and letting it sit until later when it gets rinsed off with the prep in the OR. Note: Patients will not like you if you reverse the order and place the Betadine before the block.

- Proprioception of the eyelid is lost with a good block, so manually close the patient's eye. Tape a gauze pad over the eye to keep the lid shut if it insists on remaining open.

Open Globe Emergencies

Traditionally, regional anesthesia has been considered *verboten* for open-eye injuries due to the concern that pressure from local anesthetic might lead to the extrusion of globe contents. We have found that simpler lesions (small, well-defined, linear, more anterior) and higher-risk-for-anesthesia patients do well with eye blocks and MAC. In our papers, we report no difference in visual outcomes between eyes repaired with regional versus general anesthesia.

So when you are "volunteered" to provide anesthesia for that 400-lb Pickwickian with an impossible airway, angina, *and an open globe injury*, consider an eye block.

Major Bleeding

Bleeding in the orbit can make a patient look like they just went a few rounds in the boxing ring; however, the actual hemorrhage is often of no clinical significance. Very rarely, one can encounter significant arterial-based bleeding. If the globe becomes very tense, immediate assessment is required because permanent blindness can occur from retinal ischemia. Get the ophthalmologist to measure the intraocular pressure and do a funduscopic exam to determine the perfusion status. Don't delay!

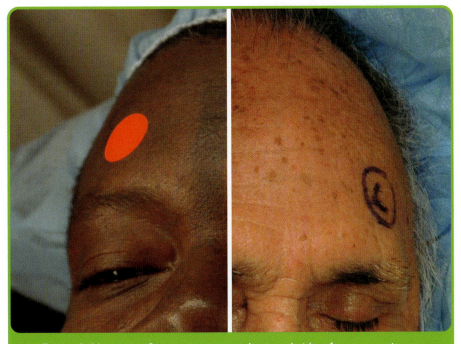

Figure 1. Always confirm patient, procedure, and side-of-surgery prior to performing regional anesthesia. The side to be marked should be clearly marked. The patient's cap should not obscure the label.

Megamajor Bleeding

Extremely uncommon. We have seen this only a handful of times in 10 years at a busy eye hospital. It may require a lateral canthotomy to relieve orbital pressure and uncompromise perfusion. What's a lateral canthotomy? It is a fancy term for inserting a scissor at the lateral corner of the eye and cutting the tissue in the direction of the ear until sufficient space is made for the globe to bulge forward and the pressure on the eye to be relieved. Don't delay! If the ophthalmologist determines that perfusion is fully compromised, then an immediately available plastic surgeon, the ophthalmologist, or you need to do this. Don't delay!

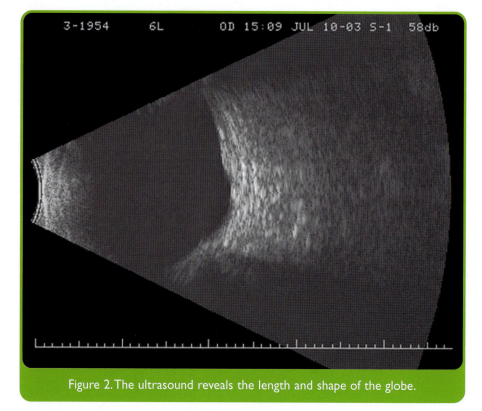

Figure 2. The ultrasound reveals the length and shape of the globe.

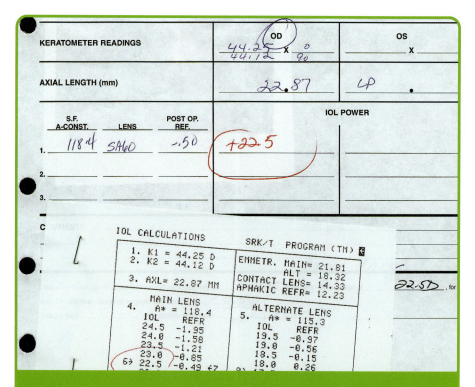

Figure 3. The ultrasound report may be handwritten or computerized. Make note of the length of the eye. Note that this patient's axial length is 22.87 mm, not 22.5 mm!

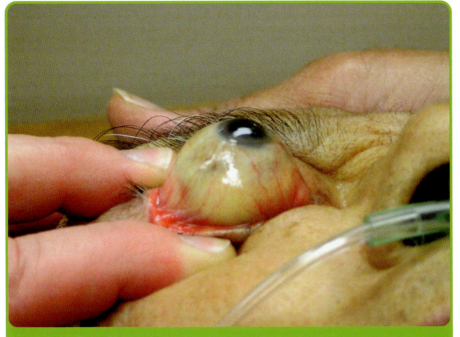

Figure 4. Examine the surface anatomy. Deeper-set eyes are more likely to be punctured.

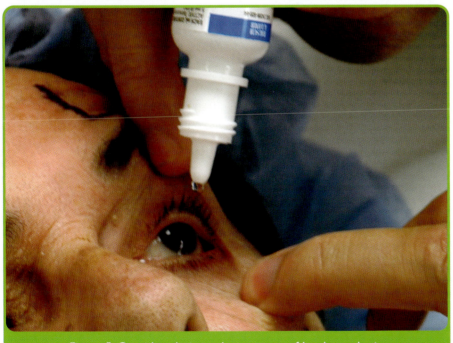

Figure 5. Consider placing a drop or two of local anesthetic.

The Unconscious Patient

Anesthesiologists and ophthalmologists often disagree about the etiology of lost consciousness or apnea after an eye block. The ophthalmologist will insist the cause is over-sedation, particularly if they did the eye block. After considering and ruling out excessive sedation, the anesthesiologist may decide brainstem anesthesia is the correct diagnosis. Everyone else around you has no idea what brainstem anesthesia is, but they all know that you often induce loss of consciousness and apnea in the OR, so the ophthalmologist is probably correct and you must have overdosed the patient with sedatives.

Your reputation is on the line! First, in a very loud and showy manner, give an appropriate dose of narcotic or benzodiazepine reversal agent. Vociferously proclaim to all that you have reversed the sedative activity, yet the patient remains unconscious! Next, open the contralateral, unblocked eye for all to see. A dilated pupil indicates flow of local anesthetic across the optic chiasm to the other eye. In addition, when the patient arouses, diminished vision or mobility of the unblocked eye are pathognomonic for brainstem anesthesia due to leakage of anesthetic agent across the optic chiasm. Irrefutable diagnosis made. You da man (or woman, as the case may be)!

Keep an Eye Out for This Problem!

A real eye-opener: The most commonly reported, permanently disabling injury from *all* regional anesthesia in the ASA Closed Claims Analysis database was associated with nerve blocks of the eye, often resulting in blindness!

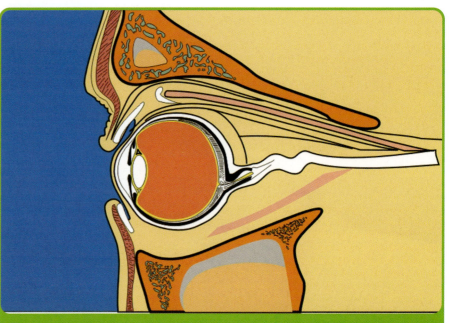

Figures 6. Ask the patient to gaze forward, placing the globe in a midline, neutral position. This allows the optic nerve to rest loosely in the posterior orbit. A taut optic nerve is easily damaged by an oncoming block needle.

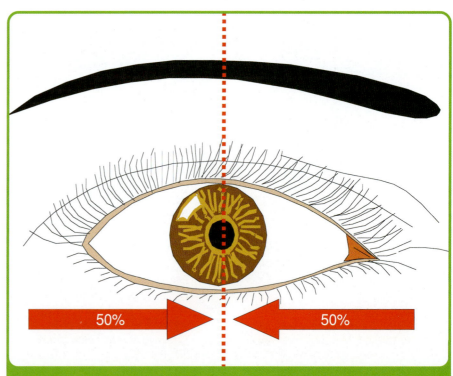

Figures 7. Ask the patient to gaze forward, placing the globe in a midline, neutral position. This allows the optic nerve to rest loosely in the posterior orbit. A taut optic nerve is easily damaged by an oncoming block needle.

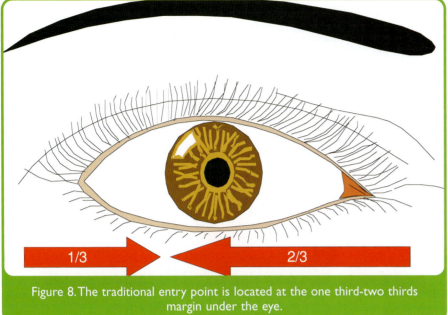

Figure 8. The traditional entry point is located at the one third-two thirds margin under the eye.

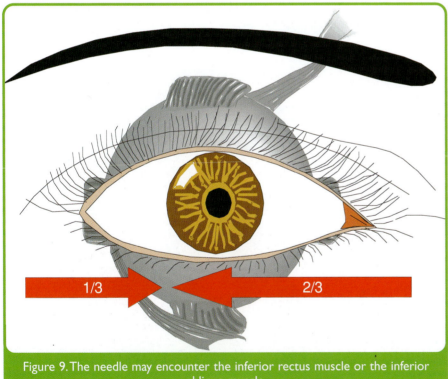

Figure 9. The needle may encounter the inferior rectus muscle or the inferior oblique muscle.

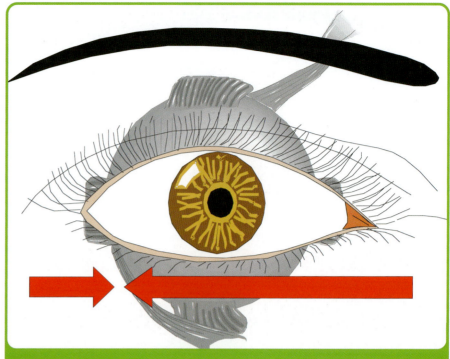

Figure 10. Moving the needle insertion point more laterally than the traditional entry point is recommended.

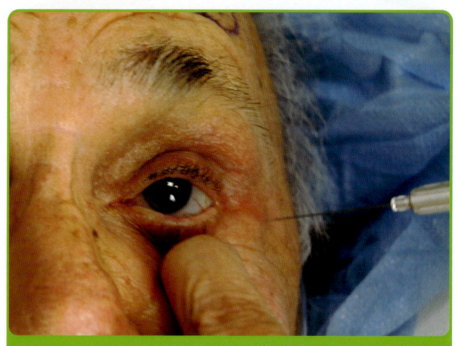

Figure 11. Ballot the globe away, creating space between inferior orbital rim and the eye.

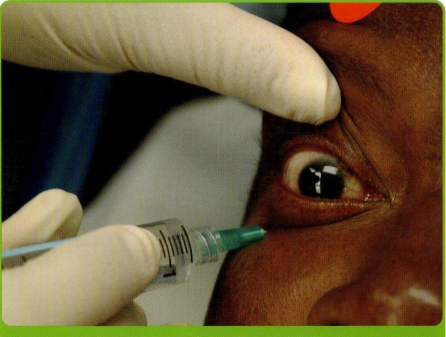

Figure 12. Decide if you will go through skin . . .

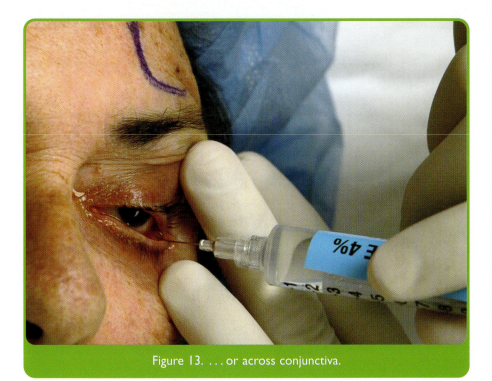

Figure 13. . . . or across conjunctiva.

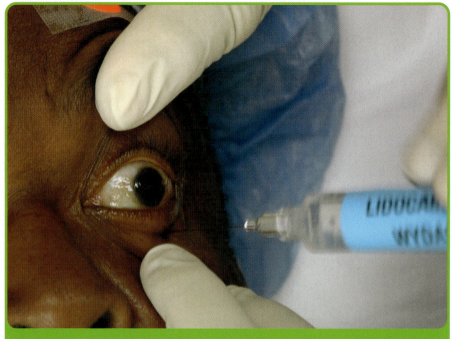

Figure 14. Angle the needle parallel to the axis of the eye such that the needle tip avoids the apex of the orbit (dangerous structures lurk there—optic nerve, cranial nerves, veins, and arteries). This is the proper direction for a peribulbar block.

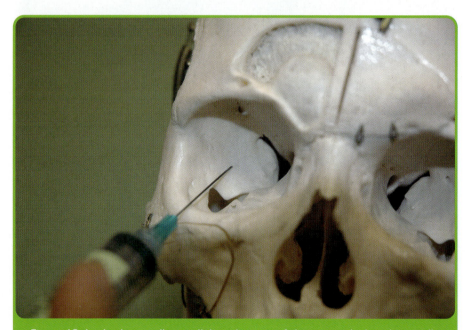

Figure 15. Angle the needle parallel to the axis of the eye such that the needle tip avoids the apex of the orbit (dangerous structures lurk there—optic nerve, cranial nerves, veins, and arteries). This is the proper direction for a peribulbar block.

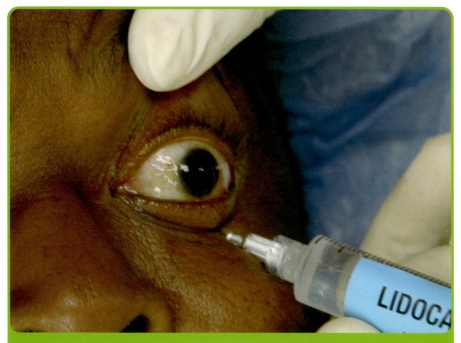

Figure 16. Alternatively, the traditional angulation of a needle has been along the axis of the orbit. This is a retrobulbar block and is associated with more complications; therefore, it is not recommended for the novitiate.

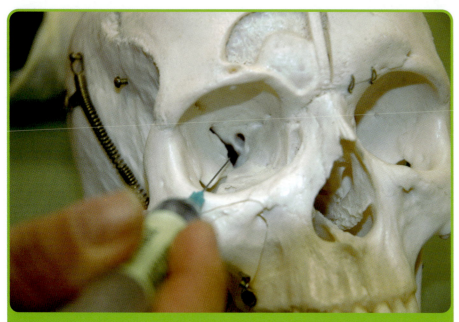

Figure 17. Alternatively, the traditional angulation of a needle has been along the axis of the orbit. This is a retrobulbar block and is associated with more complications; therefore, it is not recommended for the novitiate.

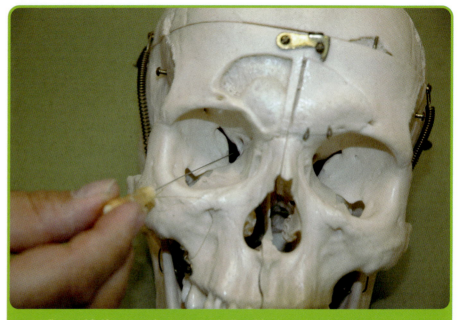

Figure 18. If you perform a retrobulbar block using a long needle, this may happen.

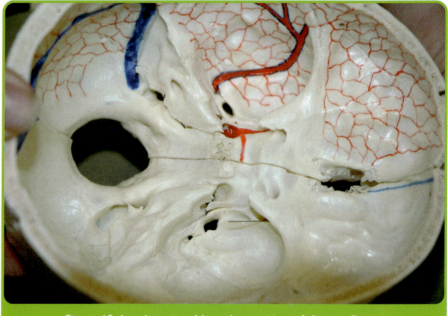

Figure 19. Another view. Note the position of the needle tip.

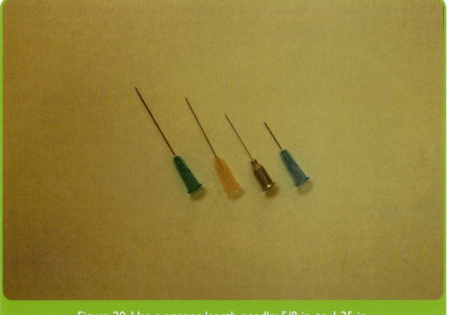

Figure 20. Use a proper length needle: 5/8 in. to 1.25 in.

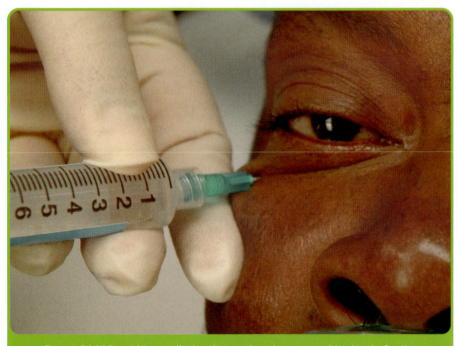

Figure 21. When the needle has been placed to a suitable depth, fix the position such that it will remain in place as anesthetic is injected or if the patient should move.

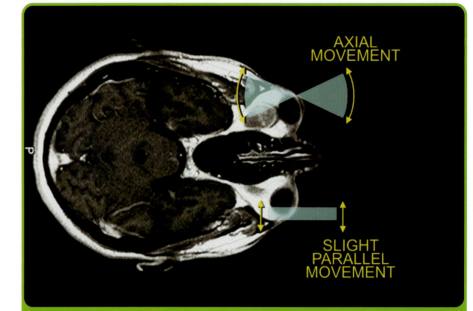

Figure 22. Prior to injecting, assure that the needle has not penetrated the globe by asking the patient to gaze to one side and then back into neutral position. Alternatively, consider gently wiggling the needle from side to side with a slight parallel motion. Do not pivot the needle about an axial point as this creates too much motion of the needle tip in the orbit.

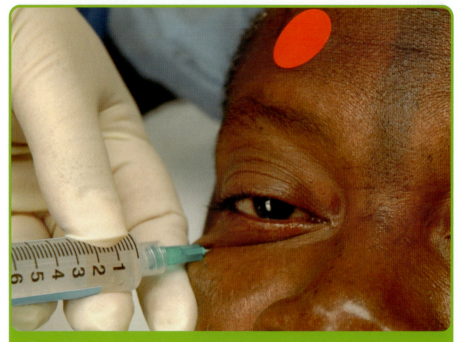

Figure 23. A sympathetic blockade of Muller's muscle should cause the upper lid to begin to droop as one injects local anesthetic.

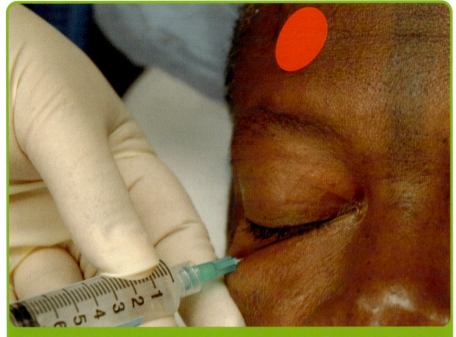

Figure 24. A sympathetic blockade of Muller's muscle should cause the upper lid to begin to droop as one injects local anesthetic.

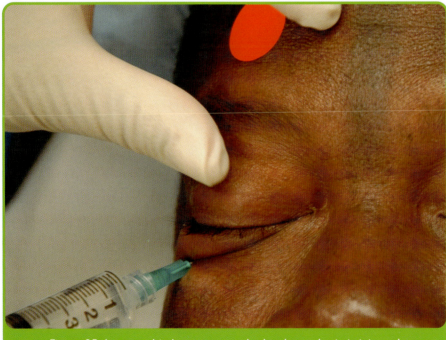

Figure 25. Assess orbital pressure as the local anesthetic is injected.

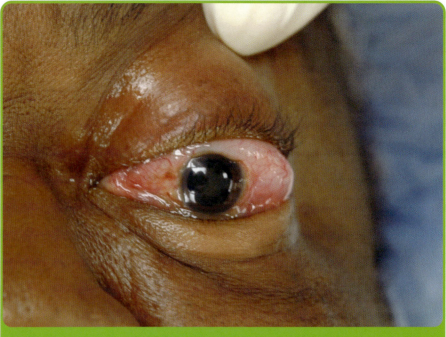

Figure 26. Chemosis may occur when local anesthetic dissects underneath the conjunctiva. This is normal.

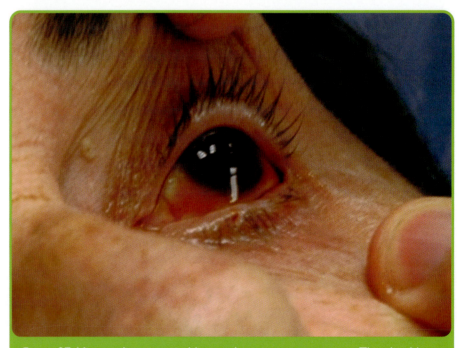

Figure 27. Minor subconjunctival hemorrhage is not uncommon. This should not be a problem.

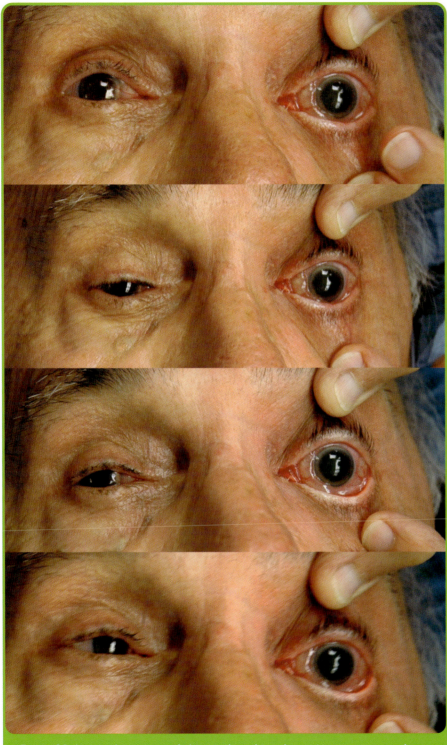

Figure 28. Assess the extent of akinesia by asking the patient to gaze up, down, right, and left.

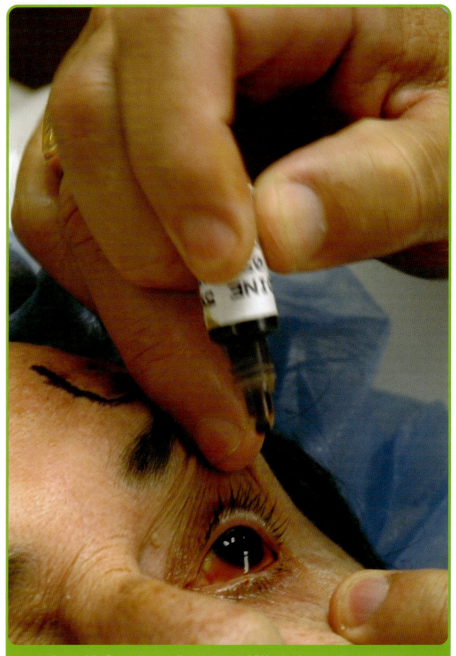

Figure 29. Consider instilling a drop of 5% povidone-iodine solution.

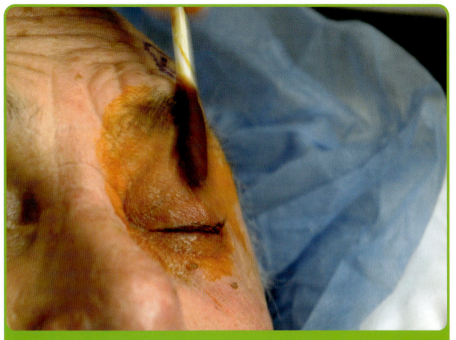

Figure 30. Consider swabbing the eyelids with povidone-iodine solution.

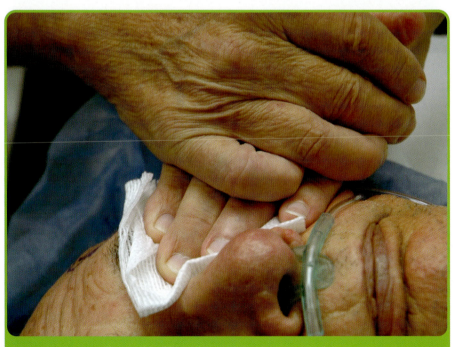

Figure 31. Close the eyelids and protect them.

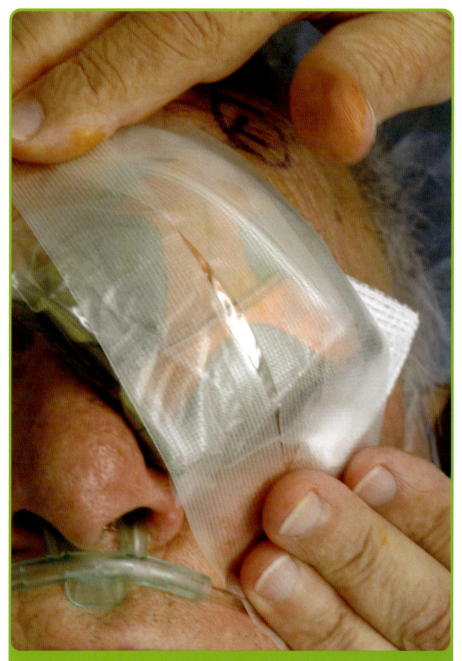

Figure 32. Consider an occulocompression device to help spread the local anesthetic and dissipate tension. Avoid prolonged use of such a device, particularly with glaucoma patients.

SUGGESTED READING

Ahmad S, Ahmad A. Complications of ophthalmologic nerve blocks: A review. J Clin Anesth 2003; 15:564–9.
• *The authors nicely categorize the complications of ophthalmologic nerve blocks in an organized review of all the potential mishaps that can result during the placement of eye blocks. A must-read for the serious ophthalmologic anesthesiologist.*

Chang WM, Stetten GD, Lobes LA Jr, Shelton DM, Tamburd RJ, et al. Guidance of retrobulbar injection with real-time tomographic reflection. J Ultrasound Med 2002;21: 1131–5.

- *Guidance of retrobulbar injection with real-time tomographic reflection seems cool but way too involved for practical application. Reportedly, the authors are still trying to perfect this science and may just be on to something, but just not yet.*

Gombos K, et al. A catheter technique in ophthalmic regional anaesthesia. Acta Anaesth Scand 2000;44:453–6.

- *This group of innovators describe a technique for continuous administration of local anesthetic as an alternative to giving general anesthesia during long cases.*

Guise PA. Sub-tenon anesthesia: A prospective study of 6,000 blocks. Anesthesiology 2003;98:964–8. Nouvellon, et al. Anesthesiology 2004;100: 370–4.

- *In a prospective study of 6000 blocks, the author argues that subtenon anesthesia is a relatively safe alternative to retrobulbar and peribulbar anesthesia. Nice photos of the technique are included. The second reference supports this, only that an "inexperienced" resident botched their almost perfect record.*

Johnson RW. Anatomy for ophthalmic anesthesia. Br J Anaesth 1995;75:80–7.

- *This jolly chap details the anatomy for ophthalmic anesthesia with more illustrations than you can shake a stick at (or even stick a needle into).*

Kallio H, Rosenberg PH. Advances in ophthalmic regional anesthesia. Best Pract Res Clin Anesth 2005;19(2):215–27.

- *A thorough review summarizes the advances in ophthalmic regional anesthesia, emphasizing the importance of having specially trained anesthesiologists in the face of potentially life-threatening complications. Great overview, including much more than just the anesthetic techniques.*

Katz J, et al. Injectable versus topical anesthesia for cataract surgery, patient perceptions of pain and side effects. The study of medical testing for cataract surgery study team. Ophthalmology 2000;107(11): 2054–60. Boezaart AP, et al. Topical anesthesia versus retrobulbar block for cataract surgery: The patient's perspective. J Clin Anesth 2000;12(1):58–60.

- *Surprisingly, both ophthalmologists and anesthesiologists agree that patients prefer injectable—as opposed to topical—anesthesia for cataract surgery.*

Ripart J, et al. Peribulbar versus retrobulbar anesthesia for ophthalmic surgery: An anatomical comparison of ettraconal and intraconal injections. Anesthesiology 2001;94(1): 56–62.

- *The authors recommend the use of peribulbar versus retrobulbar anesthesia for ophthalmic surgery. They explain that whereas retrobulbar is riskier than peribulbar block, they could not show a difference in efficacy between the two techniques.*

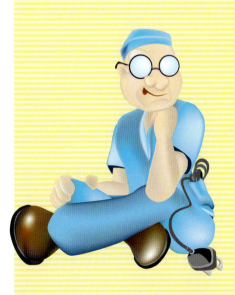

PART 7
TREASURE CHEST

CHAPTER 30

"The Lung's Not Down, You Idiot!" Lung Isolation

Lebron Cooper and
Nicholas Nedeff

Humanity with all its fears,
With all the hopes of future years,
Is hanging breathless on thy fate.

Henry Wadsworth Longfellow
The Building of the Ship, 1849

INTRODUCTION

One-lung ventilation cases take your breath away, that's for sure. And while you're struggling with that lung that keeps coming up, you'll be taking your patient's breath away, too.

Lung isolation is the most consistent pain in the neck in anesthesia. Just when you think you *finally* have the lung down, a patient will come along who didn't read the book. You'll do everything right, and that lung *will not go down*! It won't deflate for love or money. Then the next day, a patient will come down whose *lung* goes down, and in close concert with the lung, the *saturation* goes down, never to rise again.

¡Ay, caramba! What a challenge.

What's the flip side of this often "headache-plagued" procedure? If you can learn lung isolation—and really learn it well—you will be a valuable addition to whatever group (academic or private practice) that you join. You'll even be one of the most sought-after persons when everyone else has floundered in one-lung cases. What a deal, huh?

Isolating the lung is hard. If you can do the hard stuff, you will always have a job.

ABSOLUTE INDICATIONS

- Here's a mnemonic for absolute indications:
  - BPOW—blood, pus, oxygen (separate mnemonic for this), water
    - *Blood*—You don't want blood from one lung contaminating the other side.
    - *Pus*—You don't want pus from one lung contaminating the other side.
    - *Oxygen*—You don't want an oxygen leak or loss from one side making it impossible to ventilate the other side. This one has another mnemonic, SUB-T:
      - ✓ *Surgical*—If the surgeon has sectioned a bronchus and you don't have the lung isolated, you will lose all your ventilation.
      - ✓ *Unilateral lung cyst*—This rare beastie is just a giant alveolus that doesn't contribute any meaningful oxygen exchange. You must isolate it.
      - ✓ *Bronchopleural/cutaneous fistula*—The air leaking out of this will impair ventilation.
      - ✓ *Trauma*—A sectioned bronchus from trauma (call it an "amateur surgical sectioning") can also lead to lost ventilation.
    - *Water*—You don't want irrigating fluid (used to treat alveolar proteinosis) from one lung to contaminate the other side.

RELATIVE INDICATIONS

- A better view (surgical exposure)
  - Lung biopsy
  - Lobectomy
  - Pneumonectomy
  - Esophageal surgery
  - Thoracic aortic aneurysm repair/resection
  - Thoracic spine surgery
- If the lungs are in the way, and the surgeon wants them out of the way, you have a relative indication for lung isolation!
- Caveats to this:
  - Beware the surgeon who yells loud enough—they feel that they can convert a relative to an absolute indication.
  - Keep in mind that some day will come when you won't be able to isolate the lung and the surgeon, no matter how much they scream, "This is impossible! Are you incompetent?" will be forced to deal with it.
  - Guess what? The lung is really soft and squishy, so it is easy to retract. It's not like they are being asked to retract the acetabulum.
- With this in mind, learn how to do lung isolation well each and every time. Don't rely on a soft and squishy lung! Doing that will make your one-lung ventilation life a perpetual nightmare.

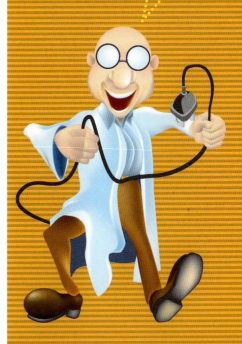

A Day at the Beach

Isolating a lung is the single most consistent pain in the ass you will face. The patient's on their side, they almost always have crummy lungs to start out with, the pulse oximeter fades in and out like a half-charged cell phone, the surgeon crawls up your butt right while they're manipulating the mediastinum and dropping your pressure, and your head is cranked around like Linda Blair in *The Exorcist* as you try to see what's going on way down yonder in the carina patch. Now the patient bucks and you're thinking of how many more decades you have to put up with this crap before you can retire.

Don't Forget the Connector

It never ceases to amaze us that no matter how many times we perform a lung isolation cases, something always seems to not work.

Take the resident who decided he'd like to place a double-lumen tube for experience yet forgets to assemble the connector ahead of time. You induce general anesthesia, give the muscle relaxant, intubate with the double-lumen tube, remove the stylet, and oops! No connector. The "Y" portion is not connected to the connector lumens and the patient is patiently holding their breath, all while you are still setting up your room. Not a good situation, mind you!

ABSOLUTE CONTRAINDICATIONS

- There are no absolute contraindications to lung isolation, but there are plenty of *precautions*:
  - If someone is absolutely near death on two lungs (such poor function that they can barely oxygenate with both lungs), attempting one-lung ventilation may just be the *coup de grace*.
  - Caveat: Don't kill someone just to isolate a lung!
  - A tracheal tear is a near damnable thing.
- *Big tubes*: If you shove a big double-lumen tube down blindly (as is typical of the procedure), you can convert a partial rent into a complete section, and then it's "Goodnight, Irene."
  - *Beware* the large esophageal cancer that can eat into the back of the trachea. Big tubes in such cases have been known to tear the trachea.
- *Big tumors*: An obstructing tumor in the upper airway or the trachea may make placement of a double-lumen tube problematic.
  - *Beware* the obstructing tumor that eats away at the trachea. You'll tear it for sure!
    - Heck, even a single-lumen or Univent® tube might not be able to make that trip.
    - As far as the double-lumen tube goes, remember that in a difficult airway, it will be extra-difficult to place. You need *such* a good view to place a double-lumen tube that you should consider alternatives (a Univent® or a regular endotracheal tube) to at least get the case started.

STUFF YOU'LL NEED TO GET STARTED

Equipment

- Stethoscope (Yep, if you've gotten used to "life without a stethoscope," it's time to steal one because this is one chest to which you'll probably need to listen.)
- Fiberoptic bronchoscope (No matter what you hear with the stethoscope, you still need to check with the scope and make sure you're in the right place. Plus, if things go awry in the case, you'll need the fiberoptic to reposition things.)
  - What size bronchoscope, you ask? A 37 French (or smaller) double-lumen

ETT will not admit an adult-sized fiberoptic bronchoscope without a fight. Make sure whatever tube you use will admit whatever fiberoptic you have.
- Best way? Test it out ahead of time. Place the bronchoscope through the lumen of the endotracheal tube *before* the tube is in the patient.
- Rules of thumb:
  - ✓ *Adult-size* bronchoscope for single-lumen ETTs or Univents® larger than 8.0 mm ID and double-lumen ETTs larger than 37 French. (You can view things *much* easier with this scope instead of an intubating scope!)
  - ✓ *Fiberoptic intubating-size* bronchoscope for ETTs smaller than 8.0 mm ID and double-lumen tubes.
  - ✓ ETT's smaller than 37 French.
- Laryngoscope—you *must* get everything out of the way for the perfect view of the cords!
  - A Mac (curved blade) just does a better job (according to many of our colleagues) than does a Miller (straight blade) at "moving aside the tongue."
  - That said, a Miller blade is better than a Mac (according to our other colleagues).
  - What does all this mean?
    - Use whatever blade makes you happy, but be able to use both kinds of all sizes!
    - You have *no* idea what you'll see and how you'll get that darned *big* double-lumen tube in, so be ready for *anything*!
- Endotracheal tubes (notice, that's plural)
  - Double-lumen endotracheal tubes
    - Have a couple of sizes available. The airway may look okay on the examination, but we've all been surprised before. Have different sizes available (just like when you do pediatric cases—you're never sure what you'll run into).
    - In general, use a 35 or 37 French for most women (depending upon their height) and a 37 or 39 French for most men (depending upon their height).
    - You may need to go one size larger than suggested if you have a really tall patient (or someone whose tracheal anatomy didn't follow the textbooks).

- Univent® Endotracheal Tube, the Arndt® Endobronchial Blocker, or the Cohen® Tip-Deflecting Endobronchial Blocker, depending upon what you want to do.
  - Prejudices abound ("I never use a double-lumen tube any more! They're just too big and dangerous! or "The Univent® stinks! It *never* works right!")
  - Like everything else in medicine, learn to use all of them and you'll have more "tools in your airway toolbox."
- A regular, single-lumen endotracheal tube
  - Just in case you can't get the fancy ones in, make sure that you can secure the airway with a plain-ol' regular tube. Don't kill a patient because you are hell-bent on isolating the lung!
  - If you are in trouble, go back to the ABCs, and that means secure the airway first and foremost, even if it's not with the exact tube you originally envisioned.
- Clamp (a Kelley Clamp, if you must be specific, but any clamp will actually work, that is, if you do the double lumen tube.) You don't need a clamp for the Univent® or endobronchial blockers.
  - Make sure when you place the clamp, that you clamp the *connector*, not the *endotracheal tube itself*. If you clamp on the endotracheal tube, the lung won't deflate, plus you won't be able to put a fiberoptic bronchoscope down the appropriate lumen.
  - Worst of all, if you tear the endotracheal tube with the clamp, you'll have to reintubate. (If you tear the connector, you just have to get another connector.)

Beware the Difficult Airway!

- If someone comes to your OR with a genuinely difficult airway, you will have a heck of a time placing a double-lumen endotracheal tube. The tube is big, clunky, hard to move, and easy to tear the tracheal cuff on the teeth.
- If someone looks like they might be a tough intubation, consider intubating them awake with a Univent® or regular endotracheal tube.
- Once you have the regular endotracheal tube in, using a tube exchanger you can then place a double-lumen or a Univent® over it using a Seldinger technique.

- If someone is already intubated and their airway looks really bad (you know, like the patient who has been intubated for three weeks, has full-body anasarca or weighs 400 pounds):
  - Either place a bronchial blocker down that ETT or use a tube exchanger.
  - Don't just pull a tube out blindly in the belief that you will be able to reintubate easily. That might not happen, and then your day just got *really* bad!
  - Caveat: Difficult airway plus lung isolation is a supreme challenge! Make sure you're ready for anything.

PHILOSOPHY OF LUNG ISOLATION

- The key in any one-lung case is keeping an open mind.
- When you initiate one-lung ventilation, the saturation can be a real problem.
  - Don't be afraid to reinflate the lungs, stabilize the patient, then reassess.
  - Don't "suffer in silence" as the patient crashes and dies. The surgeon is in this with you, and you need to work with them to make sure the patient does OK. Ego has no place in a one-lung case.
- Keep in mind *all* the options, including such exotic ones as cardiopulmonary bypass and ECMO. If, due to some wild circumstance, the patient's lungs just *absolutely cannot do it* alone, you sometimes must let a machine do it.
- Be quick to get help if you are in trouble.
  - When you are tangling with a cantankerous double-lumen endotracheal tube, Univent®, or Endobronchial Blocker, it is easier than easy to take your eye off the patient.
  - Don't let them get unstable while you are peering through the fiberoptic!
- If your partner or colleague is doing a double-lumen case, go in there and help out. You will win big brownie points, plus it's an easy way to get more lung isolation exposure.
  - You will get to look down the fiberoptic and help troubleshoot positioning.
  - Every time you do that, you learn a little. And as we all know, the more we know, the more we know we don't know!

More Exotic Quarry

In a few weird circumstances, you may need to go wild to drop the lung. To put it in proper perspective, just look at it this way: "If the lungs can't do the oxygenating, a machine will have to do it for me."

Huh?

Let's say every time you drop a lung, you just cannot maintain oxygenation, no way, no how. You do everything— you make sure the tube is properly positioned, you suction, you treat bronchospasm, you apply CPAP to the nonventilated lung and you provide PEEP to the ventilated lung. Still no soap.

OK, if this lung really needs to go down, then a machine will have to do the "breathing" for you. Stick in femfem cannulas and do a fem-fem bypass. It's ugly, it involves heparinization, you'll have to repair the vessels postoperatively but hey, what's the option?

Not do the case?

Lose the patient?

Better to "think outside the box" and go to a fem-fem bypass and get that lung down safely.

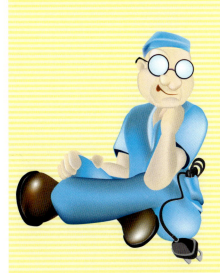

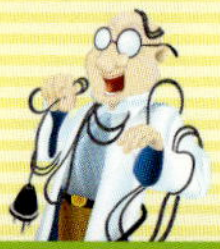

The Crack Pipe in the Trachea

Try this on for size: A patient inhaled the stem of a crack pipe and there it lay in his trachea. Nice, huh?

They couldn't, but couldn't, get it out with bronchoscopy.

I suggested fem-fem bypass while they cut it out.

Just then, a clever cuss suggested we slip the fiberoptic through the crack pipe, curl it, and pull the pipe out.

It worked—but please don't try this at home!

The Really Bad Day in Paradise!

It was just a simple thoracotomy for an esophagectomy. The anesthesiologist decided to use a double-lumen tube. No one bothered to properly check the CT scan. In went the double-lumen tube, blindly, blindly while turning, down the trachea, and low and behold, away went the bronchus. I mean, away. It ripped right off the trachea. Talk about nightmare!

We know that anecdotal stories and the practice of medicine based on them do not necessarily make the world go around, but maybe if the anesthesiologist has chosen to place a Univent® or other bronchial blocker, the placement of the blocker under direct vision with a bronchoscope may have prevented this disaster.

HISTORY AND PHYSICAL

- The H&P is even more critical in a one-lung ventilation case than in other cases.
- Airway, airway, airway. Is this person easy to intubate or just easy enough to intubate with a regular endotracheal tube? Yes, there is a difference.
- Lungs—Will they be able to tolerate one-lung ventilation? Check pulmonary function tests (preferably split-lung) for a total pneumonectomy. If it's just a lobectomy but you need one-lung ventilation during the procedure, you may "get away without" pulmonary function tests, remembering, of course, you may have issues with oxygenation and ventilation during the case.
- Heart—A bad heart with right heart failure, plus the hypoxemia of one-lung ventilation, can lead to some bad news. (Ever heard of "hypoxic pulmonary vasoconstriction? Bad news for the failing right ventricle!)
- Pathology:
  - Is this an enormous mass wrapped around the pulmonary artery? Be prepared for anything.
  - Is this a little peripheral mass easily gotten to and removed? Different story.
  - Just as the surgeon must know about your problems in a lung case, you must know about the surgical problems in a lung case.
  - Caveat: You can't do good anesthesia unless you know the surgical procedure!

OPTIONS FOR ACHIEVING LUNG ISOLATION

- Double-lumen endotracheal tube:
  - A left-sided tube is the most common, whereas a right-sided tube is less common.
  - Right-sided tubes are more difficult to position correctly because of the difficulty of positioning the right upper lobe port of the tube exactly over the right upper lobe bronchial lumen.
- Univent® Endotracheal Tube:
  - Just like a regular single-lumen endotracheal tube with an endobronchial blocker incorporated in the lumen
  - May be more difficult to place than a single-lumen ETT due to its lack of pliability (more on this later)
- Arndt® Endobronchial Blocker or Cohen® Tip-Deflecting Endobronchial Blocker:
  - Both of these devices work similarly by placing them through a single-lumen ETT and directing the blocker to the bronchus you intend to block.
  - The "tip-deflecting" blocker may have an advantage for directing the tip into a not-so-normal anatomical situation and for the inevitable need for replacing/repositioning if the blocker is inadvertently dislodged during the procedure
- Fogerty catheter:
  - Rigged to be a bronchial blocker through a single-lumen ETT
  - Unless you have some kind of connector you've previously planned to use and are familiar with, this may not be the wisest choice but it may be one of your *only* choices.
- Regular, single-lumen ETT ("mainstemmed"):
  - You can use a regular, single-lumen ETT and "mainstem" it by pushing it into the *opposite* mainstem bronchus you intend to block and inflating the cuff.
  - By doing this, you have effectively achieved one-lung ventilation, thus passively deflating the operative lung in the process.
- Faking it:
  - By placing a regular, single-lumen endotracheal tube in the trachea, you may plan "intermittent apnea."
  - You may also use *very small tidal volumes*.
    - You may have to tell the surgeon to "deal with it."
  - You may have to keep using *regular tidal volumes*.
    - You may have to tell the surgeon to "deal with it."
    - (These last two methods of lung isolation are called "not lung isolation," and your surgeon will probably hate you.)
- Cardiopulmonary bypass:
  - Guess what? Both lungs come down—that is, if you stop the ventilator.
  - Don't forget to restart the ventilator when you wean from CPB. It's the number one preventable cause of not separating from cardiopulmonary bypass!

- ECMO (Extra Corporeal Membrane Oxygenation)
  - As with CPB, both lungs come down.
  - When faced with this option, consider your day as really, really, really bad! You'll have something to tell your grandkids.
  - Caveat: These last two (CPB and ECMO) may seem a little extreme but hey, if the lungs can't do the job, *something* has to oxygenate the patient, and these "extra-pulmonic" lungs are preferable to a hypoxemic death!

THE CARINA

- Identifying the carina is the be-all, end-all of lung isolation cases. If you can see the carina, you can navigate the treacherous shoals of lung isolation.
- If you can't see the carina, or if you get faked out by a "non-carina" (a division one step "further down" the bronchial tree from the carina), then you are doomed. You are condemned to flounder about in Nowheresville for the duration of the case. You have a one-way ticket to Unhappy City and that train is leaving the station right now with you on board.
- How does an enterprising anesthesiologist make sure they can recognize the carina?
  - If you are a resident or student, get thee to the lung room every time you get a chance and ask if you can sneak a peak through the fiberoptic bronchoscope. The more carinas (carinae?) you see, the better you will be when you are ready to recognize the real deal.
- How do you tell the real deal?
  - The carina is sharp.
  - The tracheal rings (cartilages) are *organized* along the anterior aspect of the trachea (kind of like a "C"-shape).
  - A smooth, muscular, road-like band defines the posterior portion of the trachea.
  - If you are looking at a pseudo-carina, you won't see the organized Cs and smooth band along the posterior wall. You may see Cs, but they won't necessarily be organized.
- If the surgeon does a bronchoscopy first (often through a single-lumen tube before you place a double-lumen tube, or directly through a Univent®, if that's what you've placed), take a peek through the scope and get a good look at the

carina. Then later, when you're looking through the double-lumen or trying to position your blocker, you'll be looking at "familiar turf."
- This is a lot of perseveration on "carina indentification," but believe me, that carina really and truly is the difference between a good case with nice lung isolation and a miserable case with you suffering all seven circles of Dante's Purgatory at once.

CONSIDERATIONS

Double-Lumen ETT

- Good in a lot of ways. This is the "traditional" lung isolator, so most surgeons and anesthesiologists are familiar with it.
- Although it can be a pain to get in (it's so big and clunky) and it's a pain to position just right (if you get faked by a non-carina, you'll be sunk), once you get it in, it tends to stay that way. Note: this is a major plus!
- The double-lumen allows easy deflating of the lung, so the lung comes down quickly without delay.
- The relatively large bronchial lumen allows for suctioning, looking around with the fiberoptic scope, and switching back and forth between lungs (very handy and many times necessary if you do lung transplants).
- But the double-lumen has its dark side. The damn thing is so big, it can be awfully difficult to place by direct laryngoscopy.
- A small mouth, big teeth, small chin, fat jowls, and so on—all the things that make plain-ol' intubation tough—make navigating that double-lumen tube damned near impossible to place at times.
- Coupled with that is the human's inability to focus on more than one thing at a time. You look at the cords and your focal point leaves the tracheal cuff (which by now is hooking on a tooth). You advance the double-lumen tube and tear the tracheal cuff at the same time. What a nightmare!
- The next time you attempt intubation, you focus on the tracheal cuff, hoping not to tear it again, but your focal point goes off the cords and now you miss the intubation altogether. Absurd, huh? Just try it.
- One more headache with this big bastard: you can tear the hell out of the

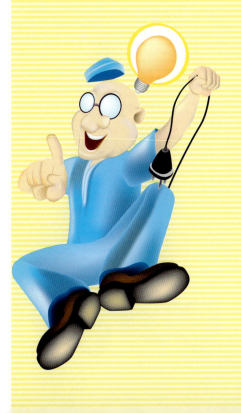

trachea itself (see relative contraindications above). Oh, wouldn't that be just ducky? Think about it—you work a case where the patient has esophageal cancer. That cancer may very well be "eating into" the trachea, which is just in front of it. In goes your double-lumen tube, and *rrriiiip*! Now you have a disrupted tracheal tree, which has been known to significantly shorten one's social calendar, may significantly shorten one's day at work, or significantly shorten your patient's lifespan, among other tragedies.

Univent®

• The groovy thing about the Univent® is that you put it in like a regular endotracheal tube.

• If you secure it at about 22 cm, you *know* when you place the fiberoptic bronchoscope that you are probably looking at the carina.

• There is a lot less confusion about "which thing is the carina?" with a Univent®.

• Also, the Univent® can be placed with the patient awake. (Try that with a double-lumen. Doable, but damned tough, and I personally dare you to try!)

• So for the difficult-intubation-lung-isolation-combo-pack, the Univent® is "da bomb."

• *However*: The Univent® is thick and stiff and sometimes it's difficult to get it through the cords. It may take a little "elbow grease" and a lot of creativity but once in, it is a cinch to use.

• The bronchial blocker sticks out the top of the tube a long way so you can hit yourself right in the face!

• So intubating with the Univent® is not necessarily a walk in the park. It's easier than a double-lumen, yes, but not as easy as a regular ETT.

Arndt® Bronchial Blocker and Cohen® Tip-Deflecting Blocker

• Whereas the Univent® has a built-in bronchial blocker in its own special tube, the Arndt® and Cohen® gizmos go through a regular ETT.

• Of note, if you try this with an ETT smaller than an 8.0 mm ID, you're going to work extra-hard as there is not enough room for everything (blocker and bronchoscope) in the smaller diameter tubes.

• The Arndt® and Cohen® blockers both have a real advantage when you already have an intubated patient and you don't want to mess around and take the risk of

changing tubes. You use what you already have, only modified.

• Not as many people use the Arndt® or Cohen® devices as use the Univent®, and in general, people find the Univent® much easier to work with.

• When faced with a choice, a lot of people would place a tube changer, use that to place a Univent®, then work with the "easier" piece of equipment. The Arndt® and Cohen® blockers take more skill than a Univent®.

TECHNIQUES

Double-Lumen Endotracheal Tube

• Do a good, and I mean good, airway exam. Look for things that will specifically gum up the works with a double-lumen tube—a jagged tooth that can tear the tracheal cuff or a small mouth that won't let you place the monster-sized double-lumen tube.

• Review the medical records for things that may bring the double-lumen to grief once past the cords—the invasive esophageal cancer, an obstructive lesion in the left mainstem bronchus that won't allow passage of the double-lumen, the enormous aortic aneurysm that may rupture as the double-lumen pushes past it (that would be a lot of fun, that is, if you're into torture and masochism).

• If your case involves first a single-lumen endotracheal tube (for bronchoscopy) followed by placement of a double-lumen endotracheal tube, then view that first intubation as a "preview of coming attractions."

• If you don't get a good view of the cords but still are able to pass the single-lumen ETT fairly easily, then trust me, there is still *no way in the world* you will be able to pass a double-lumen tube. A single-lumen placement must be *super-easy* for a double-lumen tube to be just *regular easy*.

• Left- or right-sided tube?

   • The traditional argument *against* the right-sided double-lumen tube is that the take-off of the right upper lobe bronchus is so close to the carina, you may occlude the right upper lobe. Then when you try to isolate the lung, you will end up in an imperfect world.

   • But if you look at a right-sided double-lumen tube, the bronchial cuff is manufactured on a slant, which allows you to ventilate the right upper lobe with no problem! Hey, what do you

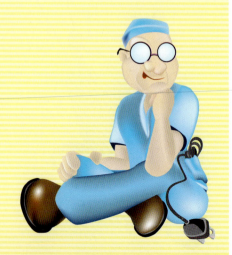

know? Somebody actually thought of things like this before they marketed this thing. So the absolute dictum, "Thou shalt not ever use a right-sided double-lumen tube," isn't really so absolute a dictum after all.

- But to tell the truth, most folks use the left-sided double-lumen tube anyway. It's just plain easier to use.

Placing the Double-Lumen Endotracheal Tube

- Do your usual good induction, do your usual good laryngoscopy. Use whatever laryngoscope blade makes you a superhero in really bad situations, and go for the gold.

- Place the tube in the mouth (carefully watching the bronchial cuff as it passes the teeth), go through the cords, and then keep on going. Turn the tube until the two openings at the top of the double-lumen tube are looking you square in the eyes. If you turn the tube so those two openings are 90° to your eyes, you've turned it around sideways and you'll have to do the whole case lying in the lateral decubitus position.

- Push the ETT in until it stops; don't force it, jam it, ram it, pound it, or jump on top of it to get it in. Just slide until the slide's done slidin'. Then pull out the stylet, hook up the connectors, and make sure you're in.

- Inflate the tracheal cuff and then inflate the bronchial cuff.

- Clamp off each lumen, in turn (on the connector, remember), and listen with your newly acquired stethoscope to get your initial impression of whether you're in the right place or not.

- Caveats:
  - Be sure to use your clamp on the connector—if you accidentally tear the connector, you get to go and get another connector; if you accidentally tear the actual ventilating double-lumen tube lumen, you get the enjoyment of reintubation. (Remember that difficult airway we talked about—you don't want to do that again!)
  - Remember, if you clamp the connector, that allows air to escape from the lung. If you clamp the endotracheal or endobronchial lumen, the lung cannot deflate.
  - If you clamp the tracheal side, you should only hear breath sounds on the bronchial side (obvious, but that means on the left for a left-sided

double-lumen tube and on the right for a right-sided double-lumen tube).

- Now go down the tracheal side with the fiberoptic bronchoscope. You should see the carina, that all-important carina, the this-above-all-else-to-thine-own-self-be-true carina.

- *Stop* here. If you are using a left-sided double-lumen tube, you'll see a little rim of blue, just to the left, just beyond the carina in the left mainstem bronchus. If you are using a right-sided double-lumen tube, you'll see that little rim of blue on the right, just beyond the carina in the right mainstem bronchus.

- If you don't see the carina, deflate the bronchial cuff—and pray. Make *absolutely sure* you are in the trachea!

- If you still don't see the carina (but you are definitely in the trachea) and you are starting to get a rising feeling of panic in your heart that this patient is an-carinic or suffers from hypo-carinaemia, relax and take a deep breath. That carina is down there somewhere.

- Pull back the entire double-lumen tube and reassess; maybe you're just in too far.
  - Caveat: If nothing seems to work, *change gears*.

- Put the fiberoptic scope down the bronchial lumen, then pull the double-lumen tube way, way, way back until you are so far out that you *must* be looking at the carina.

- Don't fret that you might extubate the patient; you have a fiberoptic scope in the trachea, after all, so you can almost always slip the tube back in. (This of course, is not an absolute—just mind your Ps and Qs.)

- Once you've pulled back a country mile and you really do see the carina, slide the scope down into the appropriate bronchus for whichever double-lumen tube you are using. (You're basically planning to do a Seldinger technique over the bronchoscope.)

- Using the fiberoptic as a makeshift guide-wire, slide the double-lumen tube down over the scope into whichever bronchial lumen the double-lumen tube is intended for (that would be the left bronchus for left-sided tubes and the right bronchus for right-sided tubes).

- Now remove the fiberoptic scope and place it in the tracheal lumen. Look for the carina (which you just saw, live and in-color) and identify the blue cuff just below the carina.

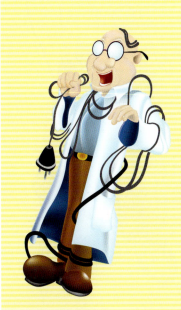

- *Key point*—When you're really lost, do this:

  - Send your bronchoscope down the bronchial lumen and pull the entire double-lumen tube way, way back.

  - This trick is the best problem-solver. It beats thrashing around for a month of Sundays in the tracheal lumen while the surgeon screams at you and you wonder why you ever got into this business!

TECHNIQUES

Univent®

- Just like the double-lumen endotracheal tube, the Univent® can be used to assure one-lung ventilation.

- Many an anesthesia provider has changed their practice since the introduction of the Univent® over a decade ago, especially after using the following techniques, seldom written about or even spoken of. You'll be hard-pressed to find someone to tell you that it can almost—once again, almost—*replace* the double-lumen tube in achieving lung isolation.

- However, if you follow the suggestions below in the *exact order in which they appear*, you will almost certainly achieve lung isolation as well, if not better than you can with a double-lumen tube.

Advantages of the Univent®

- The Univent® has several advantages over the standard double-lumen tube:

  - It is smaller, hence usually easier to place and less traumatic.

  - If you are planning a bronchoscopy before the actual procedure, you can do the bronchoscopy through the Univent® (size 8.0 mm ID or above), thus eliminating the step and risk of intubating with a single-lumen tube and reintubating with a Univent® or double-lumen tube.

  - It is placed exactly like a regular, single-lumen tube.

  - You can even do an awake, fiberoptic intubation with the Univent®. Try that with a double-lumen tube!

  - Nothing is ever advanced into a bronchus "blindly" like it is with a double-lumen tube. You get to see the lumen *before* you invade it with a foreign object.

  - What if you cannot or choose not to extubate at the end of the case? A

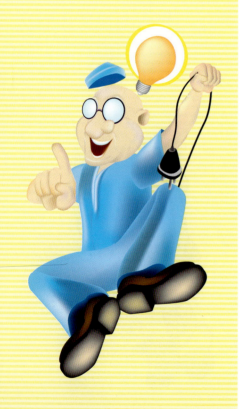

Univent® can be left in place, just like a single-lumen tube. There is *no need to reintubate*!

- Caveat: This comes in real handy when you have that bad airway, huge fluid-shift case where you are terrified of removing the tube and risking losing the airway!

Disadvantages of the Univent®

- You know if there are advantages, there must also be disadvantages, so here they are:

  - Know the *absolute indications* for a double-lumen tube (see above). These, necessarily, would be *contraindications* for placing a Univent®.

    - Remember the mnemonic: BPOW (blood, pus, oxygen, water).

    - You cannot use a Univent® anytime there may be cross-contamination between the lungs. The Univent® does *not* protect the other lung!

  - Any time you need to isolate both lungs separately at different times during the same procedure (like in a double-lung transplant without cardiopulmonary bypass), the Univent® is probably not your best choice. Although it can be done, it really can be a hassle that neither you nor I would want to deal with.

  - Occasionally, the right upper lobe bronchus lumen is so close to the carina that the Univent® bronchial blocker cannot adequately occlude the lumen, resulting in inadequate isolation of the right upper lobe.

  - In the rare patient, you'll actually find a "pig bronchus," meaning, of course, that the right upper lobe bronchus actually comes off the trachea itself, thereby making the Univent® useless in these cases.

- All that said, if you follow the procedure below *in the exact order in which they appear*, you may find that the Univent® offers superior lung isolation with much less trauma and grief than does a double-lumen tube.

Placing the Univent®

- Just as with the double-lumen tube, do a *good* airway exam. Just because the Univent® is smaller than a double-lumen tube doesn't mean it will go in as easily as a regular, single-lumen tube.

  - The Univent® is a little "stiffer" than a regular single-lumen tube, so sometimes it takes a little "creativity" to get it through the vocal cords. It may not just slide in, even if you have a good view of the cords.

- Using a stylet sometimes helps direct the Univent® through the treacherous path of the posterior pharynx.

- Also, just like with the double-lumen tube, it would probably be a good idea to review the medical record and any studies (like a CT scan) to rule out any obstructing tumor in either the posterior pharynx or the tracheal/bronchial lumens.

- Choose the correct size Univent® for the patient and procedure. If the surgeons are planning a bronchoscopy, the smallest Univent® that an adult-size bronchoscopy will pass through is an 8.0 mm ID.

- Getting the blocker down the right side is easy—placing it down the left side can be a challenge.

  - Note: Do not remove the bronchial blocker stylet. It improves your ability to direct the blocker into the bronchus you intend to block!

  - Although it is not known why the manufacturer suggests removing the stylet prior to intubation, it is assumed to be to prevent tracheal or bronchial damage; however, recent reports have shown this not to be the case, and your chances of successful placement are much greater with the stylet left in place.

  - You may have to "twist" the blocker, or you may even have to "twist" the *entire* Univent® tube to successfully direct the blocker to the bronchus you intend to block. Don't be shy.

- Before intubating, check both the tracheal *and* bronchial cuffs to make sure they are intact.

- Note: The connector to the bronchial cuff *does not fit* a Luer lock syringe! You must use a syringe with a slip lock, or place a T-piece with a slip lock on the connector, and then use a Luer lock syringe to inflate the cuff.

- The bronchial cuff almost always requires between 5 ml and 7 ml of air to completely occlude the bronchial lumen, not 3 ml to 4 ml as the manufacturer suggests.

- Intubate as you normally would (you know, laryngoscope blade of your choosing).

- Remember, these endotracheal tubes are a bit "stiffer" than a regular tube, so sometimes it takes a little creativity getting it through the vocal cords.

- Once you've determined you are *actually in the trachea*, follow these steps *in this exact order* and you will achieve lung isolation:

  - Place the blocker in the bronchus you intend to block, using the fiberoptic bronchoscope to guide your efforts.

    - Remember, leaving the blocker stylet in place will improve your chances of success.

    - Don't be afraid to "twist" the blocker or the entire Univent® to direct your blocker where you want it to go.

  - Push the blocker *all the way in* until you get mild resistance. (That's way too far in, I know, but trust me; we'll get to that later.)

  - Position the patient in the lateral decubitus position with an axillary roll, beanbags, pillows, and so on. Don't forget about safe patient positioning just because you're worried that the Univent® may not work.

  - Once positioned safely, *disconnect the ventilator circuit.*

    - This will allow the lungs to deflate passively.

    - Give them a couple of minutes or so to deflate because if these were normal lungs and had normal recoil, you probably wouldn't be doing the surgery you're about to do!

  - Using your bronchoscope, *with the ventilator circuit still disconnected*, position the blocker cuff *just past the carina* (remember the carina?), so you can just see the edge of the blue cuff.

  - Now, *with the ventilator circuit still disconnected*, inflate the blocker cuff with 5 ml to 7 ml of air.

  - Reconnect the ventilator circuit. You should now be ventilating only one lung, the one you didn't block. What a cool trick, huh?

The following *Quick Reference Guide* is included for your use in the operating room. Unless you just *hate* this book, I wouldn't suggest cutting out the page—just photocopy it, or visit the University of Miami Department of Anesthesiology website at http://www.anesthesiology.med.miami.edu, click on "Department," then "Cardiothoracic," and then "Protocols" to access this *Univent® Quick Reference Guide.*

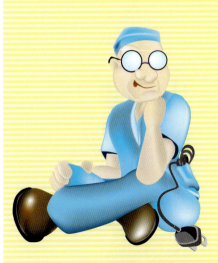

UNIVENT® PLACEMENT QUICK REFERENCE GUIDE

1. Place blocker in the correct bronchus and push *all the way in*.

2. Position the patient safely.

3. Using a bronchoscope, pull back on the blocker until you see the cuff just past the carina.

4. *Disconnect the ventilator circuit* to drop *both* lungs.

5. *Wait*.

6. Inflate the blocker cuff with 5 ml to 7 ml of air to occlude the bronchial lumen.

7. Reconnect the ventilator circuit to ventilate the other lung.

- Why, you ask, do I disconnect the circuit and stop ventilation all together?
  - Because if you inflate the bronchial cuff while you are ventilating, you will trap air *inside* the lung and the lung will *never* deflate.

- Why, you ask, do I place the blocker *before* I position the patient?
  - Because once the patient is positioned, it is almost impossible to get the blocker in the bronchus you intend to block (unless the stars are with you and you are incredibly lucky).

- Why, you ask, do I push the blocker *all the way in*?
  - Because if you place the blocker where it really *should* be before you position the patient, the blocker will almost inevitably migrate *out* of the bronchus when you turn the patient. This ensures the blocker stays in the bronchus you are planning to block.

Troubleshooting the Univent®

- Can't ventilate, high peak airway pressures:
  - Chances are your blocker has migrated out of the bronchus and the cuff has herniated over the carina, thus blocking *both* lungs.
  - Simply deflate the blocker cuff, reposition the blocker so the cuff is just past the carina, *disconnect the ventilator circuit again* to drop *both* lungs, wait, reinflate the blocker cuff with 5 ml to 7 ml of air, and then reconnect the ventilator circuit to ventilate the other lung.

- Lung begins inflating even after you've blocked the bronchus:
  - First and foremost, *look into the surgical field*! Sometimes surgeons like to

"whine." Make sure the lung is actually inflating and you don't just have a "whining surgeon."

- Keep in mind that the surgeons are working on the lung in question, so they may intentionally or inadvertently *move* the bronchus, thus dislodging the blocker.

- Just *disconnect the circuit again*, deflate the blocker cuff, wait, reposition the blocker just past the carina, reinflate the cuff, and then reconnect the ventilator circuit to ventilate the other lung. This will work about 99% of the time.

TECHNIQUES

Arndt® Bronchial Blocker and the Cohen® Tip-Deflecting Blocker

- Intubate with a regular ETT (preferably size 8.0 mm ID or above) or leave the ETT in place in a patient who is already intubated.

- Place the connector (which comes in the kit) on the ETT, place the fiberoptic through the *middle port* of the connector, slide the blocker through the *angled port*, hook up your circuit, and ventilate through the *side port*.

- Such a clever design! (Trust us, we know George Arndt. George is so smart, he's scary-smart.)

- For the Arndt® blocker, slide the tip of the fiberoptic scope through the loop at the end of the blocker. Now you're using the bronchoscope as a guide for a "Seldinger technique."

- For the Cohen® blocker, using the incorporated screw control, deflect the tip toward the bronchus you intend to block.

- Advance the bronchoscope into the target bronchus (you know, the one you intend to block).

- Slide the blocker down the scope into the bronchus. You should slide the blocker *all the way in*, just like you do with a Univent®. Yes, this is too far in but remember, we have a reason for that.

- Now position the patient in the appropriate lateral decubitus position, remembering, of course, to use an axillary roll and appropriate padding.

- Once the patient is positioned safely, *disconnect the circuit and wait*! You must drop *both* lungs so air can escape. Once the blocker cuff is inflated, you will never be able to deflate the lung!

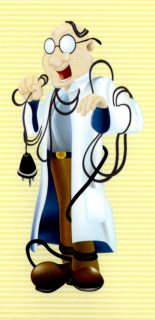

- Once both lungs have had adequate time to deflate, pull back on the blocker just to the point where you see the edge of the blue cuff. *Stop!* Unlike the Univent®, if you pull these blockers out of the bronchus you intend to block, you *may not be able to replace them*. You must get another blocker and start all over.

- Now that your blocker is positioned with the edge of the bronchial cuff just barely visible, inflate the bronchial cuff with 3 ml to 7 ml of air. You should now have successfully blocked the lung you wish to block.

- Don't forget to *reconnect the circuit* to the side port and resume ventilation of the other lung.

- With the Univent®, the Arndt® Bronchial Blocker, and the Cohen® Tip-Deflecting Blocker, the blocker is on the end of a long skinny stick. Thus with a little surgical tugging and pushing, the blocker can easily pop out. No problem when using a Univent®—just put the fiberoptic scope back down and push the blocker back in again.

- However, with the Arndt® this probably will not work. Take extra care to *not* displace the blocker from the bronchus. You may not be successful replacing it. You may have more success with the Cohen® because of its tip-deflecting feature but be careful, it may not work.

- The Univent® is like those chronically dislocating shoulders some people have. They pop out easily but they're easy enough to pop back in. On the other hand, the Arndt® is akin to an amputation—once it's gone, it is almost impossible to save.

Differences between the Arndt® and Cohen® Blockers

- As the name suggests, the Cohen® blocker has the ability to deflect the tip to the direction you wish the blocker to go. Although this is an advantage over the Arndt® design, you may still have some difficulty directing the tip into the bronchus you are trying to block.

- The Arndt® blocker has a loop at the end of the blocker that is designed to slide over the bronchoscope in a "Seldinger" manner. Once this loop is removed, the blocker itself essentially becomes unmaneuverable. If indeed you can leave the loop in place during the surgery, you may have more success replacing the blocker in the event of inadvertent dislodgement.

Advantages of the Arndt® and Cohen® Blockers

- The main advantage of either of these blockers is that you do not have to reintubate a patient who is already intubated just to achieve lung isolation.

- You also do not have to reintubate at the end of the case if, indeed, you plan to leave the patient intubated and mechanically ventilated.

Disadvantages of the Arndt® and Cohen® Blockers

- The bottom line with either of these blockers is that they're just plain harder to use.

- The Arndt® is very difficult to replace in the bronchus if it inadvertently becomes dislodged during the procedure.

- The Cohen®, although easier to replace than the Arndt® because of its tip-deflecting feature, is still more difficult to save than is a Univent®.

LUNG ISOLATION PROBLEMS

Glitches

- Almost every placement glitch ends up being one of these two things—you can't intubate or you can't see the carina.

- If you can't intubate, you didn't really consider how clunky and hard to maneuver the double lumen tube is. Maybe you'd better reconsider and use either the Univent®, Arndt®, or Cohen® blocker.

- If you can't see the carina, well, this boils down to your experience. Try pulling *way* back on the entire ETT, just in case you're in too far.

  - Do everything in your power to "see as many carinas as humanly possible." Go into the lung room on your break and "just take a peek."

  - There's no magic to it—the more you see, the better you'll be able to recognize it.

- When the lung doesn't deflate, look with the fiberoptic bronchoscope after you look in the surgical field to ensure the lung isn't deflated. Look, reposition, look, and look again.

- If the patient has a lot of adhesions, then the lungs will sometimes not "come down" because they are "held up." The surgeon will just have to deal with it. And this time, he will just "have to deal with it." You have no control over this one.

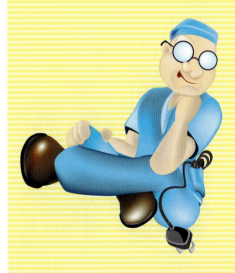

One-Lung Oxygenation Tips and Maneuvers

- If the oxygen saturation begins to drop, there are several things you must do to improve oxygenation.
- If you follow these simple maneuvers, you may never have to inflate both lungs and interfere with the surgical field.
- Caveat: If things aren't working, by all means inflate both lungs and take a (pardon the pun) breather. Killing the patient to keep the surgeon happy is *not* an option.
  - First and foremost, make sure you are ventilating with 100% FiO$_2$!
  - Make sure the ventilator is working, turned on, and the circuit is connected.
  - Make sure the ETT (doesn't matter which one you're using) is free of kinks, mucous, or other obstruction.
  - Make the ventilation match the patient! What does that mean?
    - Check your I:E ratio. A long I:E ratio is used for *restrictive* lung diseases and a short I:E ratio is used for *obstructive* lung diseases.
    - Keep in mind that most of these types of patients have *obstructive* lung disease probably due to their history. However, remember that you just positioned the patient in the lateral decubitus position.
      - ✓ They are now lying on the lung you are trying to ventilate.
      - ✓ To move the chest and ventilate with an adequate tidal volume, you may need to increase your inspiratory pressures.
      - ✓ You have, in essence, created an iatrogenic *restrictive* lung disease.
      - ✓ Now you have an *obstructive component* and a *restrictive component*!
  - If you have a newer-model anesthesia machine with the newer-model ventilators, try adding an *inspiratory pause*.
    - ✓ This maneuver is based on the same concept as PEEP—you recruit more alveoli.
    - ✓ Remember your respiratory and lung physiology—alveoli have an *opening pressure*, which is actually an opening pressure *over time*.
    - ✓ If at the end of the inspiratory phase of the ventilation cycle you add a pause, you are essentially recruiting more alveoli at the same

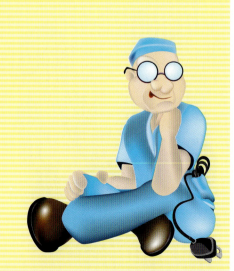

peak airway pressure that only took a couple of extra seconds to open.
  - ✓ This can *markedly* improve gas exchange!
- Add PEEP (positive end-expiratory pressure) to the "dependent" lung.
  - Some people call this the "down" lung because it is in the inferior position to the other lung. However, this terminology is somewhat confusing because the other lung—you know, the operative lung—is "down," meaning in this case, "deflated." Get in the habit now of saying the "dependent" and "nondependent" lungs.
  - How much PEEP should you add? Try starting at 5 cm H$_2$O. If that doesn't work, increase to 10 cm H$_2$O.
    - ✓ What if the O$_2$ saturation goes down? You have just increased the alveolar pressure more than the capillary closing pressure, and you have now effectively caused a huge VQ mismatch.
    - ✓ In other words, you have shunted blood *away from* the alveoli you wish to ventilate.
- Add CPAP (continuous positive airway pressure) to the "nondependent" lung.
  - Make sure you know how to do this. You'll need to know this, not only for your patient's survival, but also for the Oral Boards.
  - Use a CPAP device that is commercially available. Know where they are located in your facility and know how to set up and use them.
  - The idea is simply to connect the commercially available CPAP device to the bronchial lumen of the double-lumen ETT and the other end to an additional oxygen source (flowmeter). You can dial an amount of pressure you would like to deliver to that bronchus.
    - ✓ What if you are using a Univent®, Arndt®, or Cohen® blocker? The commercially available CPAP delivery device does not fit the port of the blocker. What to do?
    - ✓ Hint: Get a piece of oxygen tubing, connect it to an oxygen source (flowmeter at 2 l/min) and *intermittently* hold the tubing to the port opening. Do not continuously connect this to the port—

you will inadvertently inflate the lung as there is no way for the oxygen/gases to escape. However, if you hold it only for a few seconds, you just may recruit enough alveoli to improve oxygenation.

- If none of the above methods work, discuss this with the surgeon. You may consider *intermittent* ventilation of the operative (nondependent) lung as long as the surgeon will work with you on this.
  - When can you *not* bring up the "nondependent" lung?
  - Only when you are in a crisis situation—like when you're doing a dissecting thoracic aortic aneurysm and the surgeon just lost the proximal aortic cannula, leaving a big hole in the aorta. You *cannot* bring up the lung or the patient will bleed to death.
    - This is an example of a *really bad day*.
- When all of this fails to improve oxygenation, it's time to *really discuss*; I mean, be forceful with the surgeon if you have to about the need to ventilate both lungs.
- There are times when, even though you are now ventilating *both lungs again*, that the insult caused will result in an inability to oxygenate with both lungs.
  - And you just thought your day was bad so far.
  - Don't forget—there is always *cardiopulmonary bypass and ECMO (Extra Corporeal Membrane Oxygenation)*.
  - We don't wish this on anyone but, hey, we've been there, so don't think you will never have the opportunity!

TECHNIQUE

Intercostal Block

- Strictly speaking, this belongs in the regional chapter but you will most often do intercostal blocks after thoracotomies, so the technique to this block is included here.
- Intercostal blocks *do not* provide the same pain relief as a thoracic epidural, no matter how much you love them nor how much easier they are to perform.
- Intercostal blocks have a high rate of absorption of local anesthetics, so be careful with the amount of local anesthetic you give here. You really should get in the habit of calculating the toxic dose in

mg/kg of your local anesthetics, and *do not* exceed this amount, especially in intercostal nerve blocks.

- Localize the ribs in the dermatomes you want to block.
- Do yourself a favor: If you perform the blocks *after* a chest tube is already in place (as it will be after a thoracotomy or after a chest tube is placed for multiple rib fractures), you don't have to worry about the #1 complication of these blocks, the dreaded *pneumothorax*.
- Use either a 22G needle or a special "regional block" needle—these tend to be a little longer and afford you the opportunity to get into the neurovascular bundle, even in people with excess thoracic cage fat pads.
- Insert the needle, *hit* the rib, then *walk the tip of the needle off the bottom edge of the rib*.
- Advance the tip of the needle until you are just underneath the rib. (Think "below" the rib "above.")
- You might feel a "pop" as you enter the neurovascular sheath, and you might not.
- Aspirate to ensure you are not in a vein or an artery! Remember, it only takes about 3 ml to 5 ml of bupivicaine injected intravascularly to cause complete and total cardiovascular collapse!
- Inject 3 ml to 5 ml of local anesthetic per intercostal space (calculating the total toxic dose and dividing it by the number of spaces you intend to block).
- Caveat: You can effectively block only one side of the thorax because of the risk of local anesthetic toxicity.

TECHNIQUE

Setting Up the Nitric Oxide Delivery Device (INOVENT® by Ohmeda™)

- This has absolutely nothing to do with lung isolation except that it may be the only thing that saves you during lung isolation when oxygenation hits the floor.
- This is one special thing you will need to do during some heart, lung, or heart/lung transplants, not to mention a few other selected disaster cases where you can only ventilate one lung.
- Nitric oxide is an inhaled gas delivered by a specially built system. Currently, there is only one system, the Inovent® System manufactured and supplied by Ohmeda™. There are other delivery

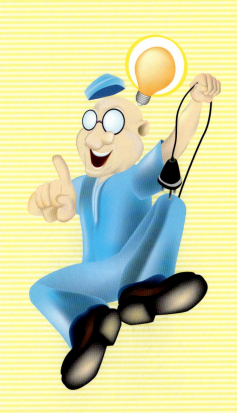

devices currently under investigation awaiting FDA approval but right now, this is the only one you've got, so you may as well know how to set it up and use it.

- The dose of nitric oxide is extremely small, in the 5 ppm to 80 ppm (parts per million) range.

- Nitric oxide is extremely expensive—about $125 per hour of use, up to 96 hours (that's nearly $5000 per day). Of course, it's free for the remainder of the month in use, but the charge recurs at the beginning on the following month if indeed you are still using it.

- Nitric oxide is an attempt to provide a "magic bullet" that can decrease pulmonary artery pressures yet not affect systemic pressures. In spite of its billing, it does not always work and it does not always "spare" the systemic pressures.

- Connect the nitric oxide tank to the Inovent® Delivery Device.

- Open the tank.

Setting Up the System

- Connect the nitric oxide delivery tube to the front of the Inovent®. (There is only one port on the front of the machine that the delivery tube will fit.)

- Connect the other end of the delivery tube to the regulator.

- Connect the electronic cable to the front of the Inovent® and to the regulator.

- Place the regulator on the *inspiratory limb* of your circuit, just as it leaves the anesthesia machine.

- Attach the sampling line to the front of the Inovent® (once again, there is only one port where it will fit).

- Place the other end of the sampling line in the *inspiratory limb* of the circuit, *at least 6 in. proximal to the "Y"*. This will allow you to measure adequately the *inspired* nitric oxide concentration without contamination from exhaled nitric oxide.

- You will need to insert an extra bit of corrugated circuit tubing into the inspiratory limb of your circuit so you can connect the sampling line. These extra pieces of circuit are provided by the manufacturer.

- Remember, you will hook each of these devices up on the *inspiratory* limb because you want to measure the nitric oxide *inspired*.

- Fortunately, each device can only plug into one place on the Inovent®, so the device setup is nearly fool-proof.

- Dial up the nitric oxide concentration you wish to deliver until you get a response you hope to achieve. Keep going until you max out at 80 ppm.

- Notice the amount of inhaled NO_2 (nitrogen dioxide). This is toxic to humans and causes methemoglobinemia. The Inovent® measures the inhaled NO_2 as well as nitric oxide, and any amount of inhaled NO_2 above 3 ppm is unacceptable. You may need to dial back your nitric oxide concentration to reduce the amount of NO_2 you are delivering to the patient.

- Keep an eye on the systemic blood pressure; this "perfect drug" is far from it.

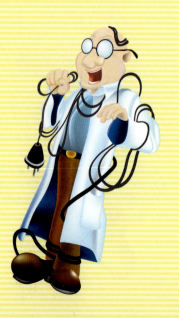

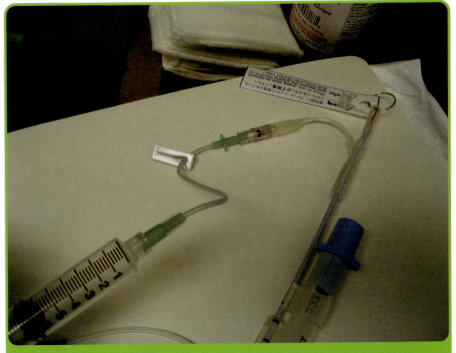

Figure 1. Univent® with T-piece for bronchial blocker inflation.

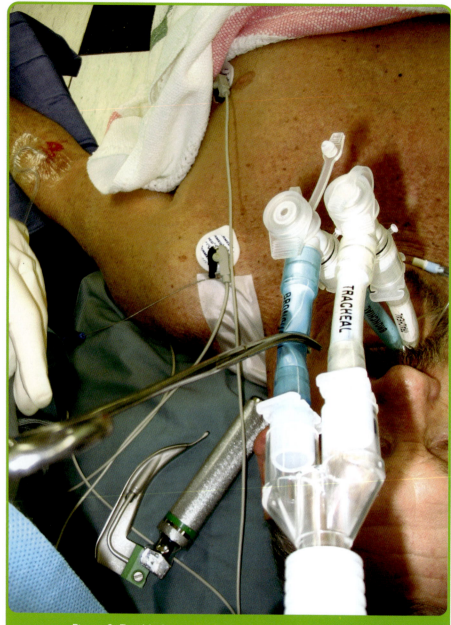

Figure 2. Double-lumen with clamp on bronchial connector.

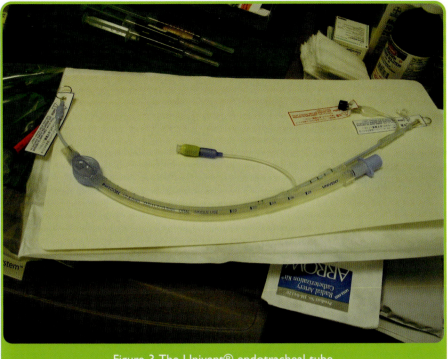

Figure 3. The Univent® endotracheal tube.

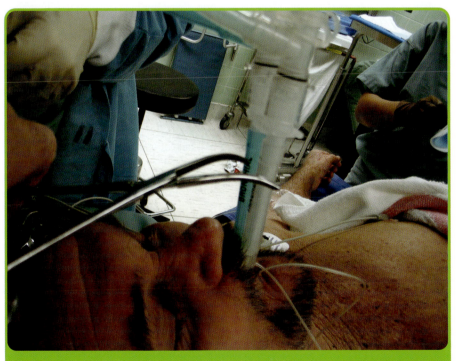

Figure 4. Incorrect double-lumen clamp position.

SUGGESTED READING ARTICLES REGARDING MULTIPLE STRATEGIES

Campos JH. An update on bronchial blockers during lung separation techniques in adults. Anesth Analg 2003;97:1266–74.
* *Review article providing a summary of commonly used bronchial blocking strategies.*

Campos JH, Kernstine KH. A comparison of a left-sided bronco-cath, with the torque control blocker Univent and the wire-guided blocker. Anesth Analg 2003;96:283–9.
* *Study of 64 patients comparing the double-lumen tube, Univent®, and Arndt® endobronchial blocker. Ease of use as well as effectiveness were compared.*

DOUBLE-LUMEN TUBES

Benumof JL. Double-lumen tube position should be routinely determined by fiberoptic bronchoscopy. J Cardiothorac Vasc Anesth 1993;7:513.
* *Editorial discussing the importance of checking position of a double-lumen tube throughout case.*

Benumof JL, Partridge B, Salvatierra C, Gibbins J. Margin of safety in positioning modern double-lumen tubes. Anesthesiology 1987;67:729.
* *Study evaluating margin of safety of both left- and right-sided double-lumen tubes.*

Brodsky JB, Benumof JL, Ehrenwerth J, Ozaki GT. Depth of placement of left double-lumen endobronchial tubes. Anesth Analg 1991;73:570.
* *Study with 101 patients looking at how far to advance a double-lumen tube.*

Cohen E, Kirschner PA, Goldofsky S. Intraoperative manipulation for positioning of double-lumen tubes. Anesthesiology 1988;68:170.
* *Correspndence discussing methods of double-lumen tube manipulation intraoperatively.*

Desiderio DP, Burt M, Kolker AC, et al. The effects of endobronchial cuff inflation on double-lumen endobronchial tube movement after lateral decubitus positioning. J Cardiothorac Vasc Anesth 1997;11: 595–8.
* *Study with 50 patients looking at the change in tube position of a double-lumen tube with the bronchial cuff inflated versus deflated.*

Saito S, Dohi S, Naito H. Alteration of double-lumen endobronchial tube position by flexion and extension of the neck. Anesthesiology 1985;62:696.
* *Correspondence discussing the change in position of a double-lumen tube in 13 patients with flexion and extension of neck.*

Wagner DL, Gammage GW, Wong ML. Tracheal rupture following the insertion of a disposable double-lumen endotracheal tube. Anesthesiology 1985;63:698.
* *Case report of what is considered a bad day at the office with a double-lumen tube.*

THE UNIVENT®

Benumof JL, Gaughan S, Ozaki GT. Operative lung constant positive airway pressure with the Univent bronchial blocker tube. Anesth Analg 1992;74:406.
* *Study with seven patients looking at the effects of CPAP on ventilation and oxygenation.*

Gayes JM. The Univent tube is the best technique for providing one-lung ventilation. Pro: One-lung ventilation is best accomplished with the Univent endotracheal tube. J Cardiothorac Vasc Anesth 1993; 7:103.
* *Article forwarding the idea that the Univent® is the best technique for one-lung ventilation.*

Kamaya H, Krishna PR. New endotracheal tube (Univent tube) for selective blockade of one lung. Anesthesiology 1985;63:342.
* *Correspondence regarding experiences with the Univent® on five patients.*

Schwartz DE, Yost CS, Larson MD. Pneumothorax complicating the use of a Univent endotracheal tube. Anesth Analg 1993;76:443.
* *Case report of a bad day at the office with a Univent®.*

Slinger P. The Univent tube is the best technique for providing one-lung ventilation. Con: The Univent tube is not the best method of providing one-lung ventilation. J Cardiothorac Vasc Anesth 1993; 7:108.
* *The article argues that Univent® is not the best technique for one-lung ventilation, but rather the reason for one-lung ventilation determines the preferred method of lung isolation.*

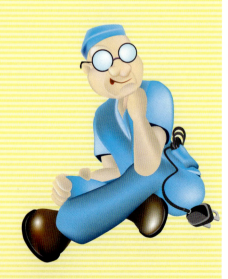

ARNDT® ENDOBRONCHIAL BLOCKER

Arndt GA, Kranner PW, Rusy DA, Love R. Single-lung ventilation in a critically ill patient using a fiberoptically directed wire-guided endobronchial blocker. Anesthesiology 1999;90:1484–6.

- *Case study and discussion of the benefits of the Arndt® Endobronchial blocker in the critically ill. Discusses issues such as ventilation, oxygenation, and ability of patient to tolerate the procedure.*

Sandberg WS. Endobronchial blocker dislodgement leading to pulseless electrical activity. Anesth Analg 2005;100:1728–30.

- *Case report of a bad day at the office with an endobronchial blocker.*

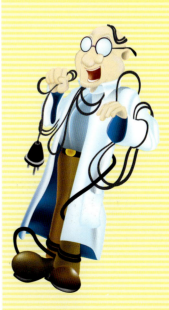

Living Better with Electricity: Pacing

Dan Castillo and Neil Anand

Yes, our lives are merely strange dark interludes in the electrical display of God.

Eugene O'Neill
Strange Interlude, Pt. I,
Act V, 1928

INTRODUCTION

Try to keep the following strange, dark interlude from occurring in your operating room.

"Quick, pace!"

The patient has flatlined and the surgeons have just thrown you a pacing line. You are holding the pacer box.

"Uh. . ."

You keep staring at the pacer box, no more able to figure it out than a Cro-Magnon man trying to figure out how to assemble a Maserati from its component parts.

Let's learn about pacers and avoid such an electrical display.

INDICATIONS

- Inadequate cardiac output due to low heart rate
- Inadequate cardiac output due to *no* heart rate (asystole is what you call bradycardia with attitude)
- Cardiology has a bewildering array of diagnoses that require pacing but they all boil down to the same thing: When the heart doesn't go fast enough, we have to make it go fast.

CONTRAINDICATIONS

- Ventricular fibrillation (Not really a contraindication, you just won't be able to pace in the face of this chaotic rhythm. You need to defibrillate, then turn your attention to pacing.)

EQUIPMENT

- Generates a pulse of current to depolarize a bit of myocardium

PULSE GENERATOR

- Battery
- Output circuit
- Sensing circuit
- Timing circuit

PACER FUNCTION

1. Stimulate cardiac depolarization
2. Sense intrinsic cardiac function
3. Respond to increased metabolic demand by providing rate-responsive pacing

4. Provide diagnostic information stored by the pacemaker

- A machine to deliver your electricity—either a handheld pacing box, an external pacer (a defibrillator machine that can also pace), or an implantable pacer (the surgeons or cardiologists will be putting those in)
- A wire, pad, or esophageal device to get your electricity from the pacing machine to the heart
- That wire can be a pacing Swan sitting in the heart, an implanted wire from an implantable pacer, a wire sewn into the heart (as during open chest procedures), or a wire slid down a pacing port into the heart.
- The pad should be a low-resistance, well-applied device that can get enough electricity through the chest wall to pace the heart. Of note, this is sufficient energy to be uncomfortable to the patient.
- There are esophageal pacers, the concept being that the device is slid down the esophagus to lie directly behind the heart. From there, it's a "short jump" to the heart and a pacing current can pace the heart from this location.
- A working source of energy—that means batteries in the pacing devices and electricity (duh, plug the thing in) for the external pacers. I can see the smirks—don't be surprised that people sometimes forget these basic ideas. In an emergency, your head gets pretty "amped up" and it *is* easy to forget this fundamental concept.

LEAD SYSTEM

Bipolar

- Lead has both negative (cathode) distal and positive (anode) proximal electrodes

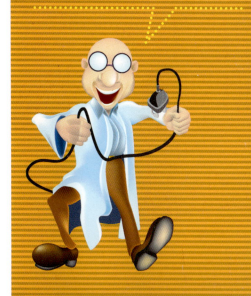

I Thought that Was Hard to Cut

The cable from a defibrillator/pacer costs a pretty penny.

At the end of a case, a technician was cutting the drapes with a scissors, and seemed to be really "gnawing away" at the last bit of drapes.

Ooops!

Cut the cable right in half.

Sort of a Pacer Story

I was called to sedate a patient for cardioversion. He had atrial fibrillation with a rapid response.

On arrival, the patient's saturation was in the mid-80s. I had the impertinence to ask whether the patient needed some ventilatory support. After intubation, his saturation picked up, and guess what?

His atrial fibrillation went away. What do you know—fix the *root* problem (hypoxemia) and you fix the symptom (atrial fibrillation).

- Separated by 1 cm
- Larger diameter: more prone to fracture
- Compatible with ICD

Unipolar

- Negative (cathode) electrode in contact with heart
- Positive (anode) electrode: metal casing of pulse generator
- Prone to oversensing
- Not compatible with ICD

BEWARE THE "CAME FROM THE CATH LAB" PACER

- This scene plays out in the cardiac room and you need to know it's "out there."
- In the cath lab, a patient has trouble with inferior ischemia (that most often implies the right coronary, and trouble with the right coronary often means trouble with the conduction system).
- The cardiologists place pacing wires in the femoral sheath.
- As the patient rolls to the OR, blankets are placed over the patient.
- This patient may be *completely* pacer dependent.
- Down they come to the OR. You move the patient over to the OR table, a blanket pulls back, hooks the pacing wire, and pulls it out. No one sees and you wonder why the patient looks so bad.
- You must be a meticulous maniac when someone comes down paced!
- See that wire, see where it goes, see that pacer box. Let no harm or evil befall it—guard it with your life!

PHILOSOPHY OF PACING

- Like everything else in anesthesia, get familiar with this stuff before you *have* to do it. Asystole and impeding death are not times to get your "first look" at a pacing box.
- There is a dizzying array of buttons and there's precious little "obvious" about some pacing boxes, so play with them ahead of time.
- Make sure you *have* a pacing box if you anticipate the need. Many a foul-up has occurred because of, "Hey, who's got the pacer? I thought you had it! I thought *you* had it!"

- In a similar vein, get used to the pacing functions on the defibrillator. An emergency is not a good time for "Um, could you in-service me on this while they do chest compressions?"
- Don't forget the basics of medicine: a rhythm disturbance usually has a cause. Treat the cause rather than the symptom. Make sure, by lab studies, that there is not some chemical imbalance contributing to rhythm troubles. The pacer is not the cure for hypoxemia, hypothyroidism, hypoglycemia, or any of a dozen other disturbances.
- In a similar way, the pacer is not the cure to coronary disease. Yes, a pacer helps re-establish a rhythm after an inferior MI, but consider revascularization as *the* cure, not just pacing.

HISTORY AND PHYSICAL

- Scour the chart and look over the patient.
- Lo and behold, you may discover a lump under the skin that is—surprise, surprise—a pacer.
- If the patient already has a pacer, make sure you know what kind it is.
- Is the pacer working? When was it last checked? Has the patient had symptoms of pacer failure (syncope, dizziness)?
- If the patient has an AICD, then you will need to have it turned off prior to an operation so it won't mistake "Bovey" for "fibrillation."
- Don't be throwing magnets on pacers and AICDs. That can screw them up and reprogram them to just about anything.
- If you turn off an AICD, remember that the patient is *still* at risk for fatal rhythms (their heart is still bad; turning off the AICD doesn't miraculously make them healthy). So place external pads and be ready to defibrillate.

TECHNIQUE

- Fortunately, pacer boxes are designed with the "doctor-standing-there-like-deer-in-headlights" in mind.
- If you just turn the dumb thing on, as done by pressing the "On" button, the pacer will automatically go to a good and reasonable setting.
- 80 beats per minute

- 10 milliamps of juice
- Inhibited mode
- So if you hook up a ventricular line only, your pacer will be in the VVI mode—*ventricular* paced, *ventricular* sensed, *inhibited*—when it "sees" a signal.
- Although you may have to adjust later, and yes, that will involve switching more buttons and dials, this initial setting will get you out of most troubles.
- Can't pace? Make sure the pacer is hooked up correctly, double-check the connections, and make sure the battery is working or the defibrillator/pacer is plugged in.
- If all is OK, then you may be in a "tough to pace" spot (scar tissue), so increase the amperage all the way to 20 mA. If by 20 mA you can't pace, think about putting the wire in a different spot.
- If the surgeon places wires in the atrium, then you have a few options.
- If there is no AV block, then you can just atrially pace.
- If there is an AV block, then an atrial rhythm won't get past the AV roadblock and you'll need to pace both atrium and ventricle.
- What if the patient is in atrial fibrillation? Then pacing atrially won't help. The paced signal will be lost in the shuffle of the chaotic atrial rhythm, so you'll need to V pace.
- You can pace through a pacing Swan. Now this can be a little trickier than directly sewn-in wires placed during cardiac surgery. With a Swan, you must hope that part of the Swan is resting on just the right spot so you can pace there. Usually, this works out fine but if the Swan is repositioned (for example, pulls back during transport), then you don't have contact in the right spot and you can lose your pacing.
- You can also slip a wire down a Swan (a Pace Port Swan) until the pacing wire hits the right ventricle, and you can pace from there.
- Zoll pacing pads go on the patient's chest. Where you place them matters because the current must get across the meat of the heart. So wherever you place them, draw an imaginary line from one pad to the other and ask yourself, "Does that path put current across enough heart meat to give me a paced beat?" (or, for that matter, a defibrillating jolt).
- Once you've placed the pads, take a good look at the controls on the machine. Just as you can be freaked out with a pacer box, you can be freaked out with the controls on an external pacer. Take the time to "get to know" the controls.
- What about a combo internal-external approach? Enter the esophageal pacer. Why pace all the way from the outside when you can jump across most of the chest and lay a pacer right behind the heart and pace away?

PACER MALFUNCTION

1. Failure to output
2. Failure to capture
3. Inappropriate sensing: undersensing or oversensing
4. Inappropriate pacemaker rate

Failure to Output
Absence of Pacemaker Spikes
- Fracture of pacemaker lead
- Dead battery
- Disconnection of lead from pulse generator unit
- Cross-talk: atrial output sensed by vent lead
- Oversensing

Failure to Capture
- Spikes on the EKG are not followed by a myocardial depolarization

Inappropriate Sensing: Undersensing
- Pacemaker incorrectly misses an intrinsic depolarization and fires
- The pacer is not seeing what the heart is doing and is pacing at times when it shouldn't
- After a native QRS, the pacer trace shows a ventricle pace (VP) and a spike appears on the EKG.
- The pacer failed to sense the native QRS and paced regardless.
- Notice that capturing may or may not occur depending on the electrical status of the myocardium.

Inappropriate Sensing: Oversensing
- There is detection by the pacer of electrical activity not of cardiac origin that will inhibit pacing activity.
- Pectoralis major: myopotentials oversensed (fasciculation from succinylcholine)
- Electrocautery

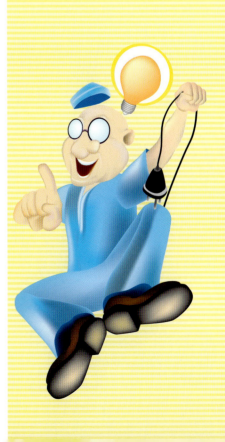

PREANESTHETIC EVALUATION

No special laboratory tests or CXRs are needed on a routine basis on patients with pacemakers, unless indicated by patient disease, medications, or planned intervention.

PERIOPERATIVE INTERROGATION

- Determine the indication for and date of initial device placement.
- Determine the last generator test date and battery status.
- Obtain a history of generator events.
- Obtain the current program information and manufacturer.
- Ensure that generator discharges become mechanical systoles.
- Ensure the magnet detection is enabled.
- Determine whether the pacing mode should be reprogrammed.

REPROGRAMMING

- Appropriate reprogramming is the safest way to reduce intraoperative complications.

ASYNCHRONOUS PACING

- Ensures that no over- or undersensing will take place
- Will not protect the device from internal damage or reset caused by electromagnetic interference (EMI)
- Rate responsiveness and other features should be disabled.
- Hysteresis, sleep rate, AV search, and so on

REPROGRAMMING INDICATIONS

- Any rate-responsive device
- Special pacing indications (HOCM, DCM, Peds)
- Pacemaker-dependent patient
- Major procedure in the chest or abdomen
- Special procedures: lithotripsy, TUR, uterine hysteroscopy, MRI, ECT, nerve stimulator testing

INTRAOPERATIVE OR PROCEDURE MANAGEMENT

- No special monitoring or anesthesia technique is required.

KEEP IN MIND

- The EKG monitor should have the ability to detect pacemaker discharges (filtering should be disabled).
- Ensure that myocardial electrical activity is converted to mechanical activity: pulse oximetry, pulse palpation, cardiac auscultation, plethysmogram, arterial waveform.

ELECTROCAUTERY

- *Avoid* if possible
- Bipolar preferred
- If monopolar is necessary, keep the pacemaker generator out of the path between the cautery and bovie pad, and use in short bursts to avoid long periods of asystole.

DO NOT USE A MAGNET WITH YOUR PACER!
WHAT DOES A MAGNET DO?

- Don't put magnets on pacers if you don't know what the magnet will do to it.
- Some pacers are magnet-disabled and must be enabled before going to the OR.
- Is part of the preoperative pacer interrogation to ask what the pacer will do in the presence of a magnet?
- In general, when a magnet is placed on a pacer it will go to an asynchronous mode.
- The most important thing to do is to be prepared in case the pacer fails, and have transcutaneous or transvenous pacing capability available in the OR.
- Use a magnet only in emergencies when the pacer fails and the patient becomes asystolic or severely bradycardic because whatever mode the pacer goes into when the magnet is applied will be better than the rhythm the patient is having.

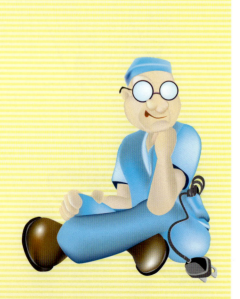

POST-ANESTHESIA PACEMAKER EVALUATION

- A pacemaker that was reprogrammed for anesthesia should be reset appropriately.
- For non-reprogrammed devices, interrogation is recommended. Ensure functioning and battery life if electrocautery was used.

IMPLANTABLE CARDIOVERTER-DEFIBRILLATOR (ICD)

- Major medical breakout for patients with ventricular tachydysrhythmias
- Prevents death from malignant ventricular tachydysrhythmias
- Superior to antiarrhythmic drugs
- Approved by US FDA in 1985

ICD INDICATIONS

- Ventricular tachycardia
- Ventricular fibrillation
- Brugada syndrome (RBBB, S-T elevations V1-V3)
- Arrhythmogenic right ventricular dysplasia
- Long Q-T syndrome
- Hypertrophic cardiomyopathy
- Prophylactic use post-MI, EF < 30%

MAGNETS AND ICDs

- Most devices will suspend tachydysrhythmia detection.
- Some devices can be programmed to ignore magnet placement (Angeion, CPI, Ventritex).

- With some CPI devices, 30 seconds of magnet placement permanently disables antitachycardia therapy.
- In general, magnets will not affect antibradycardia pacing mode or rate except ELA Defender and Telectronic Guardian.

PRE-ANESTHETIC EVALUATION

- All ICDs should have their antitachycardia therapy disabled prior to induction or procedure.

INTRAOPERATIVE MANAGEMENT

- No special monitoring or anesthetic technique
- Electrocardiography monitoring
- Ability of delivering external cardioversion or defibrillation

POST-ANESTHESIA EVALUATION

The ICD must be reinterrogated and re-enabled, all events should be reviewed, and the counter should be cleared.

GLITCHES

- Most pacer glitches are common-sense problems:
  - Didn't think to get the pacer box
  - Forgot to make sure it has batteries
  - "I never worked with this kind before, how does this work?"

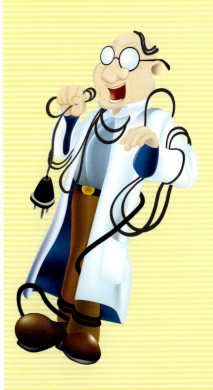

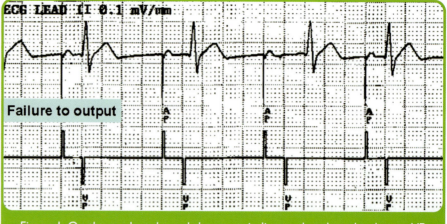

Figure 1. On the marker channel the pacer indicates that there has been a VP (ventricular pace) yet there is no spike indicating output in the EKG trace. Notice that AP (atrial pace) does present a spike corresponding with output in the EKG tracing.

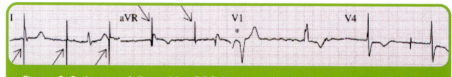

Figure 2. Spikes not followed by QRS (capturing), notice that the output of the pacer is inadequate suggesting a possible failure to sense.

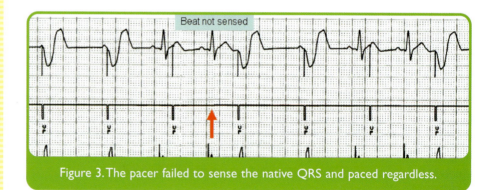

Figure 3. The pacer failed to sense the native QRS and paced regardless.

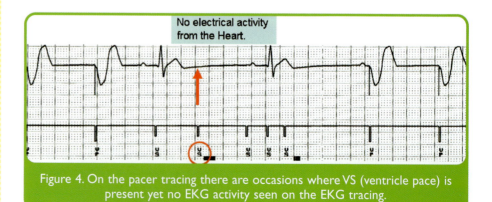

Figure 4. On the pacer tracing there are occasions where VS (ventricle pace) is present yet no EKG activity seen on the EKG tracing.

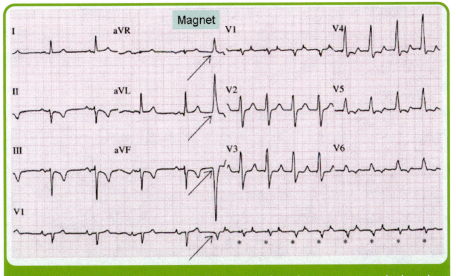

Figure 5. The arrows are pointing the moment when the magnet is applied to the pacemaker, notice that the pacer starts firing asynchronously.

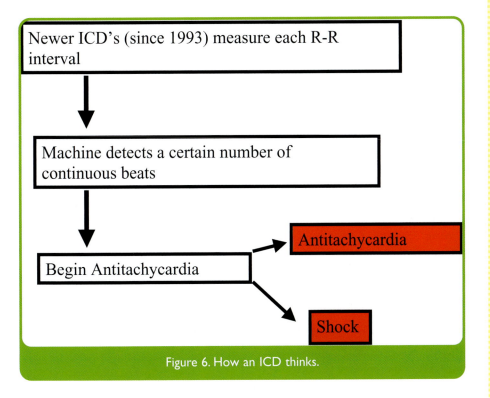

Figure 6. How an ICD thinks.

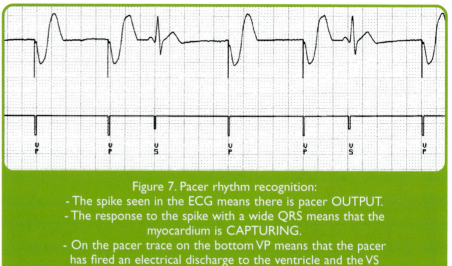

Figure 7. Pacer rhythm recognition:
- The spike seen in the ECG means there is pacer OUTPUT.
- The response to the spike with a wide QRS means that the myocardium is CAPTURING.
- On the pacer trace on the bottom VP means that the pacer has fired an electrical discharge to the ventricle and the VS means that the pacer has sensed electrical activity in the ventricle.

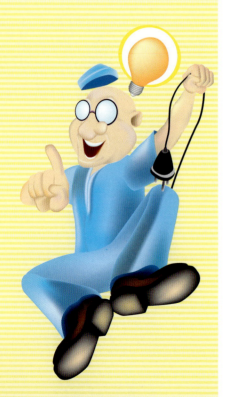

SUGGESTED READING

American Society of Anesthesiologists Task Force. Practice advisory for the perioperative management of patient with cardiac rhythm management devices: Pacemakers and implantable cardioverter-defibrillators. Anesthesiology 2005;103: 186–98.
- *A recent report that discusses the perioperative management of patients with cardiac rhythm management devices. This paper will tell you how to avoid the most common mistakes that occur during the perioperative setting.*

Anand NK, Maguire DP. Anesthetic implications for patients with rate-responsive pacemakers. Sem Cardiothor Vasc Anesth 2005;9:251–9.
- *This is a cool review article on the management of rate-responsive pacemakers.*

Atlee JL, Bernstein AD. Cardiac rhythm management devices (Part 1). Anesthesiology 2001;95:1265–80.
- *This is part one of the definitive anesthesiology article on pacemakers and ICDs from the Jedi Master of pacemaker anesthesiology. The first part discusses indications for CRMD use and describes device selection and function.*

Atlee JL, Bernstein AD. Cardiac rhythm management devices (Part 2). Anesthesiology 2001;95:1492–506.
- *This is part two of the definitive anesthesiology article on pacemakers and ICDs. The second part discusses perioperative management of cardiac dysrhythmias.*

Atlee JL, Bosnjak ZK. Mechanisms for cardiac dysrhythmias during anesthesia. Anesthesiology 1990;72:347–74.
- *This is another review article from the Jedi Master, and this paper also describes mechanisms and treatment of perioperative cardiac dysrhythmias.*

Del Nido P, Goldman BS. Temporary epicardial pacing after open heart surgery: Complications and prevention. J Card Surg 1989 Mar;4(1):99–103.
- *This report describes several clinical complications: failure of ventricular sensing, failure of ventricular capture, bleeding from a right ventricular laceration with tamponade, avulsion of a side branch from a saphenous vein coronary bypass graft, and perforation of the superior epigastric artery.*

El-Sherif N, Samet P, (eds). *Cardiac Pacing and Electrophysiology.* Philadelphia: Saunders, 1991.
- *This book gives an in-depth look at the technical functioning of pacemakers.*

Gal ThJ, Chaet MS, Novitzky D. Laceration of a saphenous vein graft by an epicardial pacemaker wire. J Cardiovasc Surg (Torino) 1998 Apr;39(2):221–2.
- *A case of cardiac tamponade following removal of an atrial pacing wire.*

Gregoratos G, Cheitlin M, Conill A, et al. ACC/AHA guidelines for implantation of cardiac pacemakers and anti-arrhythmia devices: A report of the ACC/AHA Task Force on Practice Guidelines (Committee on Pacemaker Implantation). J AM Coll Cardio 1998;31:1175–206.

- *These are practice guidelines for the insertion of pacemakers.*

Hoidal CR. Pericardial tamponade after removal of an epicardial pacemaker wire. Crit Care Med 1986 Apr;14(4):305–6.
- *A case of pericardial tamponade after removal of an epicardial pacemaker wire is presented.*

Pacifico AD. Management of temporary epicardial ventricular pacing wires. J Card Surg 1998 May;13(3):228.
- *This is a great paper and is the perfect supplemental information about epicardial pacemakers for this chapter.*

Smith JA, Tatoulis J. Right atrial perforation by a temporary epicardial pacing wire. Ann Thorac Surg 1990 Jul;50(1):141–2.
- *Cardiac perforation by an epicardial pacing wire is an extremely rare event, yet this is a case of right atrial perforation occurring 10 hours after coronary artery bypass grafting.*

Toprak V, Yentur A, Sakarya M. Anesthetic management of severe bradycardia during general anesthesia using temporary cardiac pacing. Br J Anaesth 2002;89(4):655–7.
- *A case report on a 65-year-old female patient who developed bradycardia and hypotension during surgery and was treated with epicardial pacing.*

Trankina MF, White RD. Perioperative cardiac pacing using an atrioventricular pacing pulmonary artery catheter. J Cardiothorac Anesth 1989 Apr;3(2):154–62.
- *This article explains the use of pacing pulmonary artery catheters and is a good supplement for this chapter.*

http://www.hrsonline.org
- *Heart Rhythm Society, formerly North American Society of Pacing and Electrophysiology (NAPSE) 202-464-3400.*

http://www.lhsc.on.ca/critcare/ucicu/procs/epipace.htm
- *London website on the epicardial pacemaker setup.*

http://www.medtronic.com/brady/clinician/medtronicpacing/5388dc.html
- *Medtronics website on their dual- and single-chamber epicardial pacemaker.*

Important Manufacturer Contacts

Medtronic: 800-Medtronic, http://www.medtronic.com
St. Jude: 800-PaceICD, http://www.sjm.com
Guidant: 800-Cardiac, http://www.guidant.com
Biotronik: 800-547-9001, http://www.biotronik.com

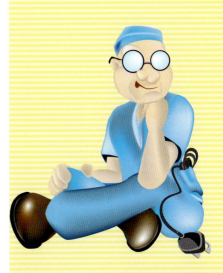

Echo, Echo, Echo: Transesophageal Echocardiography

Jay Grossman and Jonathan Katz

INTRODUCTION

Transesophageal echocardiography (TEE) is the newest and coolest thing that has happened to anesthesia since PA catheters. It's definitely a rush when your colleagues call you into the room and ask you to do the echo because no one else there knows how to use all the knobs on the machine or knows what they mean. You can be way cool and use phrases like "axial resolution" and "shift the baseline because we're aliasing here" to mystify your friends and really hotdog in front of the surgeons (who, by the way, know even less than you do).

Why is it cool? Because as anesthesiologists, we always looked at numbers (CVP, PA) and we *inferred* what we thought was going on. With TEE, we *see* everything! No inferring, no guessing: reality TV!

It's not just for open-heart surgery, either. Anytime you want to know what's going on with the heart—be it vascular surgery or transplant surgery or a patient going south—just drop a TEE probe in and check it out.

INDICATIONS

- Assessing myocardial function
- Assessing valvular function
- Assessing aortic pathology (dissection, aneurysm)
- Looking for pericardial effusion
- Seeing anomalies in the heart, like renal cell cancer crawling up the IVC into the right atrium, left atrial myxomas, clots in the atrium, and so on
- In cardiac bypass surgery, you look closely at wall function, looking for regional wall motion abnormalities—a sign of coronary insufficiency.
- If you aren't sure what's happening with the patient (in other words: if you can't make sense of the hemodynamics), put in the probe.
- Looking for intracardiac air. The TEE is exquisitely sensitive to air bubbles.

CONTRAINDICATIONS

- All contraindications have to do with the passage of the probe into the esophagus. If you rip it, you own it!
- Meckel's diverticulum
- Esophageal stricture
- Esophageal surgery (either in the past or planned today)
- Massive upper pharyngeal tumor (you might disrupt it as you pass the probe)

RELATIVE CONTRAINDICATIONS

- Cervical instability. Don't risk making the patient a cervical quadriplegic (a.k.a. "C Quad"). If you can pass the probe without extending the neck, great.
- Esophageal varices. Not a contraindication—we put them down liver transplant patients all the time (they all have varices).

EQUIPMENT

- TEE probe (adult and pediatric size)
- TEE monitor (expensive!)
- Bite block. You should use a bite block on everyone; that way, you won't forget. You can really ruin the probe if someone inadvertently bites down on this and scores the bundles inside.
- A device to record the exam. Most machines come with a VCR but digital archiving is best.
- A tip protector. As we say in Miami, *la puntica* is where the money is. The tip of the probe is seriously high-tech and you should be sure to protect it before or after the case. (Note: These probes cost anywhere from $50,000 to $75,000 each, "*con cuidado*!")
- The probe is disinfected by placing it in a disinfection solution. You don't autoclave these!

It's that same bad echo again!

Tom Petty and the Heartbreakers
"Echo"

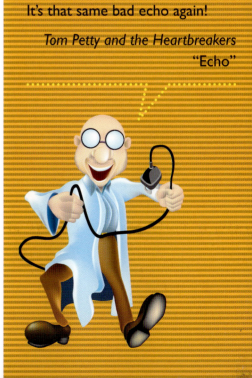

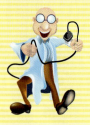

CARDIOLOGISTS

- The real reason you and not the cardiologist are now doing TEE in the OR is because it doesn't pay enough for them to want to break up their day, put on scrubs, and come to the OR to read your TEE when they could be making the big bucks in the cath lab. However, if you're not sure about something you see, most of them will come (if you beg nicely) and give their opinion as to what you're seeing.

- Pediatric cardiology is a totally different deal. These cases are very complex and most of us mere mortals need someone in there who's familiar with these inversions and other problems of congenital malformations.

THE ZEN OF TEE

- Once you get into TEE, there's a lot to learn. To pass the SCA exam, you must read and learn a lot of stuff. (If I may plug the author of this book, Dr. Gallagher's *Board Stiff TEE* is a great review for the test.)

- Having said that, there are only a few things that most anesthesiologists must know to make intelligent decisions reading TEEs.

- Is the heart empty or full? The vast majority of patients that are hemodynamically unstable can be diagnosed by this simple and easy assessment.

- Is the ventricle good or bad? Many mathematical models are used to access this stuff. If you have nothing better to do, you can study them, memorize them, and regurgitate them at cocktail parties or you can, with a minimal amount of practice, be able to eyeball these pictures and decide, "Good ventricle, bad ventricle." See, I told you this was cool!

- Is there an effusion? Once you learn to delineate the borders of the heart, you can easily see fluid around it. Is it *so* much fluid that the heart isn't filling right? (Hmmm, didn't I learn something about this in medical school? Was it *tamponade*?)

- Anything obviously wrong with the valves? Obvious regurgitation or stenosis? Is there crud hanging off the mitral or aortic? You'll see it if it's obvious. That makes sense, doesn't it?

- Aortic pathology is a bit more difficult to master. Aortic dissections can be tough to call and artifacts can fool you here.

- Artifacts are those pesky creatures that make you think you're seeing something when you're not. There are a couple different ones like "reverberations," "side lobe artifacts," "acoustic shadowing," and "mirroring." The bottom line here is that if you're not sure if it's an artifact or the real thing, look at the structure in another view. You can see just about everything from two different views. So if you have any doubts, try to find it in another view.

- TEE "sees" through fluid and tissue but can't see through air. As you pull the TEE probe up (cephalad for those who prefer anatomic terms), you run into the left mainstem bronchus and lose your signal. It's conveniently located so you can't see much of the ascending aorta or the bottom (inferior portion) of the transverse aorta.

PHYSICS OF THE TEE

- OK, this is the part no one likes. You must learn something about the physics of ultrasound to make sense of the TEE. Listen, if you learned College Physics and got into medical school, you can learn this stuff too. It isn't *that* hard!

- The TEE probe is very pricey. These cost anywhere from $50K to $75K each (!) and have a transducer at the end (which, by the way, is *very delicate*, so handle with care) and a control handle that allows you to flex/anteflex, rotate, and laterally flex the transducer. The other thing it allows is control of the multiplane angle (more on this later).

- TEE produces ultrasound waves that are above the range of human hearing, (which tops out at about 20 kHz). Clinical echocardiography uses frequencies from 2 MHz to 10 MHz. The higher frequencies are more easily manipulated and focused. Image resolution also increases with increasing frequency.

- An electrical signal is sent to the transducer, which consists of a piezoelectric crystal, a lens for focusing, and some backing material to dampen the vibrations quickly. The signal causes the piezoelectric crystal to vibrate and send out the ultrasound waves.

- These ultrasound waves strike their target, bounce back, and are received by the same crystal, which now acts as a receiver. Images are created from the reflected signal. A good analogy is radar, which acts in much the same way but uses different frequencies.

- Sound waves travel well through fluids but poorly through air. Therefore, it's a good idea to suck out the stomach with an NG tube before inserting the TEE probe.

- Sound waves are characterized by their frequency, which is the number of cycles per second, and their wavelength. Low frequencies have longer wavelengths and penetrate further. Higher frequencies have shorter wavelengths and have better resolution but don't penetrate as far.

- A sound wave loses energy as it travels through tissue. This loss of signal strength is called attenuation.

- When a sound wave hits a tissue of different density, it can refract, or bend (think: the straw sitting in a glass of water seems bent), or it can reflect, or bounce back, to the transducer.

- The reflected signal is used to create the image.

- The transducers on the TEE probe are usually set up as a "phased array" of transducers—many transducers sending out many signals that are manipulated by a computer to produce a clearer image.

- The axial resolution is the ability to tell how far apart things are along the axis of the beam. If the next line in this book is the beam, then axial resolution is telling that the first two letters are close together and the next two are far apart:

AB (close together)   A   B (far apart)

- Lateral resolution is the ability to tell two things apart in a line perpendicular to the beam:

A

B (close together)

A

B (far apart)

- TEE probes can use different modes.

- M-mode (the M stands for "motion") looks at a pencil-like shot of the heart. Cardiologists like this one because no one else can understand what's going on when you look at it.

- 2-D is the most common mode. This is the one that gives you the "picture of the heart in action" shot.

- Doppler imaging relies on the scatter of the ultrasound signal from red blood cells.

- Remember that College Physics course? Of course you do. Blood coming toward the transducer gives a higher frequency signal than blood going away from the transducer. The Doppler shift, remember?

The train whistle sounds at a higher pitch as the train is coming toward you, and the whistle sounds at a lower pitch when the train is moving away from you. Now you remember, right!

- You get the most accurate measurements form Doppler signals when the ultrasound beam is parallel to the direction of blood flow. If there's more than a 20° angle imposed, the resulting Doppler signal is inaccurate.

- Doppler signals are cool because they give you flow velocities. Flow velocities can be used to calculate pressure gradients based on the simplified Bernoulli equation:

$$\text{Pressure (in Torrs)} = 4 \times \text{velocity}^2$$

- For the Bernoulli equation to work, the velocity must be expressed in m/sec. (Note: When reading velocities off the TEE machine, they are expressed in cm/sec, so you must convert).

- When the flow velocity exceeds a certain limit (called the Nyquest limit), the transducer is "fooled" and gives an inaccurate signal. This is a problem called aliasing.

- In pulse wave Doppler imaging, the ultrasound crystal first sends out a "pulse" of ultrasound and then turns off to "receive" the returning signal. Because it must "wait" for the returning signal before it can transmit another "pulse," the number of pulses it can send at any given time is limited. This limits the flow velocities it can accurately measure without "aliasing."

- The good thing about pulse wave Doppler imaging is that you can put the cursor (or sample volume) right where you want it and measure velocities at that point.

- For things like the mitral and tricuspid valves where velocities are relatively low, this works great. For high velocity flows, like aortic stenosis, you need continuous wave Doppler imaging.

- Continuous wave Doppler imaging works by having one crystal sending out a signal continuously and another crystal in receive mode constantly receiving the return signal.

- Continuous wave Doppler imaging is great for high velocities but the transducer can't tell you exactly where that velocity is. It can't pinpoint it like pulse wave Doppler imaging. This makes it vulnerable to something called "range ambiguity," another term to make your life just a little more difficult!

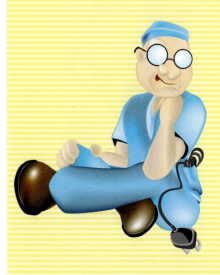

- To summarize: Pulse wave Doppler imaging is good for low-flow velocities and can pinpoint from where the "sample" is coming. It's subject to "aliasing" at higher velocities (the Nyquest limit). Continuous wave Doppler imaging can "see" high velocities but cannot pinpoint where the sample is coming from and is therefore subject to range ambiguities.

- This is not easy stuff, so if it throws you for a loop, you're not alone. This is one of the more difficult aspects of learning TEE.

- Color Doppler imaging allows you to visualize the flows and velocities. By convention, blue shows flow *away* from the transducer, red shows flow *toward* the transducer: R/T, B/A. Variance or turbulent flow is shown in green.

- In the 2-D mode, you can adjust the frequency of the transducer signal. High frequencies are good for detail but don't penetrate very far. Low frequencies are good for deeper objects (they penetrate further) but don't allow as great details.

- The depth control allows you to adjust the image so that you can magnify certain things or fit more things on the screen. Depth is indicated on the side of the screen.

- Lower depths are use to magnify parts of images. Higher depth numbers allow you to see more of the image. Don't be afraid to play with this knob.

- The multiplane angle is the angle at which the plane of the ultrasound is slicing through the heart. It ranges from 0° to 180° and is indicated on the top of the image. It is changed by a set of buttons on the handle of the probe. One button increases the angle and the other decreases it. This allows you to get multiple views at a particular depth.

IMAGES

- There are 20 standard views that the American Board of Echocardiology says you should know. You can find them and review them in agonizing detail if you wish; they are in all major echo textbooks. Or you can just learn a few that will give you what you need to know.

- The mid-esophageal four chamber view: Stick the probe in and advance to around 40 cm, then slightly retroflex the probe. Voila! There's the four-chamber view.

- Look at the right and left atrium. Big? Normal?

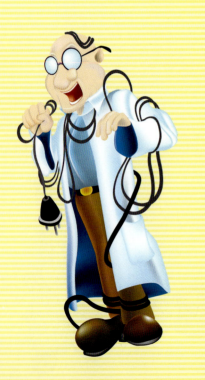

- Look at the mitral valve. Does it open and close? Any lesions (anomalies)? String-like things gyrating above the valve, as in ruptured chordae?

- Put color flow Doppler on the mitral valve. Any regurgitation?

- In the four-chamber view, advance the multiplane angle to 120°. Turn the probe slightly to the right. This is the long-axis aortic valve view.

- Look at the leaflets: Do they close OK?

- Use color flow Doppler: Is there AI?

- Use the multiplane angle to go back to around 45°. You should see the aortic valve in the short axis view (a.k.a. the Mercedes Benz sign). Move the probe in and out slightly. This will allow you to see the valve leaflets and how they're opening and closing. Are they sclerotic and laden with trash, or are they smooth and sexy like they're supposed to be?

- Go back to the four-chamber view (change the multiplane angle back to 0°).

- Advance the probe into the stomach and flex the probe. This is the transgastric short axis view (or as it's affectionately known, the donut).

- Do all the walls move? Does one wall not move very much? If that's the case, then that wall would be hypokinetic. If it doesn't move at all, it's akinetic.

- The anterior and anterior septal walls are supplied by the LAD; the lateral and posterior walls by the circumflex artery; and the inferior and septal walls by the right coronary.

- Look at the papillary muscles. Look at how far apart they are when you start the case. Check them again after bypass. Are they "kissing" now? If they're that close together, then your patient needs volume.

- Eyeball the ejection fraction: What's the difference between systole and diastole? 50%? 30%? 15%? You should be able to give a pretty good estimate of left ventricular function based on this value.

- Go back to the four-chamber view: Is the heart shaped like a football (good!) or basketball (bad!). A big dilated heart looks more like a basketball then a normal heart that's more football-shaped.

- Really, the most important thing is to look at the heart before you start and compare it to the pictures you get as you go along. That's the great thing about TEE: It's a visual thing, so you really don't have to learn all the details to be able to use it well. Just look and compare images. If you do that, you'll be amazed at how easy this becomes.

HISTORY AND PHYSICAL

- You don't want to put the probe in anyone who has any type of esophageal pathology like diverticulum, prior surgery, radiation therapy, . . . you get the picture. Esophageal tears can be deadly and you don't want to be the cause of one of those puppies.
- Don't even think about placing one of these nasally—*forget about it!*
- Empty vs. full. Many times you will be called in to settle this debate. TEE is very handy for this. You'll often get the "he can't be empty, the CVP is 24" thing. You'll be truly amazed at how often the patient *really is empty!* Look at the donut view—are the papillary muscles "kissing"? If they're smooching, he's empty!
- Be aware that you can cause a hemodynamic bump with the insertion of the probe. If you're looking for aortic dissections, this can, um, open things up a little more, as we say.

TECHNIQUE

- You want the probe in the unlocked position. You want it to be able to move easily. You don't want it stiff—the stiff TEE will do damage.
- Insert an NG tube into the *mouth* and suction the stomach/esophagus first.
- Most of your TEEs will be performed on anesthetized patients. That's a good thing! It's hard to sedate awake patients for TEE. They really don't like it! If you do have to do it, topicalize the mouth and use your favorite cocktail of sedation. Where I work, we use a lot of dexmedetomidine, which seems to work pretty well.
- Place a bite block.
- Lubricate the probe.
- Make sure the probe works before placing it in the patient.
- Lift the chin and extend the neck.
- Slide in the probe. Usually, it'll get hung up at about 15 cm to 20 cm in the posterior pharynx. Advance it slowly.
- Don't—I repeat—don't grab the probe with a fist and ram it down. Use your fingers only.

- If you're still having trouble, try putting a laryngoscope in the mouth, lift, and advance under direct vision.
- Record the study.
- When finished, withdraw the probe and put it somewhere safe so it can be cleaned. Take care of it—remember it costs a bundle and it's fragile.

GLITCHES

- The number one complication of TEE is that you forget about the patient. True story: I was once reminded by a surgeon that the pressure was very low because I was so enthralled by what I was seeing, I wasn't paying attention to the *patient*. Yeah, TEE is definitely the coolest thing to happen to anesthesia since fentanyl lollipops, *but don't forget about the patient!*
- *Don't force the probe down anyone's throat!* Esophageal tears can be fatal quickly. If it doesn't go, use an epicardial probe.
- The probe will quickly overheat and can cause burns if left in any of the Doppler modes, including color flow Doppler. Either disconnect the probe when not in use or put it in the 2-D mode and freeze the picture.
- This chapter was written for someone wishing to get a handle on TEE. It was not intended as an authoritative text on the subject. The day-to-day use of TEE really involves interpretation of basic things: full/empty, ventricle good/bad, effusion yes/no. Most importantly, practice with the device! Turn the knobs and see what they do. You won't hurt anything. The machine can't throw out death rays that evaporate the heart.

DOING THE "QUICKIE" EXAM

- First, put an NG tube in through the mouth (better known as the "OG") and suck out the stomach.
- Insert the probe.
- Go to about 40 cm to get the mid-esophageal four-chamber view.
- Look at the heart: normal or dilated? Full or empty?
- Walls move or don't? Transgastric short-axis view is the best (the donut!).
- Put color flow Doppler on the valves. Any regurgitation? Remember: red toward, blue away, green turbulence.

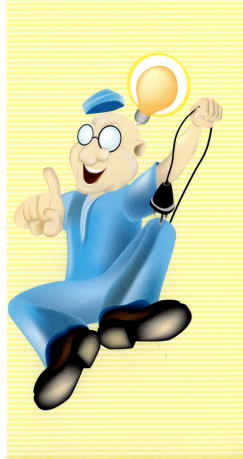

- How much? If the regurgitant jet fills more than half of the atrium or the LVOT, it's classified as 4+. All else is irrelevant.
- Stenosis? Shows up as turbulent flow on color flow Doppler imaging during systole.

REAL LIFE MISADVENTURES (NO, NOT AFFAIRS)

- Into the room we go, called in because the numbers and hemodynamics don't make sense (once again!). TEE should tell us what's up.
- Patient is having a big abdominal procedure and had huge retractors in, pulled right up against the diaphragm.
- Sure enough, the CVP was 25 but the patient had respiratory variation on the arterial line. That respiratory variation said *h-y-p-o-v-o-l-e-m-i-a*.
- We place the TEE–in the transgastric short-axis view, the ventricular walls were kissing, indicative of hypovolemia.
- The big retractors were falsely elevating the CVP but the arterial line was "true blue" (as it always is when you see respiratory variation) in letting us know that the volume status was low.
- Thank you, TEE.
- And yes, thank you, good old-fashioned arterial line.

- While running the floor one day, I'm told that there is a lower abdominal case that is having a lot of hemorrhage.
- I go into the room and find out that there is a greater than 6.5-*l* blood loss that has been kept up with by our outstanding anesthesia staff. All labs are OK and surgeons are starting to close. Cool!
- About 20 minutes later, I get called back to the room stat for Code Blue. Arrive in the room to find the patient in EMD with no forward output. CPR is in progress.
- A cardiac surgeon arrives and immediately opens the chest and prepares to put the patient on cardiac bypass.
- We get a TEE machine and drop the probe. The finding: massive amounts of air in the right and left sides of the heart and a patient foramen ovale.
- Patient ultimately dies and a postmortem exam reveals a probe patent foramen ovale and a massive right-sided pattern of infarction confirming the diagnosis.
- Why is this case important? Because it shows by TEE (don't forget to record your exams) and later by gross pathology that the insult had nothing to do with anesthesia and everything to do with surgery.
- Your surgical colleagues might not like it, but we just saved our department literally millions of dollars.

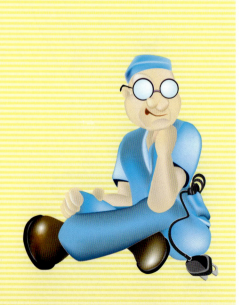

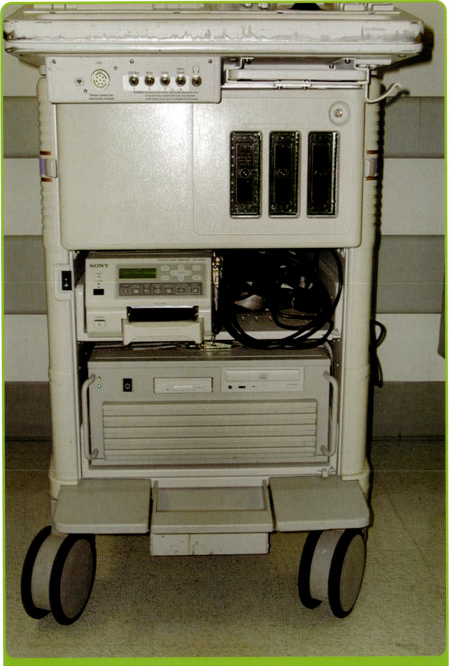

Figure 1. These damn machines are so big and clunky, it's ridiculous. But fear not: they're building newer, smaller versions that are easier to work with. Oh, and by the way, they will also be easier for people to steal. Put a Lo-Jack on your TEE machine!

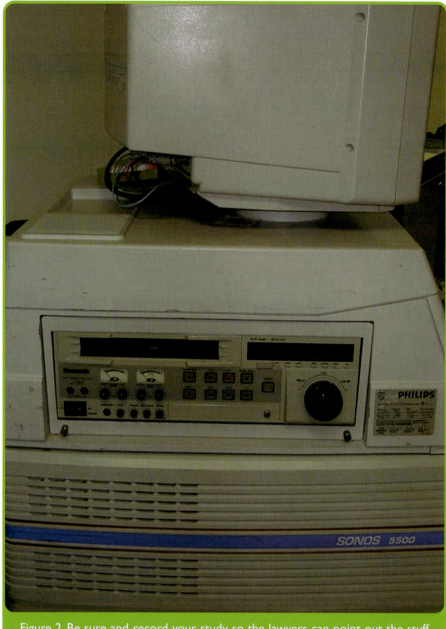

Figure 2. Be sure and record your study so the lawyers can point out the stuff you missed later on. This is an example of primitive "tape technology," right up there with eight-track cassettes for modernity. Better to record this "a la digital."

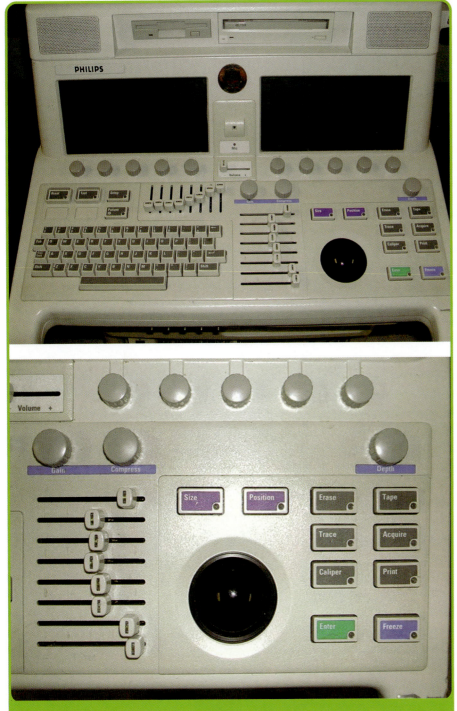

Figure 3. Millions of buttons, buttons and displays. Play with your machine—it's the only way to learn! Don't worry, none of the buttons are, "This Machine Will Self-Destruct in 60 Seconds," like in the James Bond movies.

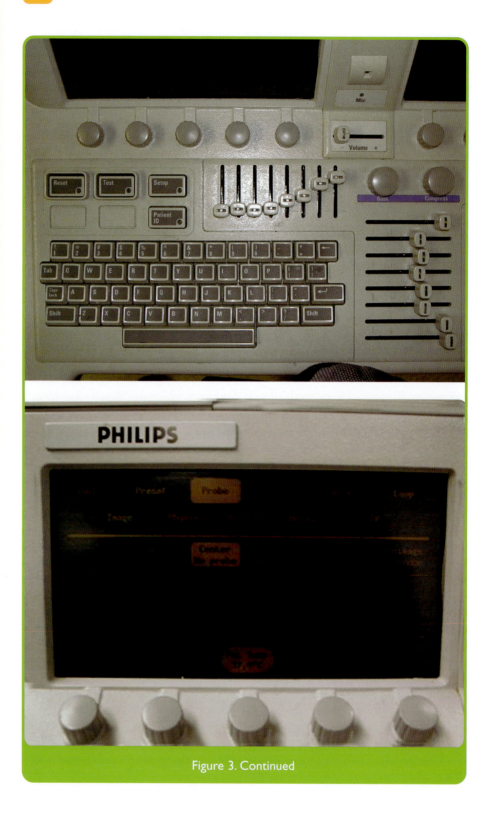

Figure 3. Continued

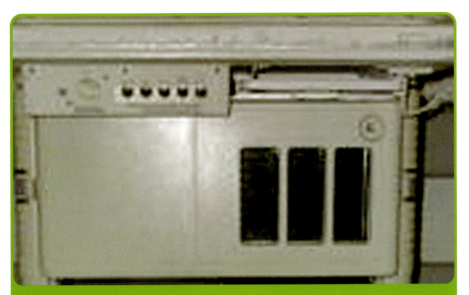

Figure 4. Where you plug in the probe. Don't force it. If you *squoink* the delicate little "pusher-inner thingies," you'll screw the pooch.

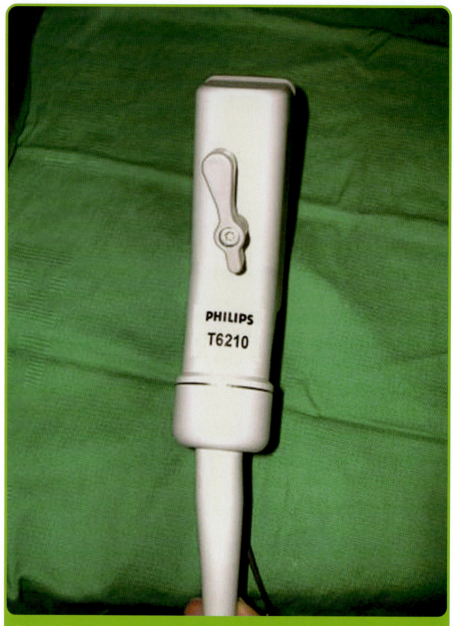

Figure 5. The plug-in end of the probe. Do not try to put this end in the patient's mouth. That would be a big mistake.

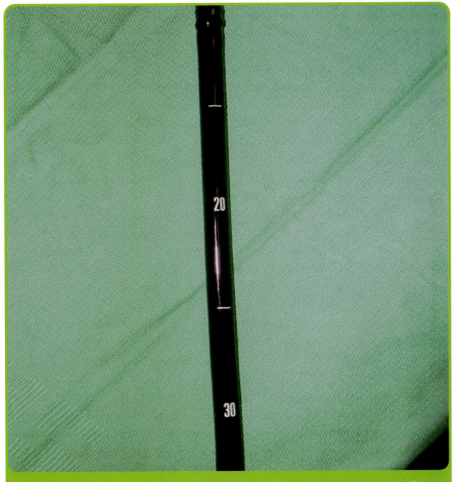

Figure 6. Depth markers. Don't go below 500 m or your submarine will get crushed.

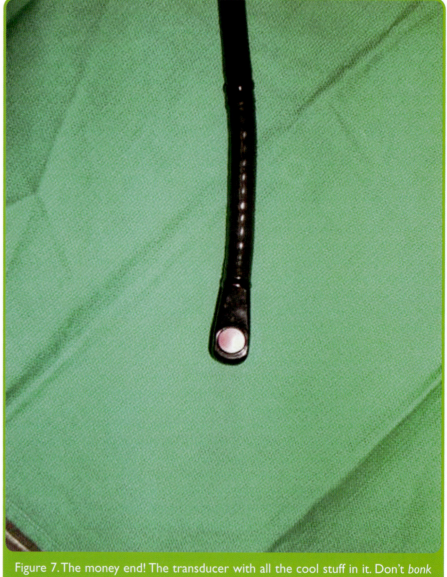

Figure 7. The money end! The transducer with all the cool stuff in it. Don't *bonk* this, it costs as much as a Lexus! That's almost as much as the Mercedes Benz that the cardiologist just parked next to you!

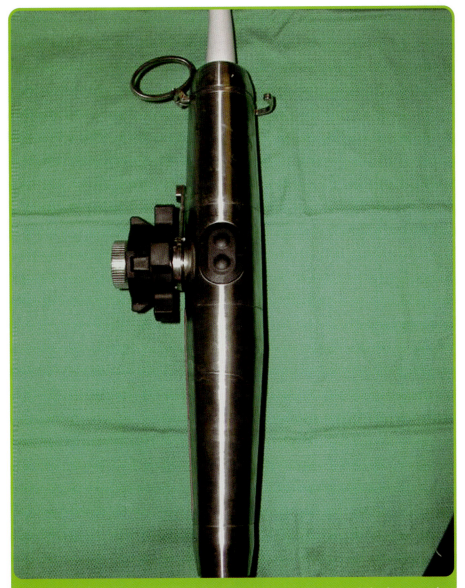

Figure 8. The control end. This is where you control the vertical, the horizontal, the omniplane, and all that "Outer Limits" kind of stuff.

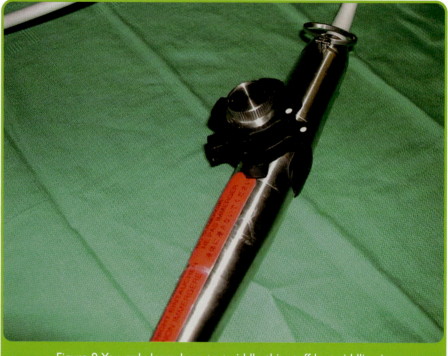

Figure 9. You only learn how to twiddle this stuff by twiddling it.

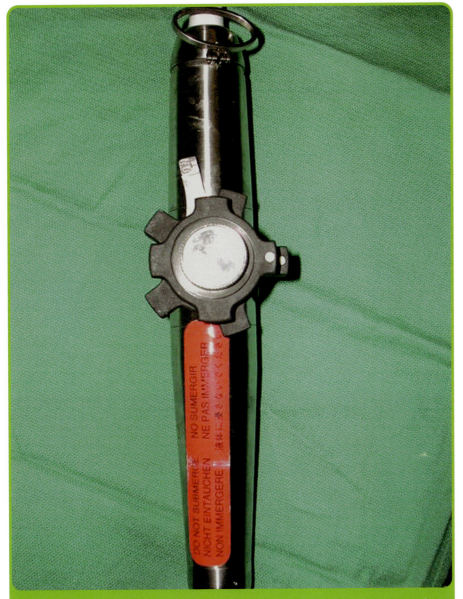

Figure 10. Make sure the probe is unlocked when you put it in. Don't turn the patient into an involuntary sword swallower!

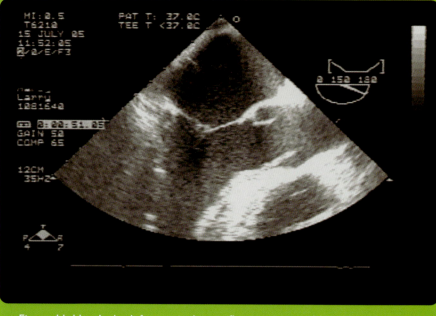

Figure 11. Here's the left ventricular outflow tract view. Note the pie shaped image. (TEE was invented by the same guy who invented pizza.)

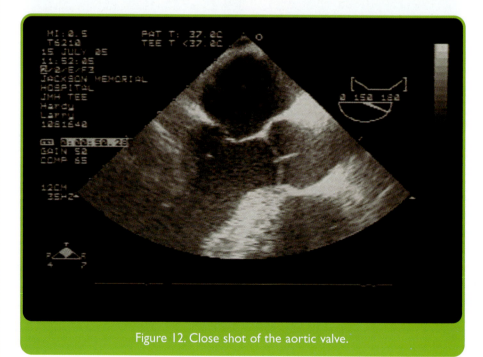

Figure 12. Close shot of the aortic valve.

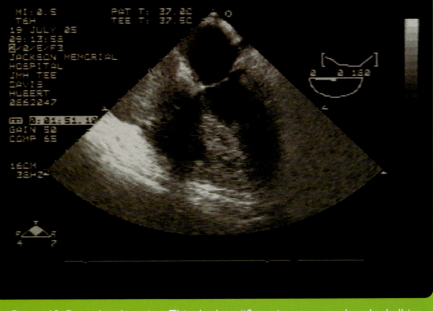

Figure 13. Four-chamber view. This the best "first view to see what the hell is going on" view.

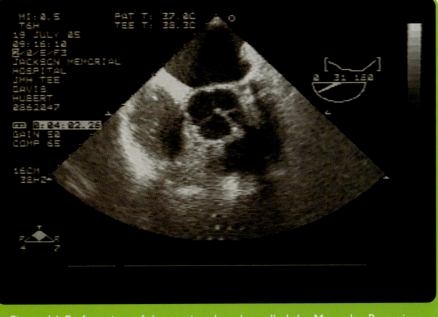

Figure 14. En face view of the aortic valve, also called the Mercedes Benz view. They call it this because all cardiologists drive Mercedes Benz.

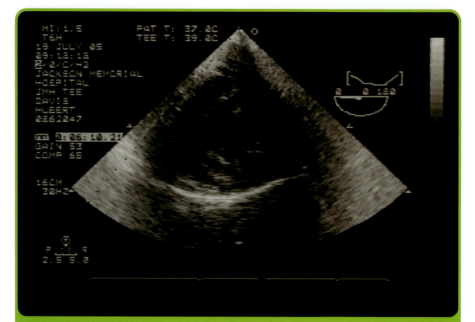

Figure 15. Transgastric short-axis view. A great view to tell you the volume. Also called the bouncing donut view. (TEE was invented by the guy who invented pizza but improved upon by the guy who invented donuts.)

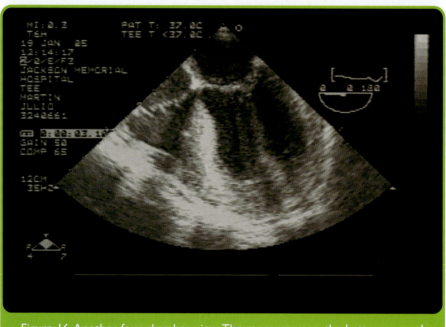

Figure 16. Another four-chamber view. The more you see, the better you get!

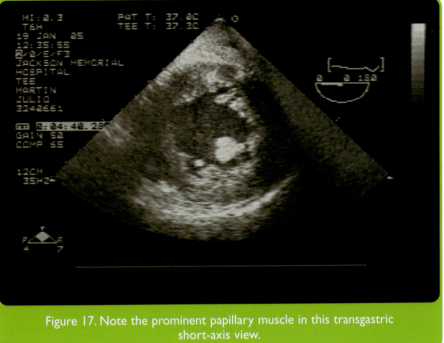

Figure 17. Note the prominent papillary muscle in this transgastric short-axis view.

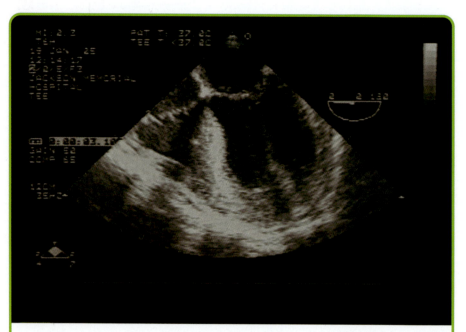

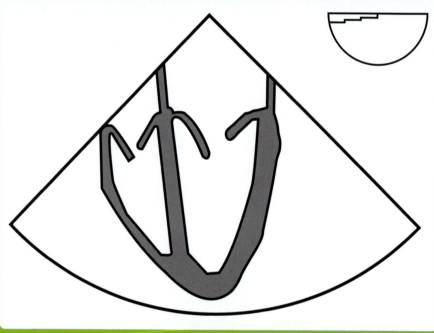

Figure 18. Now we're into pictures and drawings of the most often-used views. This is the generic four-chamber view that you should get first.

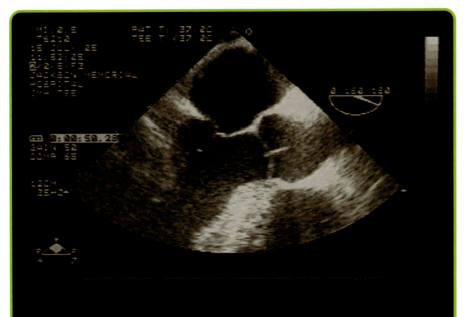

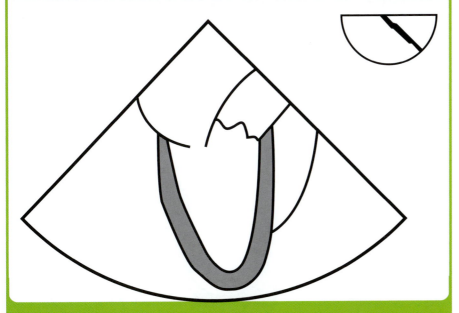

Figure 19. This is the long-axis view of the aorta. It gives a great shot of the aortic valve.

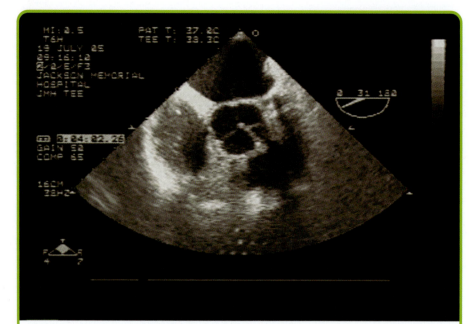

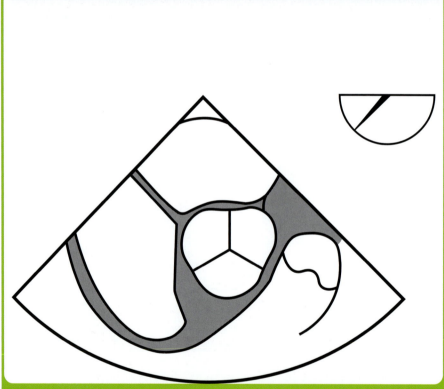

Figure 20. Back to the en face view of the aortic valve. Be sure and pronounce "en face" with a thick French accent so people think you're sort of international and vaguely exotic.

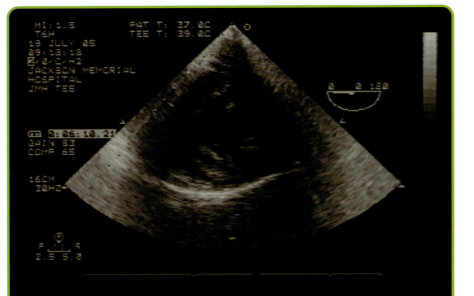

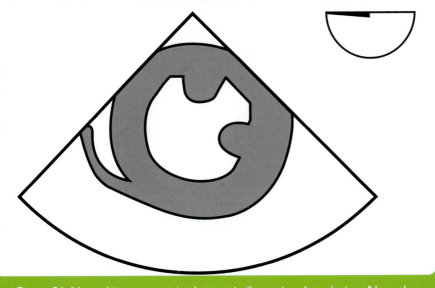

Figure 21. Note this transgastric short-axis (bouncing donut) view. Note the papillary muscles at 12 and 3 'o-clock.

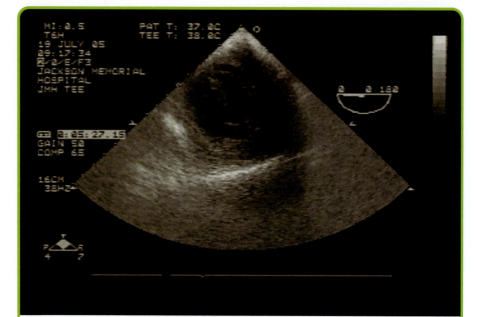

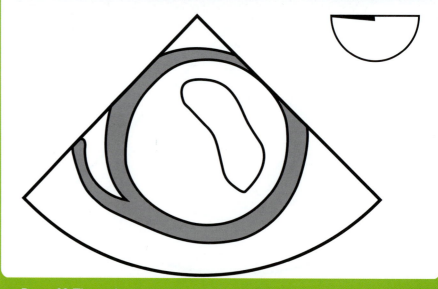

Figure 22. This is the same view as previously but a little higher up. Here the mitral valve looks like a fish mouth. (TEE was invented by a pizza guy, improved by a donut guy, and brought to perfection by a fishmonger.)

SUGGESTED READING

Botero M, Lobato EB. Advances in noninvasive cardiac output monitoring: An update. J Cardiothor Vasc Anesth 2001 Oct;15(5):631–40.

- *"From a single probe location, the anesthesiologist can monitor left ventricular regional and global wall motion using the short-axis view and measure CO, rotating the imaging plane to measure aortic flow velocities, expanding the intraoperative usefulness of TEE."*

Cheitlin MD, et al. ACC/AHA/ASE 2003 Guideline Update for the Clinical Application of Echocardiography: Summary Article. A Report of the American College of Cardiology/American Heart Association Task Force on Practice Guidelines (ACC/AHA/ASE Committee to Update the 1997 Guidelines for the Clinical Application of Echocardiography). Section XVI. Intraoperative echocardiography. Circulation 2003;108:1–17.

Gallagher C. *Board Stiff TEE: Trans-esophageal Echocardiography*. Oxford: Butterworth Heinemann, 2004.
• *Complexity made ridiculously simple.*

Kallmeyer IJ, Collard CD, Fox JA, et al. The safety of intraoperative trans-esophageal echocardiography: A case series of 7200 cardiac surgical patients. Anesth Analg 2001;92:1126–30.
• *It can be used safely, too.*

Oh JK, Seward JB, Tajik AF. *Trans-esophageal Echocardiography. The Echo Manual*, 2nd edition. Philadelphia: Lippincott-Raven, 1999.

Perrino AC, Harris SN, Luther MA. Intraoperative determination of cardiac output using multiplane transesophageal echocardiography: A comparison to thermodilution. Anesthesiology 1998;89:350–7.
• *"Multiplane TEE can provide a reliable method for intraoperative cardiac output measurement."*

Peterson GE, Brickner ME, Reimold SC. Transesophageal echocardiography: Clinical indications and applications. Circulation 2003;107:2398.
• *"TEE is used not only as a diagnostic tool but also as a monitoring adjunct for operative and percutaneous cardiac procedures."*

Savage RM, Aronson SM, Thomas JD, et al. *Comprehensive Textbook of Intraoperative Transesophageal Echocardiography*. Philadelphia: Lippincott Williams & Wilkins, 2004.
• *A heavyweight in the TEE text world.*

Shanewise JS, et al. ASE/SCA Guidelines for Performing a Comprehensive Intraoperative Multiplane Transesophageal Echocardiography Examination: Recommendations of the American Society of Echocardiography Council for Intraoperative Echocardiography and the Society of Cardiovascular Anesthesiologists Task Force for Certification in Perioperative Transesophageal Echocardiography. J Am Soc Echocardiogr 1999;12:884–900.
• *The TEE Constitution.*

PART 8

FAKING IT

Christopher Gallagher and
Christina Rankin

INTRODUCTION

But there is a damned good reason for simulating procedures on dummies before doing it to people. Just listen to the voice of our patients.

"Not on me first! No way you're going to practice on me first!"

Such is the sentiment of almost any human being.

Would *you* want to be "the first CVP," "the first intubation," or "the first bronchospasm episode" for a young doctor in training? Of course not. You want it done on someone else.

Anyone but me.

Enter the simulator.

Simulators run the gamut from "partial task trainers" (an intubating dummy, for example) to "flat screen simulators" (a computer program that walks you through a ventricular fibrillation arrest, for example) all the way to high-fidelity, programmable anesthesia mannequins (you can program one to go through the whole sequence of a malignant hyperthermia episode).

Programs using simulators now go from sea to shining sea, with huge centers in Pittsburgh (19 high fidelity mannequins!), Boston, Stanford, Chicago, Oregon—you name it.

Will a session in a simulator become mandatory for board certification one day? Maybe.

INDICATIONS

- Procedures, you name it. A "task trainer" simulator exists for almost any procedure in medicine now, from haptic (you can feel resistance) endoscopic trainers for surgeons to intubating dummies to CVP placement mock-ups.

- For anesthesia, partial task trainers are particularly good for airway tasks. An intubating dummy is the way to go with your first intubation. That same intubating dummy can help you through your first LMA placement, intubating LMA maneuver, or fiberoptic intubation.

- High-fidelity mannequins can guide an anesthesiology student through any number of crises, both commonplace (bronchospasm) and rare (malignant hyperthermia).

- Team training and communication skills are well suited to the simulator environment. With post-simulation debriefing and video review, learners can learn the fine points of crisis resource management. You can look at such issues as role clarity (who's in charge, who's in charge of the airway, who's in charge of defibrillating), global reassessment ("OK, we've shocked three times and we're not getting anywhere. Is there anything we're not thinking of here, people?"), and resource management (send the medical student to run the blood gas down and keep the anesthesiologist working on the airway, not the other way around).

- With multiple mannequins, larger groups of anesthesia providers—along with other specialties—can learn how to triage and treat mass casualties or, God forbid, victims of a terrorist bioweapon attack.

CONTRAINDICATIONS

- Can there be such a thing as a contraindication to a simulator scenario? Not unless someone is allergic to simulator equipment. There are a few cautions to note, however.

- Equipment in a scenario setting is sometimes "sabotaged" on purpose. For example, a ventilator may not work. The broken ventilator is part of a scenario that teaches residents how to troubleshoot broken equipment. For goodness' sake, don't let that broken ventilator get taken out of the simulation room and hooked up to a patient. Wouldn't that be the irony of ironies—you set up a simulation lab to promote patient safety and you kill a patient with one of the props. Oh, that would go over dandy on the front page of *The New York Times*.

- Ditto on infusion pumps, laryngoscopes, and any other "trick stuff." In the best of all possible worlds, the simulator lab is physically separated from the regular clinical arena to avoid any such glitches.

- Don't take "real stuff" that might be needed in the "real OR." A defibrillator

There is no disguise which can for long conceal love where it exists or simulate it where it does not.

Francois, Duc de la Rochefoucauld Reflection; or, Sentences and Moral Maxims, 70, 1678

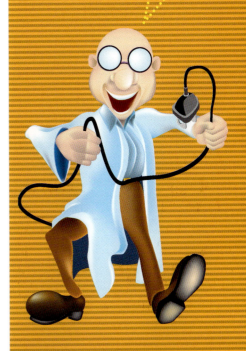

The Unsafe Safety Center

Irony is not by any stretch limited to the clinical arena.

A simulation center was opened with great fanfare. Dignitaries and poobahs from near and far descended upon this great new Center for Patient Safety.

At the last minute, it was discovered that there was some problem with the fire alarms. Somehow, the opening gala occurred but a fire marshal had to stand there in attendance "just in case."

What a great headline that could have been in the newspaper: *Safety Center Found to be Unsafe.*

serves as an example: You take it from the central core, you don't leave a note saying where it is, and then the OR is left high and dry. Someone comes down to the regular OR, goes into V-fib, and the circulator runs to the core to get the defibrillator. Surprise, surprise! No defibrillator—it's in the simulation room, but the circulator has no way of knowing that. Quick, grab the toaster from the break room, maybe you can use that!

EQUIPMENT

- The biggies in human mannequin simulation are two: METI® and Laerdal®.
- METI® is more expensive and has more stuff programmed in. You can press one button and the entire scenario will roll on its own. The METI® has a system for "recognizing drugs" using a bar code recognition system.
- Laerdal® is also programmable but doesn't have the barcode recognition system. It's easier to do stuff "on the fly" with a Laerdal®.
- Recording system. As part of the debriefing process, a video is invaluable. The individual or the team get to see exactly what happened and can talk over how to improve what they did.
- Trained debriefer. This seems odd to call a person a piece of the equipment but the person who reviews the scenario and talks over what happened is, indeed, the most important piece in the puzzle. A good debriefer asks open-ended questions and helps the learners tease out the lessons. Debriefing does not come easily and does not come naturally. A good debriefer should attend a "teach the teacher" course or at least study debriefing skills.

BEWARE THE SIMULATOR

- Simulators are good but they are not the real thing.
- Simulators can't flush or blush.
- Simulators can only "sweat" in that they can be sprayed with water ahead of the scenario.
- Masking the mechanical simulators does not have the same feel as masking a human.
- The upper airways of simulators are often breaking down and getting leaks, making mask ventilation, and assessment of mask ventilation, difficult.

- These beasts are pricey, and keeping them staffed and running is yet pricier. Upkeep and repairs are costly.
- Though simulators hold great promise as an evaluation tool, the definitive proof on this issue is still lacking.
- Clinically skilled people have flubbed a "simulator test." Clinical ninnies have excelled in "simulator tests," so no one is sure exactly where simulators stand in this issue.
- Research on simulators is slippery, with people having a hard time determining just exactly what metric to use. Residents like it? Well, yeah, OK, they like it. Residents like pizza too. Residents do better clinically after they train in the simulator? Well, maybe, but maybe not.
- Is their any outcome study to show that we truly, as a specialty, know for absolute certain that simulators make a difference? What shreds of evidence we have are scattered, inconsistent, and vary widely, according to a review of over 1000 simulator articles in the February, 2005 edition of *Medical Teacher*.
- The one thing we do know? Residents who train on simulators do better on simulators. Even the most casual of geometricians can see the circularity of that argument.

PHILOSOPHY

- The simulator is the wand but the simulator instructor is the magician. And the rule in magic is the same as the rule in the simulator—it is the *magician*, not the *wand*, that makes the rabbit jump out of the hat.
- The best simulator in the world is only as good as the instructor running it.
- Tailor the scenario to the student and modify it as you go along. You can stick to a strict script (which you need to do in a study, for example), but you're better off modifying the scenario as you go.
- At the beginning level, the simulator should test simple tasks—such as following the algorithm for a ventricular fibrillation arrest.
- At the intermediate level, the simulator should test more complex tasks with multiple branch points—such as figuring out what to do when the ST segments go up in the middle of a case.
- Once you have the earlier tasks down, then the simulator is good for testing teamwork and crisis resource

management skills. But it doesn't do any good to test "advanced skills" (role clarity, communication skills, global reassessment, group dynamics) if students don't know the basics first. It's really great that you communicate well, but if you don't know how to turn on the defibrillator and charge it, well guess what, the patient isn't getting any better, my friend!

- The chief advantage of a simulator is that you can practice without risk to a patient. Back to the defibrillator—you can flounder in the simulator until you get it right and no one gets hurt. You flounder with the defibrillator in a real cardiac arrest and the patient may very well get hurt.

- Time and chance play a big role in medical education—for example, you may or may not ever see a tension pneumothorax in your training. The simulator can "create" a pneumothorax when and where you want to, so a simulator helps education by giving you a standardized, reproducible "event" that you can show to all your residents or medical students. You don't have to sit around and "hope" the right pathology will come along.

- Simulators enjoy widespread use. Educators are hoping (though this is difficult to prove) that simulators will accelerate the learning curve. Rather than keeping residents in the hospital more and more hours for more and more years, educators hope that simulators will "bring the important lessons home early" and build more expertise in residents and medical students.

- Learning in a simulator generates emotional responses. Some would argue that you learn better when you have an emotional "tag" attached to your lesson.

- In general, people who go through the simulator like the experience and "ask to come back real soon."

- Key to the simulator is the debrief afterwards, preferably with a video to review the events as they occurred.

- Debriefing generally goes through three stages: reactions to the scenario, understanding of what occurred, and a summary lesson.

- Good debriefers refrain from using judgmental questions but rather use questions that demonstrate good judgment. For example, rather than saying, "Atropine was a bad drug to give, why the hell did you give it?" a debriefer should say, "Myself, I think atropine is not the proper drug in this setting, help me understand what you were thinking when you gave it." The

debriefer doesn't bring down the Hammer of Thor on the student's head, nor does the debriefer cagily dance around the right drug. The whole process is geared toward helping the student dissect the event, lay out their thoughts, and come up with a reasonable assessment of how to do better next time.

- Questions during a debrief should always pursue the "how can we improve" idea. Don't say, "Why the hell didn't you call for help? Things were going to hell in a handbasket!" Say, "At what point in this emergency is it appropriate to call for help? Do you recognize when events are slipping out of reach and, if not, what are the signs that things are getting out of hand?"

PHILOSOPHY OF CRISIS RESOURCE MANAGEMENT

- About 75% of sentinel events in the medical setting are problems with communication.

- In the hectic and harried setting of a hospital crisis, it's easy to fall apart or to give yourself over to shouting, waving your arms, and generally running around like a recently decapitated chicken.

- Crisis Resource Management is an attempt to create order from chaos.

- Simulators are great places to work on Crisis Resource Management—there is no risk to patients, you can go over the scenario again and again until you get it right, and you can videotape the whole process for future study.

- Crisis Resource Management might sound like a lot of fluffy, touchy-feely hooey, but it really does matter! And knowing the techniques helps you out immensely when the bottom drops out.

- The five major principles of Crisis Resource Management are:
  - Role clarity
  - Communication
  - Personnel support
  - Resources
  - Global assessment

- *Role clarity.* You establish an event manager, one person who gets all information and delivers all order. Other people get a clear assignment: "Mary, manage the airway; Joe, do chest compression; Tom, work the paddles."

- *Communication.* Don't shout orders out to the air, hoping somehow they will

Most Bang for Your Buck in a Simulator

Simulators can create a phantasmagorical menu of problems. But what does the most good? What serves residents and medical students best, seeing the weird stuff or seeing the basic stuff?

Do you run a malignant hyperthermia scenario (rare, in the 1:35,000 range) in the hope that you will train that *one* resident who will see it, somewhere in the dim and distant future?

Do you run a hypoxemia scenario (common, hell, more common than we care to admit)? Do you drill this bread-and-butter scenario in the hope that you are teaching the basic stuff that every resident and student needs to know?

Those "in the know" lean towards running the more common scenarios. Teach students and residents the basic stuff—the problems everyone sees every day. From a "number of patients helped" standpoint, you are better off training people to handle hypoxemia (common) than malignant hyperthermia (rare).

Vince Lombardi, the famous and successful football coach, emphasized blocking and tackling, the basic moves every football player needs to know. Lombardi spent little time teaching triple-reverse, flea-flicker, and fake-punt trick plays.

The successful simulator teacher also emphasizes the basics. Fix hypoxemia, fix ischemia, manage a bad airway. Don't waste a lot of time and energy on running a pseudo-pseudo-hypoparathyroidism scenario.

But Do People Really Buy into the Simulator?

No kidding, they do.

It pays to put as much "window dressing" in the simulator as possible, to make the scene look real. In an OR, have some instruments scattered around, have the usual tables, Mayos, and drapes in place. All this stuff gives the scenario the "feel" of real life.

In a simulated ICU, have blood pressure cuffs, infusion pumps, and IV poles around.

Once things get going, it may seem amazing but students and residents do actually "feel the pain" when things go wrong. You'll see the drawn look on their face and you'll hear them say, "Something's wrong," with a genuine note of alarm in their voice.

The simulator is a powerful experience.

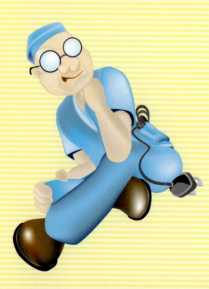

miraculously get "heard" and "completed." Look at someone, address them by name (even if you have to grab their nametag and look at it), and make sure they know exactly what to do.

- *Personnel support.* Get help early—don't wait until the 11th hour to get an extra pair of hands and an extra brain to help out. Orient new people quickly as to what's going on. "Bad airway, can't intubate," may be all you need to say.

- *Resources.* Know where stuff is and how to get it. Know which people can get stuff for you. Don't be afraid to look far afield if that's what you need to do. "Go over to trauma and get me that cordis, they'll know what I need."

- *Global assessment.* Periodically step back and think things over, avoid fixating on any one thing, and let other people voice opinions. Maybe some great suggestion that you hadn't thought of will arise from the crisis team.

SCENARIOS

Simple

- A resident walks up to a simulator, the monitor shows ventricular fibrillation.

- The resident calls for help, gets the simulator over to the patient's bedside. In the meantime, others show up at the bedside with Ambu-bag, intubating equipment, IV stuff, and drugs.

- The resident first intubates, listens for breath sounds, tapes the endotracheal tube, and then tells the assistant to start chest compressions.

- After three minutes of this, the resident tells people to apply paddles, charge to 200, synchronous, and shock.

- Nothing happens.

- The resident says go to 360 and shocks, nothing happens.

- Another student says, "Hey wait, that shouldn't be synchronous."

- First resident says, "Oh, yeah," then proceeds to shock asynchronous and gets the simulator back to sinus rhythm.

- In the debrief, the resident looks over the video and compares his performance with ACLS protocol.

- Oops! Should have gone to shock, shock, shock right away. And asynchronous at that! Oh well, lesson learned.

- The resident leaves with his tail between his legs, muttering, "I'm getting that damned protocol down cold next time!"

Ratchet It Up a Bit

- A resident shows up to a simulator is in a PACU setting and the monitor shows sinus bradycardia with a rate of 40.

- The resident grabs a syringe of atropine and gives it.

- The simulators heart rate goes up to 130 and ST segment changes occur.

- The resident starts a nitroglycerin drip, and the patient's blood pressure drops.

- The resident orders 500 cc IV bolus.

- The simulator, through its speakers, starts to complain of shortness of breath.

- The resident gives Lasix.

- A "nurse" hands the resident a recent blood gas, which shows a K of 2.3.

- The patient starts to develop ectopy.

- The resident starts to develop ectopy.

- The teacher stops the simulation before the resident codes.

- During the debrief, the resident goes over all the events while wiping their brow and wondering why they came to the simulation lab today.

- Questioning centers on the atropine. Why give it? Just because the heart rate is slow? What about checking the blood pressure? What about asking the patient for any symptoms?

- Lo and behold, over the course of the debrief, it becomes apparent that the patient had completely asymptomatic bradycardia, and the best treatment is *no* treatment.

- Once atropine was given, then you were off to the races—the heart rate got too high, now you have ischemia, then the glycerin dropped the pressure too much, then the fluids put the patient into pulmonary edema, then the Lasix exaggerated the hypokalemia and ectopy. *¡Ay, caramba!* It's just one damn thing after another!

- The resident learns the valuable lesson to "leave well enough alone."

- Each treatment created a new problem, so the resident also learned, firsthand, the "perils of pharmacology."

Advanced, Now with Crisis Resource Management Skills Included

- The resident enters a room where there are two beds with a code going on in one and people clustered around another bed.

- The resident looks things over and gets a quick report—cardiac arrest in one bed, seizure in another.

- The resident goes to the arrest, assigns an ER nurse to watch the seizure patient with instructions to keep the airway patent and keep the patient on their side in case they vomit.
- Going to the head of the bed, the resident sees the patient is intubated, listens for breath sounds, hears none, and looks for themselves.
- The esophagus is intubated.
- The resident pulls out the endotracheal tube, replaces it in the trachea, then looks at the EKG.
- Telling a respiratory therapist to ventilate with 100% oxygen by hand, the resident gets an update on the progress of the code, then administers amiodarone, directs a specific person to get a blood gas, and tells a third person to charge the paddles and shock.
- Behind the resident, the nurse watching the seizing patient yells out, "He stopped breathing."
- The resident tells the nurse to get an Ambu-bag and, while that is coming, shocks the patient with the cardiac arrest, tells a fellow doctor to continue with ACLS protocol on this patient, then turns to intubate the seizing patient.
- During the debrief, the whole team discusses the problems of managing more than one crisis at a time, how you triage needs, and how you divide up skilled personnel.

Making a Point

- Medical students cluster around a table, looking eager-beaver and smarter than smart.
- The instructor walks into the room and throws a question out into the air: "Man comes in with chest pain, a classical case. What do you think's wrong?"
- The medical students trip over themselves firing out the answer, "Heart attack!" "MI!" "Ischemia!"
- The instructor leads the medical students into the simulation room that has two mannequins, side by side, with a curtain separating them. Both mannequins have blankets over them. The mannequin on one blanket is sticking up conspicuously from his chest.
- The instructor points to the mannequin without the lump. "Go ahead, talk to him." (The mannequin has a speaker built in.)
- A medical student approaches it and asks what's the matter.

- The mannequin speaks: "I've had heart trouble for a long time. My chest feels tight, just like my last heart attack."
- The instructor looks at the medical students, "Classic."
- Now a medical student approaches the other mannequin, the one with the blanket sticking up, and asks what's the matter.
- "I was selling bibles—no, I was giving away bibles on the street corner at two in the morning," the mannequin says, "when these two dudes jumped me and stuck this knife in my chest."
- The instructor looks at the medical students, "Classic."
- "The most important part of the examination is done with your ears," the instructor intones, "talking with the patient. Chest pain that is classic can mean lots of things, not just the 'classic' chest pain of ischemia. As you can imagine, treating the older patient with chest pain involves medical or interventional management to restore the myocardial oxygen supply/demand to a more favorable level."
- "Treating the young man with a Ginsu steak knife in his chest involves something else entirely."
- The simulator does not always need to involve high-tech gadgetry to make its "point."
- You can use a simulator to deliver a graphic yet simple lesson—you must first diagnose before you treat. And the diagnosis most often comes from asking a simple question: "What happened?"

Do You Really Know How to Use the Paddles?

- Residents shuffle into the simulator room, this room set up to be an ICU.
- A defibrillator is next to the mannequin, disassembled and with all connections undone.
- "You know how to work this, right?" the instructor asks.
- "Sure," this from all and sundry.
- "Great, I want each of you to pop this mannequin," the instructor asks.
- "Uh," each resident says, looking gloomily at the spaghetti of wires.
- Once the connections are finally hooked up correctly, enough time passes for a fibrillating patient to die, decompose, and enter the nitrogen cycle.
- The simulator functions as a great "truth serum." When residents and students

Disasters: What Could be More Fun?

Eventually, you start studying disasters to learn valuable lessons.

Yes, the academic in you knows all too well that disasters present us with a unique opportunity to learn "system errors." Plane crashes, nuclear meltdowns, and industrial explosions give us great lessons.

But come on, it's damned interesting to read about this stuff just because it's *interesting*! Even if you weren't interested in simulations or medicine or education, you can't help but get fascinated by these things.

- Two 747s collide on a runway in Tenerife
- Chernobyl melts down, killing hundreds plus how many thousands from secondary effects
- Piper Alpha, an oil derrick in the North Sea, bursts into flames, killing most of the crew
- The Hindenberg blazes in the New Jersey sky
- Iceberg 1, Titanic 0, in the 1912 "Iceberg vs. Floating Palace Open"

How can you *not* want to read about this stuff?

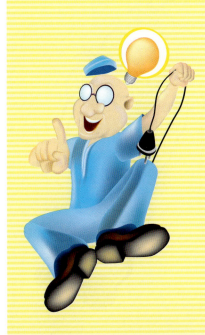

say they know something and you ask them to "prove it," you will sometimes see amazing things.

Triage

- Three residents are brought into a room with three mannequins.

- One mannequin is flatline, one is in ventricular fibrillation, one is groaning.

- Nurses in attendance confirm that the one patient is actually flatline and the one is in ventricular fibrillation, and that the third one is suffering from an abdominal wound. No artifacts here.

- Just before anyone can react, another person enters the room and says there is a fire coming down the hall and they have 30 seconds to get out.

- All eyes turn to the residents, "What do we do, doctors?"

- Like deer in headlights, they stand there, then each one tries to wheel one patient out, getting stuck in the door.

- An instructor comes in 30 seconds later with a large red blanket, waving it all around. "You're all dead, quick fried to a crackly crunch. Just like Cheetos."

- During the debrief, the instructor revisits the hard choices they had in this difficult scenario.

- Delay is death—that is not an option.

- You have to do *insta*-triage here.

- Asystole—no hope, leave that one.

- Ventricular fib—some hope, start pushing.

- Groaning—most sign of life, start pushing this one the fastest and get them out the door first. If push comes to shove, leave the fibrillating patient and run for your lives but at least get the one guy who has the best chance.

- Lesson learned—the possible scenarios you have in the simulator are limited only by your imagination. Although you want to emphasize basics (see below), there is nothing wrong with doing the occasional "out there" scenario. You can stretch the minds of students.

- Is this completely "out there"? We live in dangerous times and we might all face the unthinkable after a terrorist attack someday. So lessons in triage and mass casualties may one day prove most useful.

- If resources or time are tight, and you absolutely must let someone go, then you're better off letting the asystolic patient go than the one with at least some rhythm (you can shock V-fib, after all,

but treatment of asystole is crummy at best and most often useless).

- Plus, and this lesson must not get lost in the shuffle—save yourselves! You are a doctor, and even if you have to let *all* the patients go, then do it. Don't become a victim yourself. If you are dead, you can *never* save another patient. If you are alive, you will save someone later on.

Family Members

- A resident is in an operating room simulator setting. Your scenario focuses on a sitting craniotomy.

- Suddenly, the end-tidal CO_2 drops, the saturation drops, the blood pressure drops, and multi-focal PVCs occur.

- The resident pegs the diagnosis of venous air embolism but resuscitative efforts fail and the "patient" dies.

- In an examination room down the hall from the simulator room, a person sits—an actor playing the patient's wife.

- The resident now has to go through an "interpersonal simulation," informing a relative of an intraoperative death.

- Though you don't think of this difficult discussion as a "procedure," it is still something that every anesthesia student must experience. Operations are not done in a vacuum. Patients have relatives. And when things happen, good or bad, you have to let the relatives know.

- One approach to this extremely difficult task goes by the acronym CONES: COntext (you set the stage), Narrative (you lay out what happened in a "just the facts, ma'am" style), Emotion (you let the family members give vent to their emotions), and Summary (you sum up and go forward with a game plan).

  - *Context*—The resident says, "I'm here to talk about your husband and what happened in the OR. This is not going to be good news."

  - *Narrative*—A blow-by-blow description of the events, no editorializing, just saying what happened, what you did, and what the outcome was.

  - *Emotion*—"This must be a terrible blow to you."

  - *Summary*—You get clergy or counseling involved, help with making arrangements, and assure the wife that you will keep in touch.

- This CONES approach never goes so slick and seamless in real life, but it at least gives you some structure when you must deliver bad news.

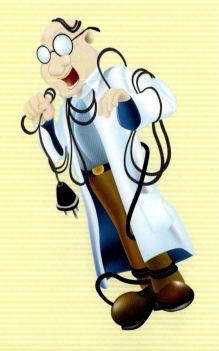

- If anyone thinks, "What a waste of time, I'll never have to do this!" then they are kidding themselves. Badness happens. Prepare for it.

Pause for a Moment to Consider What the Simulator Can Do

- As the previous scenarios demonstrate, you can use the simulator to teach just about anybody anything.
- The mannequin *itself* is limited to a certain number of vital sign permutations.
  - Blood pressure up/down
  - Heart rhythm slow, fast, irregular, fatal
  - Saturation up/down
  - End tidal CO_2 up/down
  - Temperature up/down
  - Breath sounds clear/wheezing/absent (Of note, most speaker systems transmit breath sounds poorly and you usually have to "coach" the students by telling them, "Breath sounds are absent on the left" or "Breath sounds reveal wheezing in all lung fields.")
  - Pulses present/absent
- Therefore, the mannequin has only so many tricks up its sleeve.
- But, and here is the key, the *teacher* has no such limitations. The teacher in the simulator is limited only by their *imagination*.
- So, the *simplest* mannequin maneuver (say, a drop in oxygen saturation), can give rise to *any number* of valuable lessons.
- You have a group of beginning students (CRNAs, medical students, residents)—you can go into a discussion of respiratory physiology and focus on West's three zones.
- You have some middle level students—go into depth on the differential diagnosis and treatment of common problems, such as a right mainstem intubation.
- You have advanced students, near graduation—turn the scenario into a double-lumen case with refractory hypoxemia in spite of all your tricks.
- In the controlled environment of the simulator center, you can throw in equipment glitches and see how the students react.
  - Oxygen pipeline failure
  - Oxygen crossover
  - Power failure
  - Malfunctioning ventilator
  - Missing inspiratory/expiratory valves
  - Mislabeled syringes

- Oh, the wickedness you can brew up! No wonder simulator instructors have so much fun.
- Plus, once the mannequin has "done its thing," you can move on to interpersonal issues—dealing with a hot-headed surgeon, talking with family members, discussing how miscommunication leads to disaster.
- In short, a simulator is a vehicle that puts a teacher alongside a student. Then they go for a ride.

The Difficult Surgeon

- The student walks into the simulator, where the patient is already intubated and under anesthesia.
- During the report, the student is told, "This patient is going to have a liver resection and you only have an 18G IV in. My wife is giving birth so I have to go, bye!"
- A "surgeon" is in the field.
- You say, "I need a central line for adequate volume access."
- The surgeon says, "No."
- The blood pressure drops to 80/60, the heart rate rises to 150, and ST segment depression occurs.
- A second surgeon in the field says, "We're losing some blood here."
- The student opens up the IV, says, "I need more access," and the instructor says, "The patient's arms are obese and you can't see any veins."
- "Well then I'd put in a central line, no matter what the surgeon says, no matter how much he protests."
- In the field, the surgeon goes ballistic, saying, "You can do this with a couple of 14s, now quit bothering me!"
- Blood pressure drops to 60, heart rate to 200, ST elevation now and ectopy.
- "I'd put in a cordis in the neck," the resident says.
- V-tach.
- "Get blood in the room, paddles!"
- Resuscitation gets underway.
- An ABG shows a hematocrit of 17, and a pH of 7.10.
- Resuscitation continues but to no avail.
- In the debrief room, the student sits across the table from the surgeon.
- "Just what was all this resistance to me placing the lines I needed?" the student asks.
- Over the course of the debrief, the student learns the art of talking with

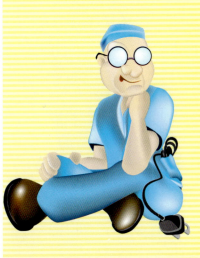

difficult people. (The book, *Difficult Conversations*, listed in the bibliography, provides a lot of information on this topic. Any medical professional should read and re-read this book.)

- The first impulse is to blame, accuse, jump across the table, rip their heart out, hold their heart in front of them while it's still beating, and take a big bite out of their heart just to make your point. Such behavior, though lauded during Aztec human sacrifices, has no place in the modern workplace.

- The student learns to disentangle the emotions, open up to the "other side's opinion," and explore the issue with an open mind.

- The surgeon had experienced trouble with anesthesia and their central lines, treating line infections and pneumothoraces. Now the surgeon was almost conditioned to oppose a central line.

- No dialogue occurred before the case, wherein the anesthesiologist could lay out their concerns (adequate venous access) while balancing the surgeon's concerns (line infections and dropped lungs).

- Though anesthesia and surgery didn't exactly "kiss and make up" after this discussion, they did get a look into each other's concerns and laid the groundwork for a better outcome next time.

- So in this setting, the simulator served as springboard to an important surgery-anesthesia discussion.

Creating Options for Mutual Gain

- A student comes into the simulator, the patient has a double-lumen endotracheal tube in place.

- A report details that the patient is undergoing a right upper lobe resection, that the patient has multiple sclerosis, and the surgeon is complaining that the lung won't come down.

- The student looks over the vital signs, then takes the fiberoptic and examines the double-lumen tube, looking to make sure the tube is in the right place.

- An exam reveals the tube is correctly located but the surgeon is still complaining that the lung is in his way.

- The student checks the connections, and everything seems OK.

- "Listen, this lung is still up!" the surgeon says.

- The student thinks about it, then says, "Is the lung actually getting inflated, or is it just not coming down."

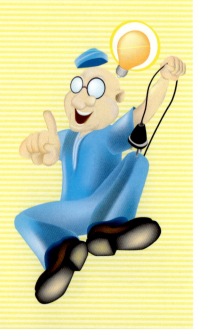

- "Oh," the surgeon says, "I guess it's not actually inflating with each breath. But it still won't come down."

- The student places a suction catheter in the right lung and exerts a little suction, allowing the lung to deflate better.

- All goes well, then as they're closing, the surgeon says, "I hope you put an epidural in this lady."

- Student looks over the chart and sees in big letters, "NO EPIDURAL, PATIENT HAS MS. DON'T WANT TO CONFUSE PICTURE WITH NEURAXIAL BLOCK."

- "Uh," the student says.

- The surgeon proceeds to rant about lazy anesthesia and how they don't care about patients in pain.

- During the debrief, the instructor lauds the student on solving the problem of "the lung that wouldn't come down." But what about the epidural and the patient's pain? The student was at a loss on that one.

- "You have to explore all the options," the instructor says. "Because one option is closed doesn't mean you have to end up at loggerheads with the surgeon about pain relief."

- The book, *Getting to Yes: Negotiating Agreement without Giving In*, listed in the bibliography, helps clarify this issue.

- Pain relief is not limited to the neuraxial route. While the chest is open, the surgeons can do intercostals blocks. Heck, there's nothing "blind" about it—they can see exactly where the nerves are!

- You yourself can do intercostal blocks at the end of the case.

- An intrapleural catheter is an option (not tremendously popular but they are a possibility).

- The key idea is to "keep the doors open." Keep thinking of ideas to solve the problem (give adequate pain relief). You don't need to surrender your viewpoint (you don't want to put an epidural in a patient with multiple sclerosis). But then again, you don't want to ignore the surgeon's concern.

- So you look for something that provides mutual gain—something that pays attention to your neural concerns but also to the patient's need for pain relief.

- Here the simulator provided a medical lesson—how to get a lung down—and an interpersonal/communication lesson—creating strategies for mutual gain.

Subspecialty Specific: Neurosurgery

- A patient is on the table, ready for induction.
- In an argument with a fellow Rhodes Scholar at a local drinking establishment, the patient had a "Close Encounter of the Barstool Kind" and now has an epidural hematoma.
- His medical history is remarkable for one persistent habit: he seems to be talking when he should be listening, as evidenced by old knife wound and bullet wound scars.
- There is a smell on his breath redolent of chardonnay, something understated, yet with raspberry and melon undertones. The kind of vintage that would complement a flaky Chilean sea bass.
- Surgery says he's near herniating and you need to get going right away.
- The student induces, correctly performing a rapid sequence induction (full-head, full-stomach) with medications to blunt the rise in ICP during induction (narcotics, lidocaine) and medication to decrease ICP (pentathol).
- Ten minutes into the case, the blood pressure suddenly goes to 240/130 and the heart rate drops to the 30s.
- The student, sharp as a tack, correctly pegs the diagnosis of herniation with Cushing's triad (increased ICP, increased BP, and reflex bradycardia).
- Hyperventilation, pentathol, mannitol—the student gives everything possible but the surgeon says, "Forget it, he's brain dead. Turn off the ventilator, he's done for."
- The student turns off the ventilator.
- During the debrief, instructor and student go over all the physiologic changes, how to induce the person with increased ICP, and how to diagnose and treat increased herniation.
- Medically, this student is a superstar!
- And heck, turn the ventilator off at the end, why not, the guys' brain dead, right?
- *Screeech!*
- The student was a physiologic and pharmacologic superstar but the student tanked on the "end of life" issues.
- The guy's brain dead, OK, but maybe he can be an organ donor. Did we forget about that aspect of the medical world?
- Family visits, notifying relatives, getting his "affairs in order." The OR is not the place to make all these decisions. You

don't just turn off the ventilator and call it a day without addressing all these issues!
- So the simulator teaches physiology and teaches, well, call it sociology.

Subspecialty Specific: Cardiac

- A patient is intubated and under anesthesia.
- The arterial trace has a mean pressure of 60 but there is no pulsatile flow.
- The EKG is flatline.
- The ventilator is off.
- The student looks at this and thinks, "Hmm, what's wrong with this picture?"
- Relax, the instructor says the patient is on cardiopulmonary bypass and you are about to come off bypass.
- A blood gas sits on the anesthesia machine. On the blood gas, the hematocrit says 20.
- "OK," the student says, "let's get ready to come off bypass."
- First, the ventilator goes on.
- Second, fix everything "chemically" that can get fixed. The student gives two units of blood to get the hematocrit out of the basement, sees that the potassium and calcium are OK, then prepares to come of bypass.
- Separation from bypass occurs but only after the student starts an epinephrine drip to support the blood pressure and the cardiac output.
- During the debrief, the student wins high praise for an organized and cogent approach to separating a patient from cardiopulmonary bypass.
- "That blood gas, that showed a hematocrit of 20—you think that needed treatment?" the instructor asks.
- "Yes," the student says, "his chart said he was 80 years old, had a poorly functioning ventricle, and I think he needed all the help he could get."
- "Did the chart mention his name?"
- "Oh, yes, his name was John Smith."
- "And what was the name on the blood gas?" the instructor asks.
- "Oh," the student admits, "I didn't look. I figured because it was on the machine, it must be . . ."
- The name on the blood gas said "Ruperto Asuncion," not even close to "John Smith."
- So the simulator teaches not just a subspecialty point—separation from

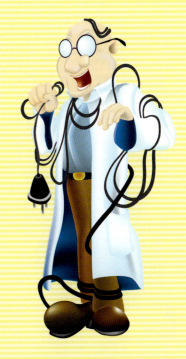

cardiopulmonary bypass—but also a basic point, check the names on the labs.

Can't Intubate, Can't Ventilate

- A student sets up to do a standard induction.
- Nothing amiss, a routine patient for a hernia repair.
- Induction, succinylcholine is used.
- The patient develops trismus (the mannequin can develop a tight, nonopenable jaw) and becomes impossible to ventilate (the mannequin can swell its upper airway so that mask ventilation is impossible).
- Saturation starts to drop.
- The student shifts into difficult airway algorithm, attempting mask ventilation then placing an oral airway (impossible), an LMA (just as impossible), then eventually going to cricothyrotomy and jet ventilation.
- During the debrief, kudos all around for following the correct sequence of events.
- Pharmacology question—does trismus mean malignant hyperthermia? Or is trismus just a question of, "You haven't waited long enough for the SUX to kick in"?
- The discussion broadens to, "Do you ever have to use SUX? What are your options?"
- Here the simulator teaches a clinical task—oxygenating via the surgical route when all else fails. And from the event, the discussion heads down the pharmacology pathway.
- A good instructor is always ready to "follow the student's lead" during the debrief session. As the instructor uncovers an area of uncertainty or curiosity, you make that the point of discussion. Because the student clearly knew what to do in a "can't intubate, can't ventilate" situation, the instructor took the discussion into another arena.
- Had the student floundered in the airway management, then the discussion would have stayed in the airway.

EXERCISE: MAKE UP YOUR OWN SCENARIOS

- The scenarios listed above are just a sampling of what craziness you can throw into your simulator scenarios.
- The goal in playing any scenario is the same—shake up the student, then make sense of it in the debrief.

- The premises listed below can all become full-blown scenarios, with technical aspects (treatment of hypotension), interpersonal aspects (dealing with a wife after the husband dies of a heart attack), and just about anything else you can think of.

PREMISES FOR MORE SCENARIOS

- A student comes into the room in the middle of a case to relieve an anesthesia provider. That provider is in a wheelchair. Has the student thought about that? What are the implications of the Americans with Disabilities Act on the anesthesia? Do you have an "obligation" to work with such a person? What if they ask for help? Is that any different than another anesthesia provider asking for help? What if the student got in a car accident and became paralyzed—would they still work? Should they? What does the law say? What does good medicine say? What does human nature say?
- In the middle of a case, the blood pressure drops and the surgeon says there is tremendous blood loss. The patient is a Jehovah's Witness. Now what? What if the patient were a minor and the parents refused "for him"?
- A case is going along routinely and all the power goes out. Do you hand-ventilate now? What are backup sources of power? What if all your invasive lines are now out? What do you do to monitor the patient?
- A patient's SAT drops, you turn up the oxygen, and the SAT drops even more, and you go to 100% oxygen and the patient codes. What's happening and what will you do about it?
- During a splenectomy, the inspiratory pressures suddenly increase and you lose breath sounds on the left. What next?
- You give a patient 2 cc from a syringe labeled succinylcholine and the patient states they can't breathe. They start making weaker and weaker breathing motions.
- You attempt to come off cardiopulmonary bypass but all the inotropes in the world can't do anything. An intra-aortic balloon pump is used—still nothing and the patient develops refractory arrhythmias and dies. You leave the simulator OR and go to an examining room where the patient's family waits to hear how it went. A 20-ish trophy wife and a

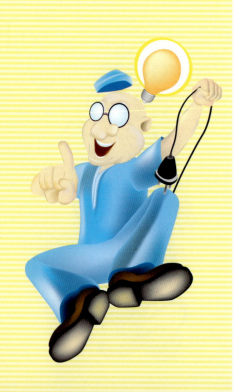

60-ish "First Wife's Club" ex-wife are both waiting in the room. What do you tell them? Do you separate the two first?

- You have a double cuff up for a Bier block. The patient has just gotten a whopping dose of local anesthetic. A "helpful" medical student undoes the tourniquet and the patient says, "I feel ringing in my ears." What next?

- You name it, you imagine it, and you can put it in the simulator.

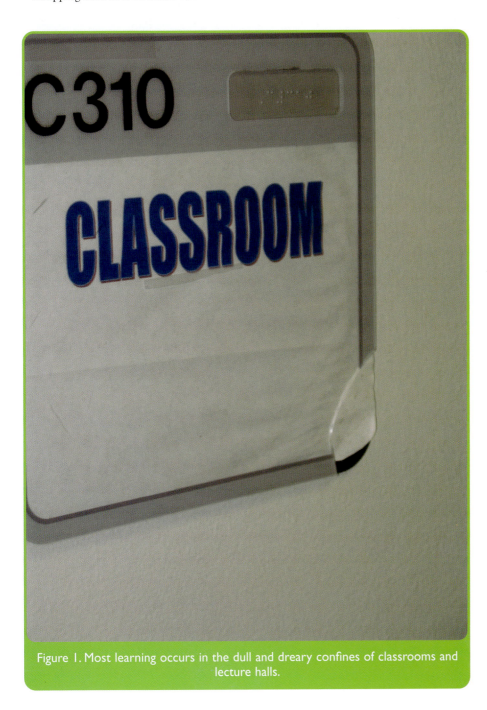

Figure 1. Most learning occurs in the dull and dreary confines of classrooms and lecture halls.

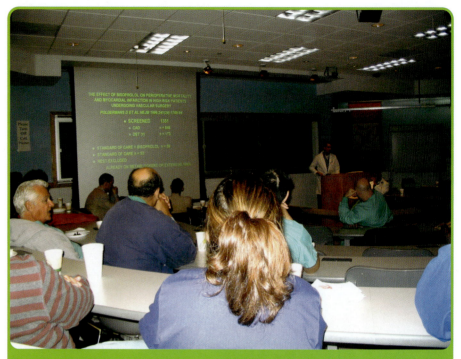

Figure 2. The emotional investment in the lecture process tends to run towards the "nil."

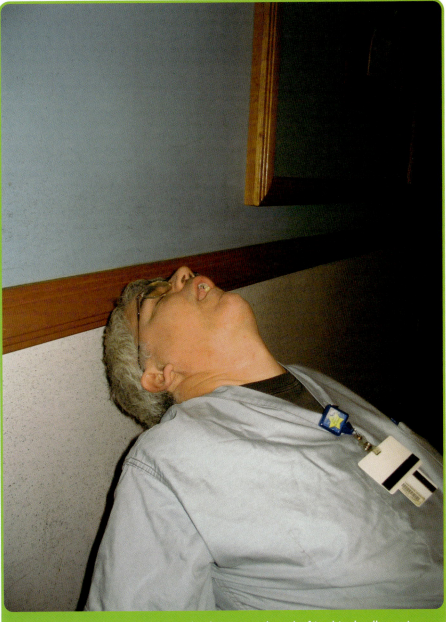

Figure 3. Airway loss and brain death is not unheard-of in this deadly setting.

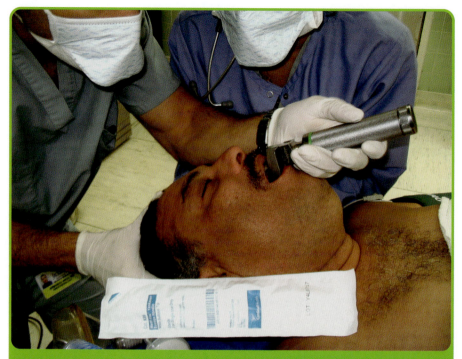

Figure 4. On the other hand, "practicing" on live patients runs the risk of hurting someone.

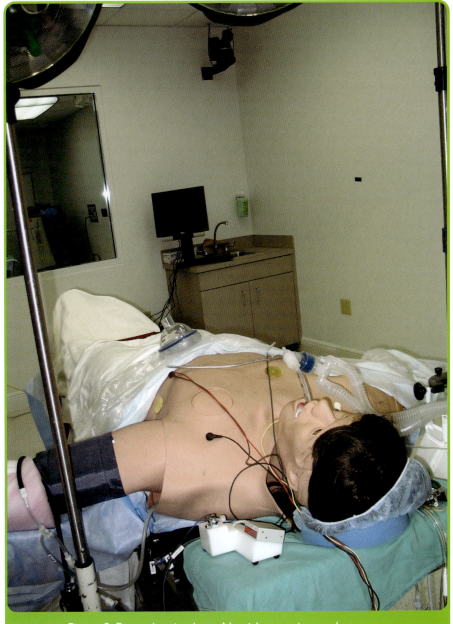

Figure 5. Enter the simulator. No risk to patients whatsoever.

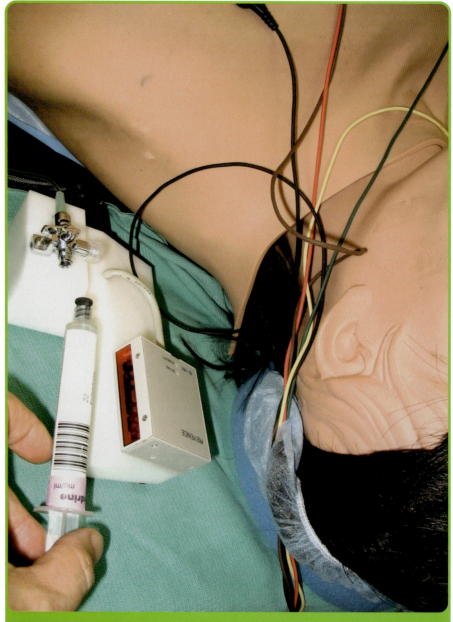

Figure 6. High fidelity mannequins allow you to inject drugs and see the response on the monitors. Here, the infrared sees the bar code, recognizes an inotrope, and the mannequin's blood pressure goes up.

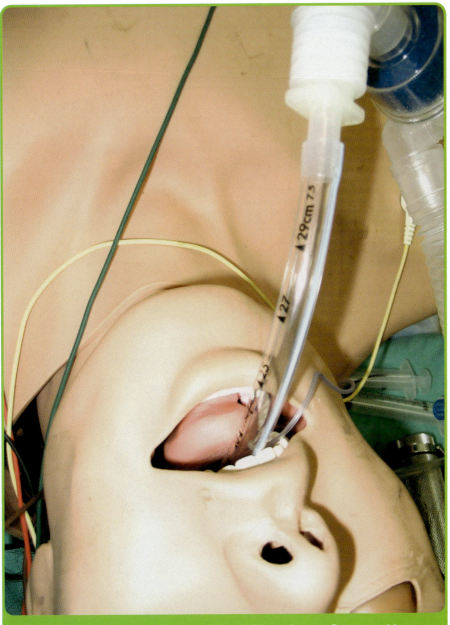

Figure 7. Practice the most dangerous stuff—intubation. Create problems galore—shunts leading to hypoxemia, tension pneumothorax, obstruction. All at no risk to any patient. And you can standardize the scenario and repeat it so all residents learn these important points.

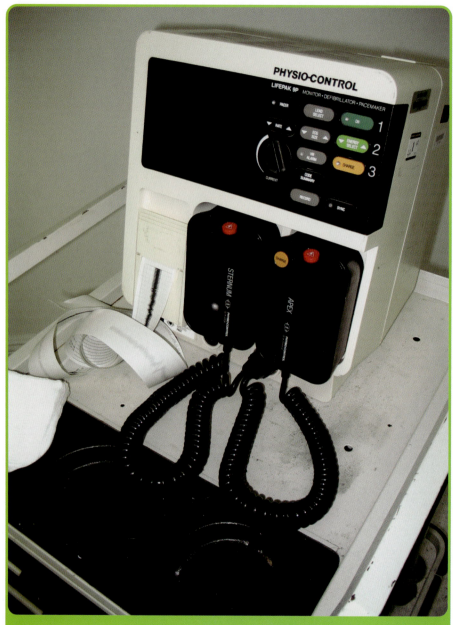

Figure 8. Practice defibrillation. Can't exactly do that on a living patient! By the by, it's amazing how often residents mix up the mechanics of the paddles.

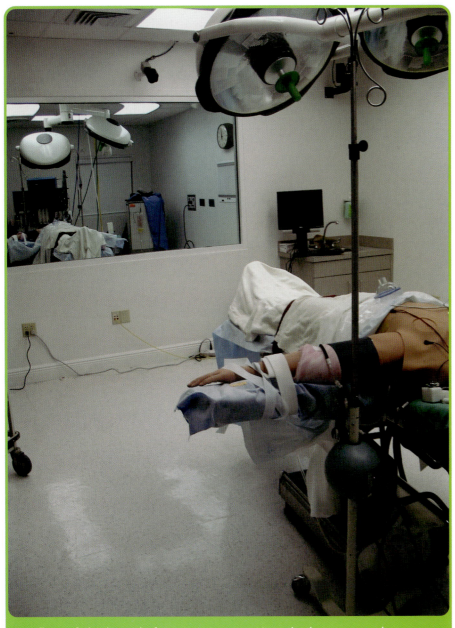

Figure 9. At the end of room, a one-way mirror leads to a control room.

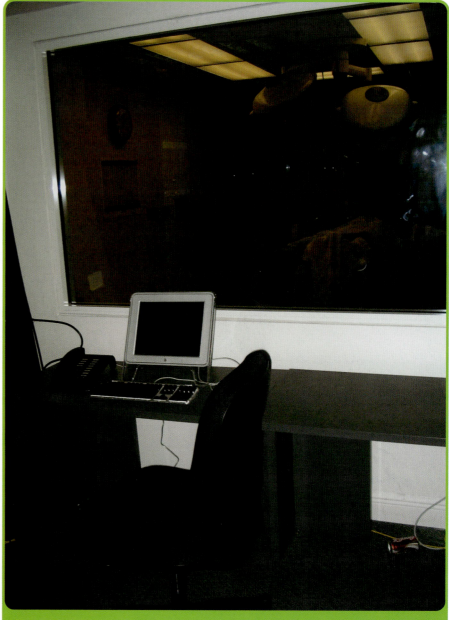

Figure 10. From the control room, you can observe the scenario and manipulate the variables.

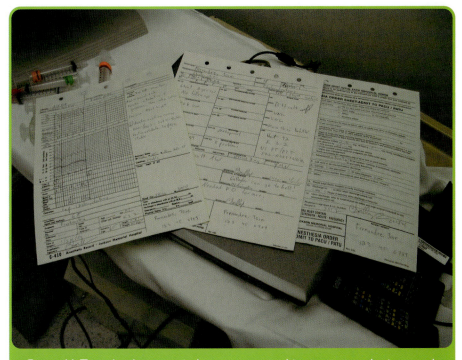

Figure 11. To make the scenario happen, create a history, an anesthetic record, some orders. All the information feeds into creating the "reality" of the scenario.

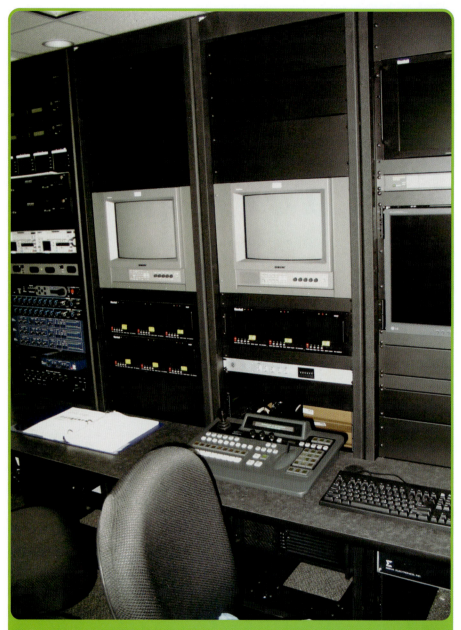

Figure 12. Videotaping the scenario helps during the debrief period. Scenarios don't have to be super complex. Most important during the scenario is "tuning in" the students, reacting to what they are doing, and making sure *something* gets taught.

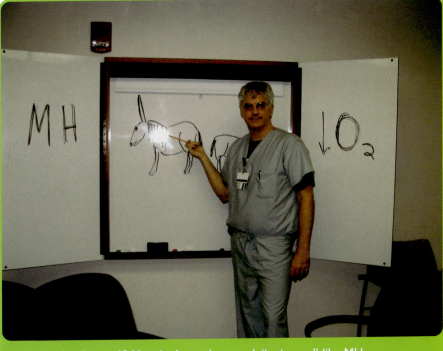

Figure 13. You don't need to teach "unicorns" like MH.

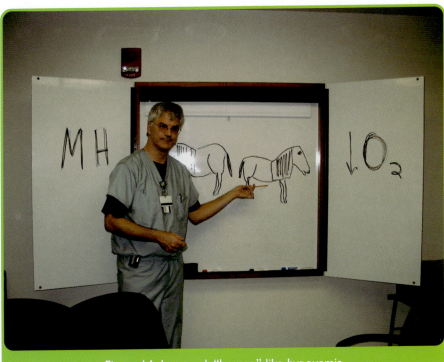

Figure 14. Just teach "horses," like hypoxemia.

SUGGESTED READING

BOOKS

Covey SR. *The 7 Habits of Highly Effective People*. New York: Free Press, 2004.
- *Another great book for building communication and coping skills. This is one pop psychology book that actually works! No wonder it sold a bazillion copies.*

Fisher R, Ury W, Patton B. *Getting to Yes: Negotiating Agreement without Giving In*, 2nd edition. Boston: Houghton Mifflin, 1991.
- *This book helps build your skills for one aspect of simulation—communicating effectively. For example, in a simulation you might have to smooth over a "fight with a surgeon." This book will give you an effective approach.*

Henson LC, Lee AC (eds). *Simulators in Anesthesiology Education*. London: Plenum Press, 1998.
- *This book consists of the proceedings of a meeting on anesthesia simulators held in Rochester, New York, in 1996, so it's a little long in the tooth. Tedious reading, you have to really love this stuff to slog through this book. Still, it is focused on anesthesia only.*

Kletz T. *Learning from Accidents*. Oxford: Gulf Professional Publishing, 2001.
- *This book looks at industrial accidents and how you thread together exactly what happened. Their method of analyzing systemic mistakes applies just as well to anesthesia mishaps. Big plus to this book: there's a voyeuristic and horrible thrill to read about these monstrous events. Sort of like slowing down to look at an accident on the highway—you hate to admit it, but we all do it.*

Loyd GE, Lake CL, Greenberg RB (eds). *Practical Health Care Simulations*. Philadelphia: Elsevier Mosby, 2004.
- *A monster book, nearly 600 pages. Comprehensive as hell, even has stuff on veterinary simulations! Go figure. A little dry, truth to tell. That's what happens, I think, when 50 or so smart people get together and write a book.*

Stone D, Patton B, Heen A. *Difficult Conversations*. New York: Penguin Books, 1999.
- *More on the communication front.*

DVD

Buckman R. "Anger and Other Emotions in Adverse Event and Error Disclosure" (2 DVD set). http://www.cinemedic.com.

- *Absolutely fantastic series of filmed vignettes where you learn how to "break the bad news." These lessons should be part of any simulator experience.*

WEBSITES

With computer and simulator developments, change occurs so fast that books become outdated even as they're printed, so check out these simulator websites to stay current. The "simulator community" is chock full of educators eager to share ideas, scenarios, and teaching strategies. So if you can sniff around on the World Wide Web, you can find a wealth of "simulator savvy."

Lots of individual anesthesia departments have valuable simulator information. Go to the anesthesia department's homepage and snoop around—you'll find great stuff. Pittsburgh, Duke, Stanford, Rochester—there's a smorgasbord of simulator coolness out there, all available at the click of a mouse.

For starters, just type "anesthesia simulators" into your search engine. At the time of this writing, that coughed up 13,721 sites. No doubt more are coming.

http://www.socmedsim.com
- *This is the web site of the Society for Medical Simulation, the Mac Daddy of this entire field. They have two extremely useful links on this website, "simblog" and "Ask the Wizards." "Simblog" is a kind of "simulator chat room" where you can knock around ideas. "Ask the Wizards" is just that, a place to ask your simulator questions (technical and educational).*

http://www.laerdal.com
- *The web site for the Laerdal® simulators.*

http://www.meti.com
- *The web site for the METI® simulators.*

ARTICLES

OK, there's a trillion articles on simulators and each article has a bibliography as long as your arm. Where do you start? Start with a "Review of the Articles Review":

Issenberg B, et al. Best evidence medical education. *Medical Teacher* 2005;27(1).
- *This is an online journal. This "look at what's out there" reviewed over 1000 articles from 1969 (when modern simulators arose like Venus from the sea) through 2003. To give an idea of how fast simulator articles are proliferating, since the article was finished until now, over 300 more*

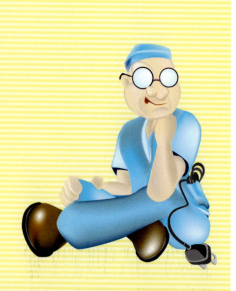

articles came out! You can't keep up with this stuff!

Now, as to individual articles—no attempt to be all-inclusive here, the bibliography itself would triple the size of this chapter.

Berkenstadt H, Gafni N, Incorporating simulation-based Objective Structured Clinical Examination (OSCE) into the Israeli National Board Examination in Anesthesiology (in press).

- *No kidding, simulation as assessment tool has arrived. In Israel, simulator technology "has gradually progressed from being a minor part of the oral board examination to a prerequisite component of the test. Haim Berkenstadt runs a great simulation (I've been lucky enough to see him in person). Plus, it doesn't hurt that he's about the funniest guy I've ever met in my entire life. Is Israel the only place doing this?*

  - New York used a simulator in "rehabbing" an anesthesiologist with lapsed skills.

  - In Heidelberg, they use a simulator to accredit nurse anesthetists.

  - In Rochester, residents have to pass muster in the simulator before they take overnight call. (Hmmm, that sounds like a good idea.)

  - Difficult airway management in the simulator is mandatory at the University of Pittsburgh.

If anyone is still wondering whether the simulator is coming, I've got news for you. It's already here.

Boulet JR, Murray D, Woodhouse J, et al. Reliability and validity of a simulation-based acute care skills assessment for medical students and residents. Anesthesiology 2003 Dec;99(6) 1270–1280.

- *Again, the authors are zooming in on the question in simulation-ness: is the simulator really a good way to know if people "know their stuff"? Here's the setting—ask faculty, "What should your people know how to treat? When a patient rolls through the door with condition X, your medical students and residents should know how to treat condition X. Give us 10 condition Xs."*

Here are the 10 *condition Xs:*

1. Femur fracture—big bleed, hypotension

2. MI—tachycardia, hypertension, PVCs

3. Pneumothorax—fell off bike, dyspnea, tachycardia, hypoxemia

4. Ectopic pregnancy—bleeding, hypotensive

5. Cerebral hemorrhage—blown pupil, Cushing's triad, unresponsive

6. V tach—chest pain, unstable

7. Respiratory failure—bronchitis progressing to respiratory insufficiency

8. Asthma—hypoxemia, tachypnea, heading toward respiratory insufficiency

9. Rupturing abdominal aortic aneurysm—abdominal mass, pain, tachycardia

10. Syncope—heart block, hypotension

Hey, that's a pretty good list! I would hope that *any doctor* would know how to handle those bad boys. Result? Another "Whew!"—residents did better than medical students. Another result? Few people did well on the cerebral bleed with herniation. (To my mind, not the *purpose* of this study but an extremely important "side result" of the study.) As primarily a clinical teacher, I like anything that exposes gaps in our teaching. If a simulator shows that our residents can't handle a cerebral herniation, then we should go back and teach more about cerebral herniation!

Chopra V, Gesink BJ, De Jong J, et al. Does training on an anesthesia simulator lead to improvement in performance? Br J Anesth 1994;73:293–7.

- *Twenty-eight anesthetists were trained on the simulator to handle anaphylactic shock. Later, the group was divided in two, half getting training in treatment of anaphylactic shock (again) and half getting trained in treatment of malignant hyperthermia. All the training was on the simulator. Four months passed, then all 28 were tested on malignant hyperthermia on the simulator. Those who had seen malignant hyperthermia before did better. Conclusion? The simulator is a good training device for teaching malignant hyperthermia. Great! Alas, we have proven the simulator's worth, beyond a shadow of a doubt. Let all rejoice who ever carried the banner of simulation! Um, that is, unless you ask yourself, "Did the simulator train someone to handle a real malignant hyperthermia crisis, or did the simulator train someone to handle a simulator malignant hyperthermia crisis?" Are we just teaching people to "game" the simulator?*

DeAnda A, et al. Unplanned incidents during comprehensive anesthesia simulation. Anesth Analg 1990;71:77–82.

- *DeAnda and Gaba smoked out a few human errors while running their simulators. What did those silly residents do? They forgot to turn the ventilator back on after hand-ventilating; they did syringe swaps; they turned the stopcock the wrong way. You name it, the residents found a way to mess it up. The simulator uncovered resident mistakes galore. When you see the mistakes they*

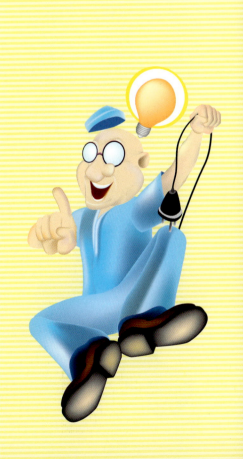

made, it does not become such a gigantic leap of faith to think you could run the simulator, see the mistakes made, correct the mistakes, prevent a repeat of the mistake, and protect a patient from harm.

Gaba DM, et al. A comprehensive anaesthesia simulation environment: Recreating the operating room for research and training. Anaesthesiology 1988;69:387–94.

• *Way back in 1988, Gaba laid out how to do a simulation and he made clear the argument that it just plain "stands to reason" that simulation is a good way to teach.*

He ran 21 people through the simulator and they all judged the experience as highly realistic. This paper did not actually do any kind of study—it just laid out how simulations are done, how much the participants liked it, and proposed that simulation has "major potential for training, continuing education, certification and research." Amen to that, Dr. Gaba.

Good ML. Patient simulators for training basic and advanced clinical skills. *Medical Education* 2003;37(Suppl 1):14–21.

• *For the "historian of all things simulationalogic," this article is great. It goes over the early days of Sim One, the very first simulator way back in the 1960s. Then this article describes the University of Florida and Stanford's work in the 1980s and brings us up to date. One-third of medical schools in America have simulators now! To learn basic skills, the simulator is the rage. You can teach first-year medical students basic pulmonary mechanics or you can teach fourth-year medical students how to manage congestive heart failure. For residents, the simulator can ease that first jump into the operating room. For advanced residents, simulators can show you the rare bird you might never see in your training (anaphylaxis, oxygen line crossover, malignant hyperthermia). Of course, we live in an outcome-based world—outcome based medicine, forget some meaningless intermediate variable, is someone alive now who would otherwise be dead but for the simulator. This is the ultimate question of "simulator worth." The answer is a resounding, unmistakable, and incontrovertible, "Maybe." Juuust maybe.*

Helmreich RI, et al. Anaesthetic simulation and lessons to be learned from aviation. Can J Anaesth 1997;44:907–12.

• *This editorial points out that simulators have a lot of potential for serving as tests. All the usual arguments hold—you don't put a patient at risk, you can reproduce the scene. But this editorial goes on to point out a crucial problem with using a simulator as a*

"test vehicle." A key problem is the idea of "equifinality," that is, different techniques can give you the same end result. (The article does not mention the following example; I made it up just to illustrate the point.)

For example, one anesthesiologist may use epinephrine to achieve a goal whereas another may use dobutamine to achieve a goal. Both achieve the same goal—better cardiac output. So in the simulator, what do you do, grade someone wrong who uses epinephrine because the "simulator grade book" says you should use dobutamine? The editorial finishes up by saying, "There is a need to provide opportunities for practice and assessment until the culture supports the fairness of the assessment process." In other words, it "stands to reason" that a simulator is a good way to test, but we haven't quite gotten there yet.

Holzman RS, Cooper JB, Gaba DM, et al. Anesthesia Crisis Resource Management: Real-life simulation training in operating room crises. J Clin Anesth 1995;7:675–87.

• *Sixty-eight anesthesiologists (a gemisch of attendings and residents at various levels) and four nurse anesthetists went into Harvard's Simulation Center to undergo training in Anesthesia Crises. The training lasted a few hours per week over a 10-week course. They handled:*

• Overdose of anesthetic vapors
• Oxygen delivery failure
• Cardiac arrest
• Malignant hyperthermia
• Tension pneumothorax
• Power failure

Think about it: If you were a program director, wouldn't you want your people to know how to handle those things? The result? The participants loved it! The people that go train in simulators think simulators are the greatest! (OK, detractors say, people like riding Space Mountain at Disney World, too. Maybe we should send our residents to Orlando.) Did anything good come of this "groovy experience in the simulator" or is this all just yummy cotton candy? Six months later, a questionnaire was sent out. Eight of the trainees reported that the simulator had helped, in *real life.* Course participation helped them handle possible malignant hyperthermia, low oxygen pressure, a trauma case, and a subclavian laceration. Four others didn't specify the crisis but said that the course had definitely helped. Think about it: Could the observations of those eight "simulation grads" be the Holy Grail? Is this the *"Simulation Does Save Lives"* proof

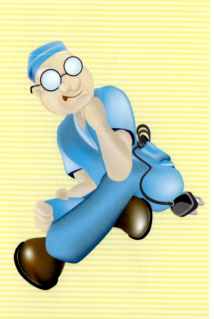

that everyone has been looking for? Well, uh, maybe, kind of.

Issenberg SB, McGaghie WC, Hart IR, et al. Simulation technology for health care professional skills training and assessment. JAMA 1999 (Sep 1);282(9):861–6.

- *Dr. Issenberg runs the Harvey cardiology simulator at the University of Miami. In this Special Communication, Issenberg touches on all the different simulation technologies available in 1999: laparoscopy simulators to train surgeons, his own mannequin Harvey to train students in 27 different cardiac conditions, flat-screen computer simulators and, finally, anesthesia simulators. What does the good Dr. Issenberg have to say about the anesthesia simulators? "The high cost and requirements for accompanying equipment, space, and personnel have resulted in research to justify the installation of such devices." (Hence, so many "Justification of Simulators" articles in this bibliography.) If you look at "intermediate" benefits of Simulators, Issenberg points out:*

- Simulators are highly realistic.

- Training on a simulator can improve the acquisition and retention of knowledge compared with sitting in a lecture hall.

- If ever used as a certification tool, "They allow the examinee to demonstrate clinical skills in a controlled clinical environment while still exhibiting cognitive and language skills."

So, as study after study comes out, *hinting* that simulators will make us better practitioners, do we have to wait for proof positive? No. Issenberg quotes David Gaba (you've seen his name popping up), "No industry in which human lives depend on the skilled performance of responsible operators has waited for unequivocal proof of the benefit of simulation before embracing it." I say we embrace it, too.

Kapur PA, Steadman RH. Patient simulator competency testing: Ready for takeoff? Anesth Analg 1998;86:1157–9.

- *Drs. Kapur and Steadman ask the important question, "Does performance in the simulator translate into competence in the real world?" In the simulator, problems tend to happen one at a time. In the cold, cruel world, problems come "not as single spies, but in battalions." The simulator is theater, and theater is not the real world. So as simulators take a bigger and bigger place at the educational table, we must ask the question—if you are good in the simulator, are you good "for real"? And the flip side of the question also applies—if you are bad in the simulator, are you bad "for real"?*

Morgan PJ, et al. Identification in gaps in the achievement of undergraduate anesthesia educational objectives using high fidelity patient simulation. Anesth Analg 2003;97:1690–4.

- *What did the simulator unmask?*

  - Students couldn't manage the airway.

  - Students didn't check the blood pressure.

  - Students didn't call for help.

  - Students didn't do an H&P.

  - Students didn't prepare the airway equipment.

Um, this study begs the question. Just what, precisely, *did* the students do? Did the students *themselves* have a pulse?

Murray WB, et al. The first three days of residency: An efficient introduction to clinical medicine. Acad Med 1998;73: 595–6.

- *Dr. Murray and the fine folk at Penn State (you can almost smell the chocolate from the Hershey factory) describe the first three days of their anesthesia residency. Rather than just shoveling a ton of stuff at their residents, they make the learning more active, using (what else) the simulator. Result: a questionnaire showed "improvement in the residents' confidence in their ability to carry out clinical tasks." So it "stands to reason" that if a simulator increases the confidence of a resident, a simulator must be a good thing. A hard-nosed scientific drudge could look at this and say, "This is no rigorous proof," and a skeptic could look at this and say, "So what, what difference does that make, a little more confidence?" But I'll bet to those Penn State residents, that confidence made all the difference in the world when they walked into the OR the first day.*

Shwid H, Rooke A. Evaluation of anesthesia residents using mannequin-based simulation. Anesthesiology 2002 Dec;97(6): 1434–44.

- *Jan Carline and a cast of thousands in this multicenter masterpiece. A total of 99 residents at 10 different teaching programs jumped through four flaming hoops:*

  - Esophageal intubation

  - Anaphylaxis

  - Bronchospasm

  - Myocardial ischemia

The residents were taped and graded. More senior residents did better than junior residents, which generated a nationwide, "Whew!" from anesthesia attendings all across America. (*We must be teaching something, for God's sake.*)

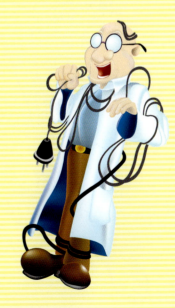

Something of additional interest pops out of this article. The residents didn't know bupkis from bronchospasm. No matter how far along their training, a lot of residents appeared to suffer from adult-onset anencephaly when it comes to the wheezing patient. Are we missing the boat here? Are we not teaching our residents right? Should the beatings increase until our residents get the message? To me, that alone was worth the price of admission on this article. Forget Schwid's elegant design, rigorous mathematics, and large numbers. He uncovered a *glaring defect* in our teaching! Damnation, tomorrow, I'm going over bronchospasm with my resident and I hope you do too!

Schwid HA, et al. Anesthesiologists' management of simulated critical incidents. Anesthesiology 1992;76:495–501.

- *This article ramps it up a little bit. We're not looking at residents making glitches during routine cases—we're looking at much more serious stuff. How do residents and faculty manage nonroutine cases?*

  - Esophageal intubation—Residents misjudged esophageal intubations.

  - Anaphylaxis—Less than half of everybody (residents *and* faculty) treated anaphylaxis correctly.

  - Myocardial ischemia—A quarter of all comers treated ischemia correctly.

  - Cardiac arrest—If your ACLS training was more than six months old, *fugetaboudit*! Less than a third knew what they were doing.

Seropian MA. General concepts in full scale simulation: getting started. Anesth Analg 2003;97:1695–705.

- *Dr. Seropian pays the most attention to the person running the simulator, not so much the simulator mannequin itself. It's the live component in the simulator that makes it happen, so Seropian emphasizes the need to "train the trainer," especially in the delicate art of debriefing.*

Shapiro MJ, et al. Simulation based teamwork training for emergency department staff: Does it improve clinical team performance when added to an existing didactic teamwork curriculum? Qual Saf Health Care 2004;13:417–21.

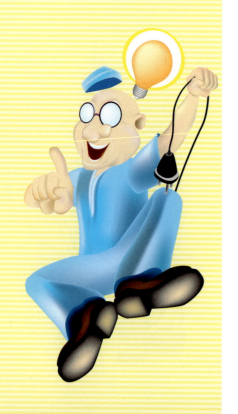

- *This was the first look at real "team simulator training" using nurses, techs, ER residents, and attendings. Of special interest in this study, teams are what actually take care of patients! This study mimics the real world rather than just how one person performs. Bravo to the people who took on this study. Guess what? Teams that practiced on the simulator did better in the (admittedly elusive) area of "team behavior." The killer here is the "metric itself." How in hell do you measure "team behavior"?*

They looked for specific things—the very things that save or lose a patient's life during a crisis:

- Assigning roles and responsibilities
- Engaging team members in the plan
- Providing situational updates
- Cross-monitoring actions of others
- Conducting event reviews

If a team does all those important tasks, then, for example, someone *specific* is told to get, send, and bring back the results of a blood gas, rather than someone just shouting out, "Hey, we need a gas!" Team behavior does make a difference. Simulators teach good team dynamics. Good stuff, that.

Weller J, et al. Survey of change in practice following simulation-based training in crisis management. Anaesthesia 2003;58:471–3.

- *A survey went out to 96 anesthesia personnel who did a simulator course the year before. Sixty-six out of 96 responded (and yes, there is always "questionnaire response bias"). The respondents valued the course, perceived a change in their practice as a result of the simulator training, and found it useful in subsequent crises. Forty-two respondents dealt with a host of critical events—cardiac arrests, big hemorrhages, anaphylaxis, amniotic fluid emboli, air emboli, airway emergencies. A total of 70% of the respondents felt "their management of the crisis was improved as a result of participation in the simulation course." That sentence is it. That sentence is the closest we can come so far to the Golden Fleece, the winning Lotto ticket, the Blue Ribbon of "Simulator Worthiness." "Their management of the crisis was improved as a result of participation in the simulation course." Oh, sweet salvation!*

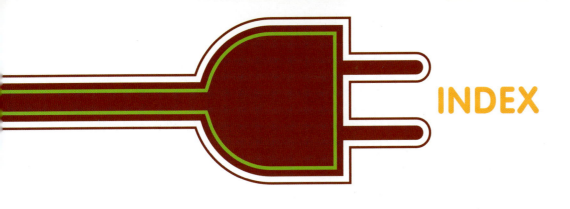

INDEX

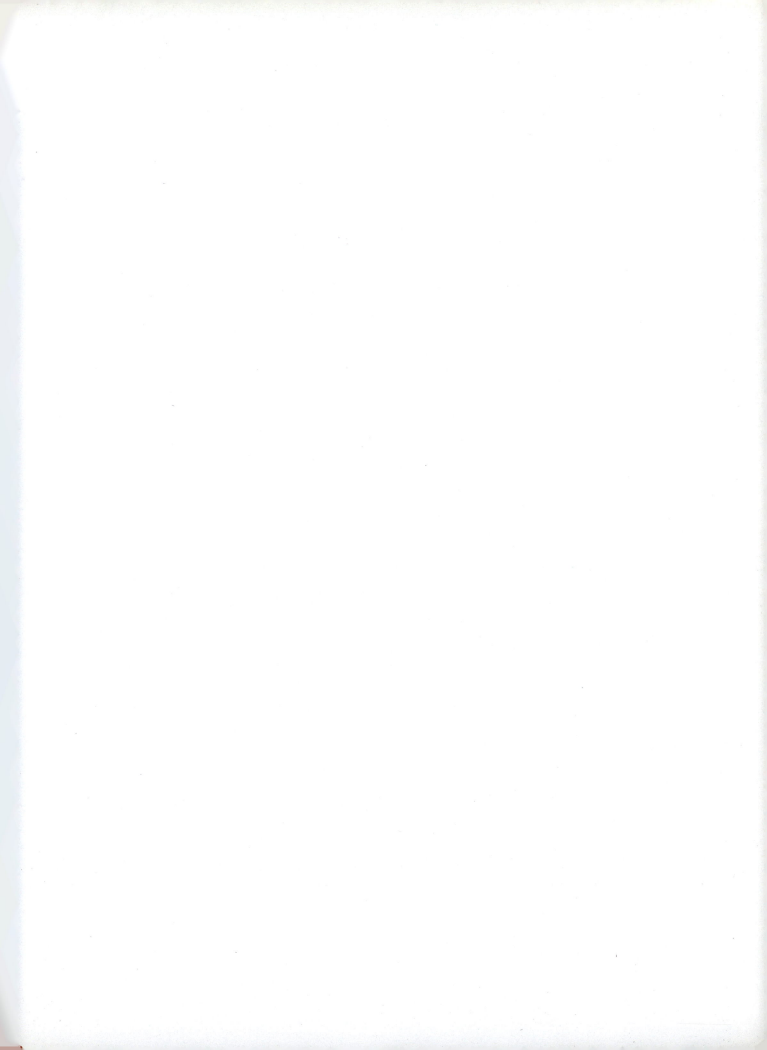